# Dimensional Analysis for Meds

## FOURTH EDITION

## Anna M. Curren

**Former Associate Professor of Nursing**

**Long Beach City College**

**Long Beach, California**

DELMAR
CENGAGE Learning

Australia • Brazil • Japan • Korea • Mexico • Singapore • Spain • United Kingdom • United States

**DELMAR**
CENGAGE Learning

**Dimensional Analysis for Meds,
Fourth Edition**
Anna M. Curren

Vice President, Career and Professional
  Editorial: Dave Garza

Director of Learning Solutions: Matthew Kane

Senior Acquisitions Editor: Maureen Rosener

Managing Editor: Marah Bellegarde

Senior Product Manager: Elisabeth F. Williams

Editorial Assistant: Samantha Miller

Vice President, Career and Professional
  Marketing: Jennifer Ann Baker

Marketing Director: Wendy Mapstone

Senior Marketing Manager: Michele McTighe

Marketing Coordinator: Scott Chrysler

Production Director: Carolyn Miller

Production Manager: Andrew Crouth

Senior Content Project Manager: Stacey Lamodi

Senior Art Director: Jack Pendleton

Senior Product Manager, Digital Solutions
  Group: Mary Colleen Liburdi

Technology Project Manager: Ben Knapp

For product information and technology assistance, contact us at
**Cengage Learning Customer & Sales Support, 1-800-354-9706**
For permission to use material from this text or product,
submit all requests online at **www.cengage.com/permissions**
Further permissions questions can be emailed to
**permissionrequest@cengage.com**

Library of Congress Control Number: 2008942905

ISBN-13: 978-1-4354-3867-5

ISBN-10: 1-4354-3867-1

**Delmar**
Executive Woods
5 Maxwell Drive
Clifton Park, NY 12065-2919
USA

Cengage Learning is a leading provider of customized learning solutions with office locations around the globe, including Singapore, the United Kingdom, Australia, Mexico, Brazil, and Japan. Locate your local office at **www.cengage.com/global**

Cengage Learning products are represented in Canada by Nelson Education, Ltd.

To learn more about Delmar, visit **www.cengage.com/delmar**

Purchase any of our products at your local bookstore or at our preferred online store **www.cengagebrain.com**

**Notice to the Reader**

Publisher does not warrant or guarantee any of the products described herein or perform any independent analysis in connection with any of the product information contained herein. Publisher does not assume, and expressly disclaims, any obligation to obtain and include information other than that provided to it by the manufacturer. The reader is expressly warned to consider and adopt all safety precautions that might be indicated by the activities described herein and to avoid all potential hazards. By following the instructions contained herein, the reader willingly assumes all risks in connection with such instructions. The publisher makes no representations or warranties of any kind, including but not limited to, the warranties of fitness for particular purpose or merchantability, nor are any such representations implied with respect to the material set forth herein, and the publisher takes no responsibility with respect to such material. The publisher shall not be liable for any special, consequential, or exemplary damages resulting, in whole or part, from the readers' use of, or reliance upon, this material.

Printed in the United States of America
3 4 5 6 7 14 13 12 11

# CONTENTS

Preface / vii

Introduction for the Learner / x

Introduction for the Instructor / xi

Using the Learning Package / xii

Using the In-Book Practice Software / xiv

Refresher Math PreTest / xvi

## 1 Refresher Math

### Chapter 1: Relative Value, Addition, and Subtraction of Decimals / 2

Relative Value of Decimals / 2

Addition and Subtraction of Decimals / 7

Summary / 8

Summary Self-Test / 9

### Chapter 2: Multiplication and Division of Decimals / 11

Multiplication of Decimals / 11

Division of Decimal Fractions / 13

Elimination of Decimal Points / 13

Reduction of Fractions / 14

Reduction of Numbers Ending in Zero / 16

Using a Calculator / 17

Expressing to the Nearest Tenth / 17

Expressing to the Nearest Hundredth / 18

Summary / 19

Summary Self-Test / 20

### Chapter 3: Solving Common Fraction Equations / 22

Whole-Number Equations / 22

Decimal Fraction Equations / 25

Multiple-Number Equations / 28

Summary / 31

Summary Self-Test / 31

## 2 Introduction to Drug Measures

### Chapter 4: Metric/International (SI) System / 36

Basic Units of the Metric/SI System / 36

Metric/SI Prefixes / 37

Metric/SI Abbreviations / 38

Metric/SI Notation Rules / 39

Conversion Between Metric/SI Units / 40

Common Errors in Metric/SI Dosages / 43

Summary / 44

Summary Self-Test / 44

**Chapter 5: Unit, Percentage, Milliequivalent, Ratio, Household, and Apothecary Measures / 46**

International Units (units) / 46

Percentage (%) Measures / 47

Milliequivalent (mEq) Measures / 47

Ratio Measures / 48

Household and Apothecary Measures / 49

Summary / 49

Summary Self-Test / 50

**3** **Reading Medication Labels and Syringe Calibrations**

**Chapter 6: Oral Medication Labels and Dosage Calculation / 52**

Tablet and Capsule Labels / 53

Tablet/Capsule Dosage Calculation / 57

Oral Solution Labels / 62

Measurement of Oral Solutions / 64

Summary / 66

Summary Self-Test / 66

**Chapter 7: Safe Medication Administration / 75**

Medication Administration Records / 75

The Six Rights of Medication
  Administration / 77

The Seventh Right: Partnering with
  the Patient / 80

Common Medication Errors / 81

Errors in Abbreviations and
  Drug Names / 81

Errors in Writing Metric Dosages / 81

Action Steps When Errors Occur / 82

Summary / 83

Summary Self-Test / 84

**Chapter 8: Hypodermic Syringe Measurement / 85**

Standard 3 mL Syringe / 85

Safety Syringes / 89

Tuberculin (TB) Syringe / 90

5 and 10 mL Syringes / 93

20 mL and Larger Syringes / 96

Summary / 97

Summary Self-Test / 98

**Chapter 9: Parenteral Medication Labels and Dosage Calculation / 100**

Reading Metric/SI Solution Labels / 100

Percent (%) and Ratio Solution
  Labels / 103

Solutions Measured in
  International Units / 105

Solutions Measured as Milliequivalents
  (mEq) / 106

Summary / 108

Summary Self-Test / 108

**Chapter 10: Reconstitution of Powdered Drugs / 122**

Reconstitution of a Single Strength
  Solution / 122

Reconstitution from Package Insert
  Directions / 128

Reconstitution of Multiple Strength
  Solutions / 129

Summary / 131

Summary Self-Test / 132

**Chapter 11: Measuring Insulin Dosages / 138**

Types of Insulin / 138

Insulin Label Identification / 139

Insulin Action Times / 145

Insulin Syringes / 146

Combining Insulin Dosages / 151

Insulin Injection Sites and Techniques / 152

Summary / 153

Summary Self-Test / 153

# 4 Dosage Calculations

## Chapter 12:  Dimensional Analysis/Units Conversion  /  160

Clinical Ratios  /  160
The Basic DA Equation  /  161
Equations Requiring Metric
  Conversions  /  166

Summary  /  169
Summary Self-Test  /  170

# 5 Dosage Calculation from Body Weight and Body Surface Area

## Chapter 13:  Adult and Pediatric Dosages Based on Body Weight  /  188

Converting lb to kg  /  188
Converting kg to lb  /  189
Calculating Dosages from
  Drug Label Information  /  190

Calculating Dosages from Drug Literature  /  192
Summary  /  196
Summary Self-Test  /  197

## Chapter 14:  Adult and Pediatric Dosages Based on Body Surface Area  /  203

Calculating BSA from kg and cm  /  203
Calculating BSA from lb and in  /  205
Dosage Calculation Based on BSA  /  206

Assessing Orders Based on BSA  /  206
Summary  /  210
Summary Self-Test  /  211

# 6 Intravenous Calculations

## Chapter 15:  Introduction to IV Therapy  /  214

Primary Line  /  214
Secondary Line  /  216
Volume-Controlled Burettes  /  219
Indwelling Infusion Ports/
  Intermittent Locks  /  219
Volumetric Pumps  /  221
Syringe Pumps  /  223

Patient-Controlled Analgesia (PCA) Devices  /  223
Introduction to IV Fluids  /  225
Percentages in IV Fluids  /  226
Parenteral Nutrition  /  226
Summary  /  227
Summary Self-Test  /  227

## Chapter 16:  IV Flow Rate Calculation  /  229

IV Tubing Calibration  /  229
Calculating gtt/min Flow Rates
  from mL/hr Ordered  /  231
Formula and Division Factor Methods
  of Flow Rate Calculation  /  234

Division Factor Method  /  237
Regulating Flow Rate  /  240
Correcting Off-Schedule Rates  /  241
Summary  /  244
Summary Self-Test  /  245

**Chapter 17: Calculating IV Infusion and Completion Times / 247**

Calculating Infusion Time from
mL/hr Ordered / 247
Calculating Infusion
Completion Times / 249
International/Military
Time Calculations / 249

Standard Time Calculations / 250
Labeling Solution Bags with Infusion
and Completion Times / 252
Summary / 256
Summary Self-Test / 256

**Chapter 18: IV Medication and Titration Calculations / 262**

Calculating mL/hr Rate for
Dosage Ordered / 263
Calculating mL/hr Rate for
Dosage per kg Ordered / 264

Calculating Infusion Titrations / 270
Summary / 272
Summary Self-Test / 272

**Chapter 19: Heparin Infusion Calculations / 276**

Heparin IV and Vial Labels / 276
Calculating mL/hr IV Flow Rate from
units/hr Ordered / 278
Calculating units/hr Infusing from
mL/hr Flow Rate / 280

Heparin Flush Dosage / 281
Summary / 282
Summary Self-Test / 282

**7 Pediatric Medication Calculations**

**Chapter 20: Pediatric Oral and Parenteral Medications / 286**

Oral Medications / 286
Intramuscular and Subcutaneous
Medications / 288

Summary / 289
Summary Self-Test / 289

**Chapter 21: Pediatric Intravenous Medications / 292**

Methods of IV Medication
Administration / 292
Medication Administration via
Burette / 294

Comparing IV Dosages Ordered with
Average Dosages / 297
Summary / 301
Summary Self-Test / 301

**Appendix A: Apothecary Measures / 306**

**Appendix B: ISMP's List of *Error-Prone Abbreviations, Symbols,* and *Dose Designations* / 307**

**Index / 311**

# PREFACE

*Dimensional Analysis for Meds,* fourth edition, is your best partner for success in the dosage calculations arena. With a growing record of positive instruction with hundreds of thousands of users, its fully self-instructional approach fosters achievement and confidence as the ideal choice for both learners and instructors.

A large part of the credit for this successful journey lies in the fact that *Dimensional Analysis for Meds,* fourth edition, has kept up with the times, while never losing sight of the beginning students it was designed to teach. *Dimensional Analysis for Meds* is the only calculations text of its kind that is completely focused to teach from simple to complex. It eliminates the unnecessary, keeps instruction consistently geared toward clinical realities, and offers a solid and seamless learning process from day one until program completion.

## ORGANIZATION

*Dimensional Analysis for Meds* allows for self-paced study, progressing from basic to more complex information. All learners are invited to complete the Refresher Math Pretest on page xvi to determine their competence in basic math skills. Section 1, Refresher Math, is also recommended for all learners, as the numerous shortcuts and memory cues included in this section are used in examples throughout the text. Calculators are used routinely in clinical facilities and on the NCLEX exam, and their use is encouraged in this text. Bear in mind that fractional variations in answers due to rounding of numbers may occur and should be considered correct.

Once the fundamental skills are mastered, the learner will move on to the basics needed for calculating dosages and administering medications; metric system units and milliequivalent dosages; reading dosage labels and syringe calibrations; and working with reconstituted drugs and insulin. Hundreds of sample dosage problems will cement these learnings.

With these basic skills solidified, students are prepared for the advanced calculations presented in the second half of the text. Body weight and body surface area dosage calculations, as well as intravenous and heparin calculations, are thoroughly covered and tested. Pediatric medication calculations round out the learner's education.

## FEATURES

*Dimensional Analysis for Meds,* fourth edition, offers examples and review tests throughout to enhance comprehension, and running answers allow the learner to receive immediate feedback on deficits and strengths. A key icon 🔑 is used throughout the chapters to allow learners to easily identify important information. The most up-to-date equipment and safety devices are depicted in color, and real, full-color drug labels and syringes are included with explanations and dosage problems. With the goal of helping students become safe and effective practitioners, *Dimensional Analysis for Meds* works through basic and advanced calculations in detail, including intravenous and pediatric calculations, so that students are fully equipped to safely prepare and administer medications in a clinical setting.

## NEW TO THIS EDITION

- All **new syringe photos** with enhanced readability and clarity make the medication administration experience mirror reality.

- Many **new, current drug labels** reflect the most up-to-date information on the market.

- **New Chapter 7: Safe Medication Administration** highlights the newest regulations on medication abbreviations, the six rights of medication administration, tips on reducing dosage errors, and guidelines for safe medication practices.

- An exciting **in-book CD** with tutorials, problems, and self-tests allows study and testing in an interactive environment.

- **New online WebTutor Advantage courses** (WebCT and Blackboard) include questions, links, quizzes, flash cards, and other valuable resources, all designed to enhance classroom learning.

- A **new** *Instructor Resources (IR) CD-ROM* with teaching aids and calculation solutions is now offered to instructors who adopt the text.

## ANCILLARY SUPPORT MATERIALS

This fourth edition of *Dimensional Analysis for Meds* offers a wealth of electronic resources to support both students and instructors. These interactive learning partners will guide, test, challenge, and help increase proficiency in dosage calculations.

### Tutorial Software

Engaging *Student Practice Software* is available *free* to each user of *Dimensional Analysis for Meds*, fourth edition. The CD-ROM packaged within the book features:

- A user-friendly menu structure invites immediate access to the program's items.

- Five modules of content, each containing three to six lessons, are supported by problem sets to test understanding.

- Audio and visual tracks enhance interactive exercises that allow calculation and measurement of dosages.

- A drop-down calculator, as used on the NCLEX-RN® examination, is available at the click of a button.

### Instructor Resources (IR) CD-ROM (ISBN 1-4354-3868-X)

An innovative new *Instructor Resources CD-ROM* offers a wealth of useful tools to facilitate teaching and support of goals for student success. The following components are included in this invaluable digital resource, which is free to adopters of *Dimensional Analysis for Meds*, fourth edition:

- **Lecture slides,** created in Power Point®, facilitate classroom instruction by offering ready-made presentation outlines, tools, and procedures.

- A **Computerized Test Bank** offers several hundred new questions designed for testing and evaluation.

- An **Instructor's Manual** offers review questions with solutions, additional practice problems with solutions, drug label exercises, syringe exercises, and teaching tips.

- A **Solutions Manual** includes step-by-step solutions to all problems and self-tests included in the text.

- An **Image Library** of dozens of figures, labels, and syringes from the text facilitates searching for, copying, and saving images into Microsoft PowerPoint® presentations or other learning tools.

## WebTutor Advantage on WebCT (ISBN 1-4354-3869-8) and Blackboard (ISBN 1-4354-3870-1)

WebTutors (both **WebCT** and **Blackboard** formats) accompany this new edition of *Dimensional Analysis for Meds*. These online resources offer must-have classroom management tools, such as chats and calendars, as well as additional content resources, including class notes, videos, student quizzes, frequently asked questions, an audio glossary, and more.

## Online Companion

An exciting, new, robust online companion is available to adopters of this textbook. This valuable resource includes instructor support materials, exercises, and more. To access the site, simply point your browser to http://www.delmar.cengage.com/companions. Select the nursing discipline.

# INTRODUCTION FOR THE LEARNER

Welcome to what we anticipate will be one of the more enjoyable texts in your bookbag. *Dimensional Analysis for Meds,* fourth edition, is about to reassure you that math is nothing to be afraid of, and that on completion of your instruction you will have the calculation skills you need to practice safely in your profession. You don't have to be a math expert to be successful in dosage calculations; what you do need is a desire for accuracy and a motivation to learn. If you have not used your math skills for a number of years, Section 1, Refresher Math, will quickly bring you up to date. *Dimensional Analysis for Meds* is fully self-instructional and lets you move at your own pace through the content. Hundreds of examples and problems will keep your learning on track. Here are some tips to help you get started.

1.  Gather a calculator, pencil or pen, and plenty of scratch paper.

2.  Start by completing the Refresher Math Pretest on page xvi. This will alert you to those areas in Section 1, Refresher Math, that will need your particular attention. Some of the items in the Pretest and Refresher Math section were designed to be completed without using a calculator, but the choice is entirely yours; when you need a calculator, use one. You must remember, however, that calculator settings vary. All answers in this text were checked with a calculator set to hundredths. If you use one with a different setting, you may experience small differences in your answers in the tenths or hundredths.

3.  Record the answers to calculations on the scratch paper as well as in your text. This makes checking your answers against those we provide much easier.

4.  As you work your way through the chapters, do exactly as you are instructed to do. Programmed learning proceeds in small steps, and jumping ahead may cause confusion. All chapters are designed to let you move at your own speed, and if you already know some of the basics, you will move through them more quickly than you can imagine.

5.  Once you have completed your instruction, keep *Dimensional Analysis for Meds* in your personal library. As you move to different clinical areas during your career, you will encounter different types of calculations. A quick refresher with *Dimensional Analysis for Meds* will be invaluable when that occurs.

# INTRODUCTION FOR THE INSTRUCTOR

Welcome to the fourth edition of *Dimensional Analysis for Meds*. Whether you are a seasoned user of this text or are becoming acquainted with it for the first time, we would like to share a few ideas on how to most effectively incorporate this bestselling text into your curriculum. *Dimensional Analysis for Meds* is designed to be used starting early in the students' beginning semester. Many instructors assign the entire Section 1, Refresher Math, to be completed before the semester starts, and test on it within the first two weeks. Or, chapters can be assigned on a weekly basis at a pace fitting your students' profiles.

Students have many pressures on their time, and experience has shown that they learn best when their progress is routinely both encouraged and monitored. A short weekly test of about ten questions on the content assigned is the ideal way to do this. If a student struggles with the first test, provide a makeup opportunity. If a second test is unsuccessful, you will need to delve more deeply to determine the exact problem and help the student establish a study plan. The content in Section 1 is ideally suited to bring students up to the level of math skills required for success in dosage calculations.

Because testing and reinforcement are such vital components of learner success, encourage learners to use the CD-ROM located in the back of the textbook. Each module in this valuable electronic resource opens with a short tutorial designed to reinforce text concepts. Interactive problems and self-tests for each module reinforce accuracy and offer feedback as the student works at an individual pace. Another valuable electronic resource for learners is the WebCT and Blackboard courses accompanying *Dimensional Analysis for Meds*; these include class notes, frequently asked questions, additional quizzes, and much more, all of which offer excellent reinforcement of concepts presented in the text.

As an instructor, you will also have access to valuable electronic resources that will enhance your students' success. Lecture slides created in PowerPoint®, calculation solutions, images, instructor strategies, and a test bank are all included on our *Instructor Resources CD-ROM*, with the goal of facilitating classroom preparation and allowing you to focus as much time as possible on student interaction and competence. With *Dimensional Analysis for Meds*, both you and your students are prepared for success!

# USING THE LEARNING PACKAGE

The gtt/min flow rate can be calculated for mL/hr IV orders in one step by dividing the mL/hr to be infused by the division factor of the administration set.

A **Key** icon designates important reminders to help with calculations and to highlight important safety considerations. As you study for your exams, locate these **Keys** and make sure you know and understand them. Consider making flash cards of the Keys to be certain you know them.

**EXAMPLE 1** The available dosage strength is **750 mg in 2.5 mL**. How many mL will be needed to prepare a **600 mg** dosage?

Write the mL unit of measure being calculated, followed by an equal sign.

mL =

There are two important reasons for identifying the unit of measure being calculated first: it eliminates any confusion over exactly **which** measure is being calculated, and it dictates how the first or "starting" clinical ratio is entered in the equation.

**Example** icons walk you through each concept in a step-by-step manner, showing the calculation and mathematical processes. Focus on these areas to be sure you understand how to do each different type of calculation.

## Problems 9.2

Refer to the gentamicin label in Figure 9-5 to answer the following questions.

1. What is the total volume of this vial?
2. What is the dosage strength?
3. If 80 mg were ordered, how many mL would this be?
4. If 60 mg were ordered, how many mL would this be?
5. How many mL would you need to prepare a 20 mg dosage?

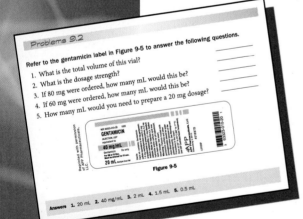

Figure 9-5

Answers  1. 20 mL  2. 40 mg/mL  3. 2 mL  4. 1.5 mL  5. 0.5 mL

**Problems** are sprinkled throughout each chapter. This is your opportunity to put your skills to the test, to identify your areas of strength, and to also acknowledge those areas where you need additional study. Answers to all problems are printed in the accompanying shaded box. Double-check your calculations if you have difficulty, or talk to your instructor for additional help.

Store below 25°C (77°F).
**Protect from light.**
Dispense in tight, light-resistant, child-resistant containers (USP).
**DOSAGE AND USE:**
See accompanying prescribing information. Each tablet contains 100 mg spironolactone.

NDC 0025-1031-31
**Rx only**
100 Tablets
**Aldactone®**
spironolactone
tablets, USP
**100 mg**
Distributed by
**Pfizer** **G.D. Searle LLC**
Division of Pfizer Inc, NY, NY 10017

2137

Used with permission from Pfizer Inc.

Actual **full-color labels** are used to support the problems and examples. Challenge yourself to read the labels carefully and accurately; are you able to understand the quantity, strength, form, dosing, and administration guidelines for every label you encounter?

New **photos of syringes** are depicted in actual size so that you can gain confidence in perfecting the real-life skill of accurately reading and interpreting syringe calibrations and medication levels.

**Summary Self-Tests** round out each chapter. Complete these as you finish studying the material, identify areas where you need to focus, and review the content again until you are confident in your calculating ability. Many of these tests include combined label and syringe questions, where you must calculate a dosage and then measure the dosage on a syringe. This is an excellent tool to test how well you apply your knowledge.

**Figure 8-6** | A 5 mL and a 10 mL syringe.

*Online Resources* are available at your fingertips. Visit the **online companion** and **web tutor** components for valuable course content, exercises, tutorials, class notes, glossaries, and more.

# USING THE IN-BOOK PRACTICE SOFTWARE

We are pleased to present the fourth edition of the *Dimensional Analysis for Meds Learning Program* CD-ROM. The CD-ROM is a proven tool for reinforcing important instructional content in your text in a unique and interactive way, using audio and visual presentation and animations. You will enjoy the following features:

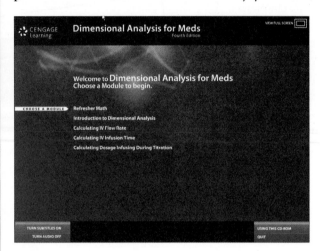

## Main Menu

The *Learning Program* presents five modules of content, each of which contains three to six lessons. The modules are:

- Refresher Math
- Introduction to Dimensional Analysis
- Calulating IV Flow Rate
- Calulating IV Infusion Time
- Calulating Dosage Infusing During Titration

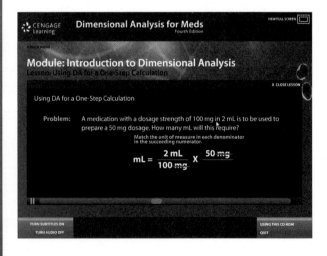

## Problems

Each didactic presentation is followed by a series of problems. Audio and visuals are used together to explain each step of solving the problem.

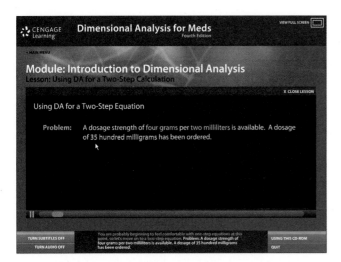

## Subtitles

The audio presentation clearly describes each step in solving problems using the dimensional analysis approach. You can listen to the narration or read it in subtitles at the bottom of the screen. Simply click a button to turn subtitles on or off.

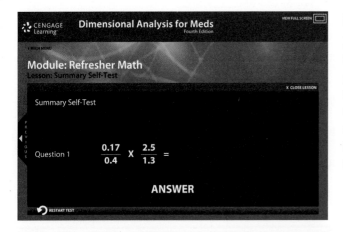

## Summary Self-Tests

Each module includes a brief test of all of the concepts presented. You have the option to print the test and complete it on the hard copy, or take the test on the screen. You can also view the answers on a separate screen to check your work.

# REFRESHER MATH PRETEST

If you can complete the Pretest with 100% accuracy, you are off to an exceptional start. However, don't be alarmed if you make some errors becuse the Refresher Math section that follows is designed to bring your math skills up-to-date. **Regardless of your proficiency, it's important that you complete the entire Refresher Math Section.** It includes memory cues and shortcuts for simplifying and solving many of the clinical calculations that are included in the entire text, and you will need to be familiar with these.

### Identify the decimal fraction with the greatest value in each set.

1. a) 4.4  b) 2.85  c) 5.3  _____
2. a) 6.3  b) 5.73  c) 4.4  _____
3. a) 0.18  b) 0.62  c) 0.35  _____
4. a) 0.2  b) 0.125  c) 0.3  _____
5. a) 0.15  b) 0.11  c) 0.14  _____
6. a) 4.27  b) 4.31  c) 4.09  _____

### Add these decimals.

7. 0.2 + 2.23  =  _____
8. 1.5 + 0.07  =  _____
9. 6.45 + 12.1 + 9.54 =_____
10. 0.35 + 8.37 + 5.15 =_____

### Subtract these decimals.

11. 3.1 − 0.67  =  _____
12. 12.41 − 2.11  =  _____
13. 2.235 − 0.094  =  _____
14. 4.65 − 0.7  =  _____
15. If tablets with a strength of 0.2 mg are available and 0.6 mg is ordered, how many tablets must you give? _____
16. If tablets are labeled 0.8 mg and 0.4 mg is ordered, how many tablets must you give? _____
17. If the available tablets have a strength of 1.25 mg and 2.5 mg is ordered, how many tablets must you give? _____
18. If 0.125 mg is ordered and the tablets available are labeled 0.25 mg, how many tablets must you give? _____

### Express these to the nearest tenth.

19. 2.17  =  _____
20. 0.15  =  _____
21. 3.77  =  _____
22. 4.62  =  _____
23. 11.74  =  _____
24. 5.26  =  _____

### Express these to the nearest hundredth.

25. 1.357  =  _____
26. 7.413  =  _____
27. 10.105  =  _____
28. 3.775  =  _____
29. 0.176  =  _____
30. Define "product."

### Multiply these decimals. Express your answers to the nearest tenth.

31. 0.7 × 1.2  =  _____
32. 1.8 × 2.6  =  _____
33. 5.1 × 0.25 × 1.1 =  _____
34. 3.3 × 3.75  =  _____

### Divide these fractions. Express your answers to the nearest hundredth.

35. 16.3 ÷ 3.2 = _____
36. 15.1 ÷ 1.1 = _____
37. 2 ÷ 0.75  = _____
38. 4.17 ÷ 2.7 = _____
39. Define "numerator."

_____

40. Define "denominator."

_____

41. Define "greatest common denominator."

_____

### Solve these equations. Express your answers to the nearest tenth.

42. $\dfrac{1}{4} \times \dfrac{2}{3} =$ _____

43. $\dfrac{240}{170} \times \dfrac{135}{300} =$ _____

44. $\dfrac{0.2}{1.75} \times \dfrac{1.5}{0.2} =$ _____

45. $\dfrac{2.1}{3.6} \times \dfrac{1.7}{1.3} =$ _____

46. $\dfrac{0.26}{0.2} \times \dfrac{3.3}{1.2} =$ _____

47. $\dfrac{750}{1} \times \dfrac{300}{50} \times \dfrac{7}{2} =$ _____

48. $\dfrac{50}{1} \times \dfrac{60}{240} \times \dfrac{1}{900} \times \dfrac{400}{1} =$ _____

49. $\dfrac{35,000}{750} \times \dfrac{35}{1} =$ _____

50. $\dfrac{50}{40} \times \dfrac{450}{40} \times \dfrac{1}{900} \times \dfrac{114}{1} =$ _____

**Answers**

| | | | |
|---|---|---|---|
| **1.** c | **18.** ½ tab | **33.** 1.4 | **42.** 0.2 |
| **2.** a | **19.** 2.2 | **34.** 12.4 | **43.** 0.6 |
| **3.** b | **20.** 0.2 | **35.** 5.09 | **44.** 0.9 |
| **4.** c | **21.** 3.8 | **36.** 13.73 | **45.** 0.8 |
| **5.** a | **22.** 4.6 | **37.** 2.67 | **46.** 3.6 |
| **6.** b | **23.** 11.7 | **38.** 1.54 | **47.** 15,750 |
| **7.** 2.43 | **24.** 5.3 | **39.** The top number in | **48.** 5.6 |
| **8.** 1.57 | **25.** 1.36 | a common fraction | **49.** 1633.3 |
| **9.** 28.09 | **26.** 7.41 | **40.** The bottom | **50.** 1.8 |
| **10.** 13.87 | **27.** 10.11 | number in a | |
| **11.** 2.43 | **28.** 3.78 | common fraction | |
| **12.** 10.3 | **29.** 0.18 | **41.** The greatest | |
| **13.** 2.141 | **30.** The answer | number that can | |
| **14.** 3.95 | obtained from the | be divided into | |
| **15.** 3 tab | multiplication of two | two numbers to | |
| **16.** ½ tab | or more numbers | reduce them to | |
| **17.** 2 tab | **31.** 0.8 | their lowest terms | |
| | **32.** 4.7 | (values) | |

# 1

SECTION

# Refresher Math

**CHAPTER 1**
Relative Value, Addition, and
Subtraction of Decimals / 2

**CHAPTER 2**
Multiplication and Division of
Decimals / 11

**CHAPTER 3**
Solving Common Fraction
Equations / 22

# RELATIVE VALUE, ADDITION, AND SUBTRACTION OF DECIMALS

## Objectives

**The learner will:**

1. identify the relative value of decimals.

2. add decimals.

3. subtract decimals.

## Prerequisites

Recognize the abbreviations mg, for milligram, and g, for gram, as drug measures.

In the course of administering medications, you will be dealing with decimal fraction dosages on a daily basis. The first two chapters of this text provide a complete refresher on everything you need to know about decimals, including safety measures when you do calculations both manually and with a calculator. We'll start with a review of the range of decimal values you will see in dosages. This will enable you to recognize which of two or more numbers has the greater (or lesser) value—a skill you will use constantly in your professional career.

### RELATIVE VALUE OF DECIMALS

The most helpful fact to remember about decimals is that **our monetary system of dollars and cents is a decimal system**. The whole numbers in dosages have the same relative value as dollars, and decimal fractions have the same value as cents: **the greater the number, the greater the value**. If you keep this in mind, you will have already learned the most important safety measure of dealing with decimals in dosages.

The range of drug dosages, which includes decimal fractions, stretches from millions on the whole number side, to thousandths on the decimal side. Refer to the decimal scale in Figure 1-1, and locate the decimal point, which

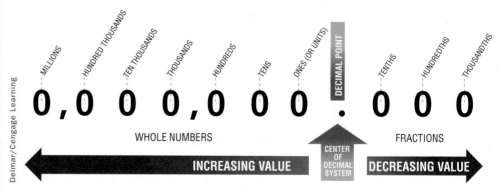

Figure 1-1

is slightly to the right on this scale. Notice the whole numbers on the left of the scale, which rise increasingly in value from ones (units) to millions, which is the largest whole-number drug dosage in current use.

 The first determiner of the relative value of decimals is the presence of whole numbers. The greater the whole number, the greater the value.

**EXAMPLE 1**   10.1 is greater than 9.15

**EXAMPLE 2**   3.2 is greater than 2.99

**EXAMPLE 3**   7.01 is greater than 6.99

## Problems 1.1

**Choose the greatest value in each set.**

| | | | |
|---|---|---|---|
| 1. a) 3.5 | b) 2.7 | c) 4.2 | _____ |
| 2. a) 6.15 | b) 5.95 | c) 4.54 | _____ |
| 3. a) 12.02 | b) 10.19 | c) 11.04 | _____ |
| 4. a) 2.5 | b) 1.75 | c) 0.75 | _____ |
| 5. a) 4.3 | b) 2.75 | c) 5.1 | _____ |
| 6. a) 6.15 | b) 7.4 | c) 5.95 | _____ |
| 7. a) 7.25 | b) 8.1 | c) 9.37 | _____ |
| 8. a) 4.25 | b) 5.1 | c) 3.75 | _____ |
| 9. a) 9.4 | b) 8.75 | c) 7.4 | _____ |
| 10. a) 5.1 | b) 6.33 | c) 4.2 | _____ |

**Answers  1.** c  **2.** a  **3.** a  **4.** a  **5.** c  **6.** b  **7.** c  **8.** b  **9.** a  **10.** b

If, however, the whole numbers are the same—for example, **10.**2 and **10.**7—or there are no whole numbers—for example, **0.**25 and **0.**35—**then the fraction will determine the relative value**. Let's take a closer look at the fractional side of the scale (refer to Figure 1-2).

Figure 1-2

It is necessary to **consider only three figures after the decimal point on the fractional side,** because drug dosages measured as decimal fractions do not contain more than three digits; for example, 0.125 mg. Notice that a **zero is used to replace the whole number** in this decimal fraction and in all dosages that do not contain a whole number.

 If a decimal fraction is not preceded by a whole number, a zero is used in front of the decimal point to emphasize that the number is a fraction.

**EXAMPLE**    **0.**125    **0.**1    **0.**45

Look again at Figure 1-2. The numbers to the right of the decimal point represent **tenths, hundredths,** and **thousandths,** in that order. When you see a decimal fraction in which the **whole numbers are the same,** or there are **no whole numbers,** stop and look first at the number representing **tenths.**

 The fraction with the greater number representing tenths has the greater value.

**EXAMPLE 1**    0.3 is greater than 0.27

**EXAMPLE 2**    0.4 is greater than 0.29

**EXAMPLE 3**    1.2 is greater than 1.19

**EXAMPLE 4**    3.5 is greater than 3.2

## Problems 1.2

**Choose the greatest value in each set.**

| | | | |
|---|---|---|---|
| 1. a) 0.4 | b) 0.2 | c) 0.5 | _____ |
| 2. a) 2.73 | b) 2.61 | c) 2.87 | _____ |
| 3. a) 0.19 | b) 0.61 | c) 0.34 | _____ |
| 4. a) 3.5 | b) 3.75 | c) 3.25 | _____ |
| 5. a) 0.3 | b) 0.25 | c) 0.4 | _____ |
| 6. a) 1.35 | b) 1.29 | c) 1.4 | _____ |
| 7. a) 2.5 | b) 2.7 | c) 2.35 | _____ |
| 8. a) 4.51 | b) 4.75 | c) 4.8 | _____ |
| 9. a) 0.8 | b) 0.3 | c) 0.4 | _____ |
| 10. a) 2.1 | b) 2.05 | c) 2.15 | _____ |

**Answers**   **1.** c.   **2.** c   **3.** b   **4.** b   **5.** c   **6.** c   **7.** b   **8.** c   **9.** a   **10.** c

If in decimal fractions the numbers representing **the tenths are identical**—for example, 0.25 and 0.27—then **the number representing the hundredths will determine the relative value.**

 When the tenths are identical, the fraction with the greater number representing hundredths will have the greater value.

**EXAMPLE 1**   0.27 is greater than 0.2**5**

**EXAMPLE 2**   0.1**5** is greater than 0.1 (0.1 is the same as 0.1**0**)

 Extra zeros on the end of decimal fractions are omitted in drug dosages because they can easily be misread and lead to errors.

**EXAMPLE 3**   2.2**5** is greater than 2.2 (same as 2.20)

**EXAMPLE 4**   9.7**7** is greater than 9.7 (same as 9.70)

## Problems 1.3

Choose the greatest value in each set.

| | | | |
|---|---|---|---|
| 1. a) 0.12 | b) 0.15 | c) 0.17 | _____ |
| 2. a) 1.2 | b) 1.24 | c) 1.23 | _____ |
| 3. a) 0.37 | b) 0.3 | c) 0.36 | _____ |
| 4. a) 3.27 | b) 3.25 | c) 3.21 | _____ |
| 5. a) 0.16 | b) 0.11 | c) 0.19 | _____ |
| 6. a) 4.23 | b) 4.2 | c) 4.09 | _____ |
| 7. a) 3.27 | b) 3.21 | c) 3.29 | _____ |
| 8. a) 2.75 | b) 2.73 | c) 2.78 | _____ |
| 9. a) 0.31 | b) 0.37 | c) 0.33 | _____ |
| 10. a) 0.43 | b) 0.45 | c) 0.44 | _____ |

**Answers  1.** c  **2.** b  **3.** a  **4.** a  **5.** c  **6.** a  **7.** c  **8.** c  **9.** b  **10.** b

## Problems 1.4

**Which fraction has the greater value?**

a) 0.125          b) 0.25

**Answer**   If you chose 0.125, you have just made a serious drug dosage error. Look again at the numbers representing the tenths, and you will see that 0.**2**5 is greater than 0.**1**25. Remember that extra zeros are omitted in decimal fraction dosages because they can lead to errors. In this fraction, 0.25 is the same as 0.250, which is exactly double the value of 0.125. **Check the tenths carefully, regardless of the total of numbers after the decimal point.**

| EXAMPLE 1 | 0.15 (same as 0.150) is greater than 0.125 |
| EXAMPLE 2 | 0.3 (same as 0.30) is greater than 0.15 |
| EXAMPLE 3 | 0.75 (same as 0.750) is greater than 0.325 |
| EXAMPLE 4 | 0.8 (same as 0.80) is greater than 0.16 |

 The number of figures on the right of the decimal point is not an indication of relative value. Always look at the figure representing the tenths first, and if these are identical, check the hundredths to determine which has the greater value.

This completes your introduction to the relative value of decimals. The key points just reviewed will cover all situations in dosage calculations in which you will have to recognize greater and lesser values. Test yourself more extensively on this information in the following problems.

## Problems 1.5

**Choose the greatest value in each set.**

1. a) 0.24        b) 0.5        c) 0.125        _____
2. a) 0.4         b) 0.45       c) 0.5          _____
3. a) 7.5         b) 6.25       c) 4.75         _____
4. a) 0.3         b) 0.25       c) 0.35         _____
5. a) 1.125       b) 1.75       c) 1.5          _____
6. a) 4.5         b) 4.75       c) 4.25         _____
7. a) 0.1         b) 0.01       c) 0.04         _____
8. a) 5.75        b) 6.25       c) 6.5          _____
9. a) 0.6         b) 0.16       c) 0.06         _____
10. a) 3.55       b) 2.95       c) 3.7          _____

**Answers**   **1.** b   **2.** c   **3.** a   **4.** c   **5.** b   **6.** b   **7.** a   **8.** c   **9.** a   **10.** c

## ADDITION AND SUBTRACTION OF DECIMALS

Complex addition and subtraction of decimals should be done with a calculator, but, on occasion, time can be saved by doing simple calculations without one. Let's start by looking at a few key points that will make manual solution safer.

**When you write down the numbers, line up the decimal points.**

**EXAMPLE**   To add 0.25 and 0.27

0.25             0.25
+0.27 is safe    +0.27 is unsafe; it could lead to errors.

**Always add or subtract from right to left.**

If you decide to write down the numbers, **do not confuse yourself by trying to "eyeball" the answer.** Also, write any numbers carried or rewrite those reduced by borrowing if you find this helpful.

**EXAMPLE 1**   When adding 0.25 and 0.27

```
    1
  0.25
+ 0.27    Add the 5 and 7 first, then the 2, 2, and
  0.52    the 1 you carried; work from right to left
```

**EXAMPLE 2**   When subtracting 0.63 from 0.71

```
    61
  0.71    Borrow 1 from 7 and rewrite as 6
- 0.63    Write the borrowed 1; subtract 3 from 11
  0.08    Subtract 6 from 6; work from right to left
```

**Add zeros as necessary to make the fractions of equal length.**

Adding zeros to make the fractions of equal length does not alter the value of the fractions, and it helps prevent confusion and mistakes.

**EXAMPLE**   When subtracting 0.125 from 0.25

0.25              0.250
0.125   becomes   0.125              Answer = **0.125**

If you follow these simple rules and make them a habit, you will automatically reduce calculation errors. The problems on the following page will give you an excellent opportunity to practice addition and subtraction.

## Problems 1.6

**Add decimals.**

1. $0.25 + 0.55$ = _____
2. $0.1 + 2.25$ = _____
3. $1.74 + 0.76$ = _____
4. $1.4 + 0.02$ = _____
5. $2.3 + 1.45$ = _____

6. $3.75 + 1.05$ = _____
7. $6.35 + 2.05$ = _____
8. $5.57 + 4.03$ = _____
9. $0.33 + 2.42$ = _____
10. $1.44 + 3.06$ = _____

**Subtract decimals.**

11. $1.25 - 1.125$ = _____
12. $3.25 - 0.65$ = _____
13. $2.3 - 1.45$ = _____
14. $0.02 - 0.01$ = _____
15. $5.5 - 2.5$ = _____

16. $7.33 - 4.03$ = _____
17. $4.25 - 1.75$ = _____
18. $0.07 - 0.035$ = _____
19. $0.235 - 0.12$ = _____
20. $5.75 - 0.95$ = _____

**Answers** **1.** 0.8 **2.** 2.35 **3.** 2.5 **4.** 1.42 **5.** 3.75 **6.** 4.8 **7.** 8.4 **8.** 9.6 **9.** 2.75 **10.** 4.5 **11.** 0.125 **12.** 2.6 **13.** 0.85 **14.** 0.01 **15.** 3 **16.** 3.3 **17.** 2.5 **18.** 0.035 **19.** 0.115 **20.** 4.8
**Note:** If you did not add a zero before the decimal point in answers that do not contain a whole number, or failed to eliminate unnecessary zeros from the end of decimal fractions, your answers are incorrect.

## Summary

**This concludes the refresher on relative value, addition, and subtraction of simple decimal fractions. The important points to remember from this chapter are:**

- If a decimal fraction contains a whole number, the value of the whole number is the first determiner of relative value.

- If a fraction does not include a whole number, a zero is placed in front of the decimal point to emphasize that it is a fractional dosage.

- If there is no whole number, or if the whole numbers are the same, the number representing the tenths in the decimal fraction will be the next determiner of relative value.

- If the tenths in decimal fractions are identical, the number representing hundredths will determine relative value.

- When manually adding or subtracting decimal fractions, first line up the decimal points, then add or subtract from right to left.

- Extra zeros on the end of decimal fractions can be a source of error in drug dosages, and are routinely eliminated.

## Summary Self-Test

**Choose the decimal with the greatest value.**

1. a) 2.45        b) 2.57        c) 2.19        _____

2. a) 3.07        b) 3.17        c) 3.71        _____

3. a) 0.12        b) 0.02        c) 0.01        _____

4. a) 5.31        b) 5.35        c) 6.01        _____

5. a) 4.5         b) 4.51        c) 4.15        _____

6. a) 0.015       b) 0.15        c) 0.1         _____

7. a) 1.3         b) 1.25        c) 1.35        _____

8. a) 0.1         b) 0.2         c) 0.25        _____

9. a) 0.125       b) 0.1         c) 0.05        _____

10. a) 13.7       b) 13.5        c) 13.25       _____

11. If you have medication tablets whose strength is 0.1 mg and you must give 0.3 mg, you will need

    a) 1 tablet.     b) less than 1 tablet.     c) more than 1 tablet.     _____

12. If you have tablets with a strength of 0.25 mg and you must give 0.125 mg, you will need

    a) 1 tablet.     b) less than 1 tablet.     c) more than 1 tablet.     _____

13. If you have an order to give a dosage of 7.5 mg and the tablets have a strength of 3.75 mg, you will need

    a) 1 tablet.     b) less than 1 tablet.     c) more than 1 tablet.     _____

14. If the order is to give 0.5 mg and the tablet strength is 0.5 mg, you will give

    a) 1 tablet.     b) less than 1 tablet.     c) more than 1 tablet.     _____

15. The order is to give 0.5 mg and the tablets have a strength of 0.25 mg. You must give

    a) 1 tablet.     b) less than 1 tablet.     c) more than 1 tablet.     _____

**Add the decimals manually.**

16. 1.31 + 0.4   = _____          20. 1.3 + 1.04   = _____

17. 0.15 + 0.25  = _____          21. 4.7 + 3.03   = _____

18. 2.5 + 0.75   = _____          22. 0.5 + 0.5    = _____

19. 3.2 + 2.17   = _____          23. 5.4 + 2.6    = _____

24. You have just given two tablets with a dosage strength of 3.5 mg each. What was the total dosage administered?     _____

25. You are to give your patient one tablet labeled 0.5 mg and one labeled 0.25 mg. What is the total dosage of these two tablets?     _____

26. If you give two tablets labeled 0.02 mg, what total dosage will you administer?     _____

27. You are to give one tablet labeled 0.8 mg and two tablets labeled 0.4 mg. What is the total dosage? _____

28. You have two tablets: one is labeled 0.15 mg and the other 0.3 mg. What is the total dosage of these two tablets? _____

**Subtract the decimals manually.**

29. 4.32 − 3.1  = _____
30. 2.1 − 1.91  = _____
31. 3.73 − 1.93  = _____
32. 5.75 − 4.05  = _____

33. 1.3 − 0.02  = _____
34. 0.2 − 0.07  = _____
35. 3.95 − 0.35  = _____
36. 1.9 − 0.08  = _____

37. Your patient is to receive a dosage of 7.5 mg and you have only one tablet labeled 3.75 mg. How many more milligrams must you give? _____

38. You have a tablet labeled 0.02 mg and your patient is to receive 0.06 mg. How many more milligrams must you give? _____

39. The tablet available is labeled 0.5 mg, but you must give a dosage of 1.5 mg. How many more milligrams will you need to obtain the correct dosage? _____

40. Your patient is to receive a dosage of 1.2 mg and you have one tablet labeled 0.6 mg. What additional dosage in milligrams will you need? _____

41. You must give your patient a dosage of 2.2 mg, but you have only two tablets labeled 0.55 mg. What additional dosage in milligrams will you need? _____

**Determine how many tablets will be needed to give the dosages.**

42. Tablets are labeled 0.01 mg. You must give 0.02 mg. _____
43. Tablets are labeled 2.5 mg. You must give 5 mg. _____
44. Tablets are labeled 0.25 mg. Give 0.125 mg. _____
45. Tablets are 0.5 mg. Give 1.5 mg. _____
46. A dosage of 1.8 mg is ordered. Tablets are 0.6 mg. _____
47. Tablets available are 0.04 mg. You are to give 0.02 mg. _____
48. The dosage ordered is 3.5 mg. The tablets available are 1.75 mg. _____
49. Prepare a dosage of 3.2 mg using tablets with a strength of 1.6 mg. _____
50. You have tablets labeled 0.25 mg and a dosage of 0.375 mg is ordered. _____

| **Answers** | **11.** c | **22.** 1 | **33.** 1.28 | **44.** ½ tab |
|---|---|---|---|---|
| **1.** b | **12.** b | **23.** 8 | **34.** 0.13 | **45.** 3 tab |
| **2.** c | **13.** c | **24.** 7 mg | **35.** 3.6 | **46.** 3 tab |
| **3.** a | **14.** a | **25.** 0.75 mg | **36.** 1.82 | **47.** ½ tab |
| **4.** c | **15.** c | **26.** 0.04 mg | **37.** 3.75 mg | **48.** 2 tab |
| **5.** b | **16.** 1.71 | **27.** 1.6 mg | **38.** 0.04 mg | **49.** 2 tab |
| **6.** b | **17.** 0.4 | **28.** 0.45 mg | **39.** 1 mg | **50.** 1½ tab |
| **7.** c | **18.** 3.25 | **29.** 1.22 | **40.** 0.6 mg | |
| **8.** c | **19.** 5.37 | **30.** 0.19 | **41.** 1.1 mg | |
| **9.** a | **20.** 2.34 | **31.** 1.8 | **42.** 2 tab | |
| **10.** a | **21.** 7.73 | **32.** 1.7 | **43.** 2 tab | |

**Note:** If you did not add a zero before the decimal point in answers that did not contain a whole number, or failed to eliminate unnecessary zeros from the end of decimal fractions, your answers are incorrect.

# MULTIPLICATION AND DIVISION OF DECIMALS

Multiplication and division are integral parts of dosage calculations. As is the case with addition and subtraction, some multiplication and division problems involving dosages can be done manually, so the basic steps in multiplication and division are reviewed in this chapter. In addition, a number of shortcuts will be introduced that can make numbers easier to work with, especially those containing decimal fractions. And for those calculations that are more safely handled with a calculator, safety in calculator use will be discussed.

## MULTIPLICATION OF DECIMALS

The main precaution in multiplication of decimals is the **placement of the decimal point in the answer**, which is called the **product**.

The decimal point in the product of decimal fractions is placed the same number of places to the left in the product as the total of numbers following the decimal points in the fractions multiplied.

**EXAMPLE 1**   Multiply 0.35 by 0.5

It is safer to begin by lining up the numbers to be multiplied on the right side. Then, disregard the decimals during multiplication.

$$\begin{array}{r} 0.35 \\ \times\ \underline{0.5} \\ 175 \end{array}$$

The product/answer is 175; 0.35 has two numbers after the decimal and 0.5 has one. Place the decimal point three places to the left in the product to make it .175, then add a zero (0) in front of the decimal to emphasize the fraction.

Answer = **0.175**

## Objectives

The learner will:

1. define product, numerator, and denominator.
2. multiply decimal fractions.
3. divide decimal fractions.
4. simplify common fractions containing decimal numbers.
5. reduce fractions using common denominators.
6. reduce common fractions that end in zeros.
7. express answers to the nearest tenth and hundredth.
8. use a calculator to multiply and divide.

## Prerequisite

Chapter 1

EXAMPLE 2    Multiply 1.61 by 0.2

$$
\begin{array}{r}
1.61 \\
\times\ \underline{0.2} \\
322
\end{array}
$$
Line up the numbers on the right

The product is 322; 1.61 has two numbers after the decimal point and 0.2 has one. Place the decimal point three places to the left in the product so that 322 becomes .322, then add a zero in front of the decimal to emphasize the fraction.

Answer = **0.322**

If the product contains insufficient numbers for correct placement of the decimal point, add as many zeros as necessary to the left of the product to correct this.

EXAMPLE 3    Multiply 1.5 by 0.06

$$
\begin{array}{r}
1.5 \\
\times\ \underline{0.06} \\
90
\end{array}
$$
Line up the numbers on the right

The product is 90; 1.5 has one number after the decimal point and 0.06 has two. To place the decimal three places to the left in the product, a zero must be added, making it .090. Eliminate the excess zero from the end of the fraction, and add a zero in front of the decimal point.

Answer = **0.09**

EXAMPLE 4    Multiply 0.21 by 0.32

$$
\begin{array}{r}
0.21 \\
\times\ \underline{0.32} \\
42 \\
\underline{63\phantom{0}} \\
672
\end{array}
$$
Indent second number multiplication
Add the totals

In this example, 0.21 has two numbers after the decimal point and 0.32 also has two. Add a zero in front of 672 to allow correct placement of the decimal point, making it .0672, then add a zero in front of the fraction to emphasize it.

Answer = **0.0672**

EXAMPLE 5    Multiply 0.12 by 0.2

$$
\begin{array}{r}
0.12 \\
\times\ \underline{0.2} \\
24
\end{array}
$$

In this example, there are a total of three numbers after the decimal points in 0.12 and 0.2. Add a zero in front of 24 for correct decimal placement, making it .024, then add a zero in front of .024 to emphasize the fraction.

Answer = **0.024**

## Problems 2.1

**Multiply the decimal fractions without using a calculator.**

1. 0.45 × 0.2   = _____
2. 0.35 × 0.12  = _____
3. 1.3 × 0.05   = _____
4. 0.7 × 0.04   = _____
5. 0.4 × 0.17   = _____

6. 2.14 × 0.03  = _____
7. 1.4 × 0.4    = _____
8. 3.3 × 1.2    = _____
9. 2.7 × 2.2    = _____
10. 2.1 × 0.3   = _____

**Answers  1.** 0.09  **2.** 0.042  **3.** 0.065  **4.** 0.028  **5.** 0.068  **6.** 0.0642  **7.** 0.56  **8.** 3.96
**9.** 5.94  **10.** 0.63

## DIVISION OF DECIMAL FRACTIONS

A calculator may also be used for division of complex decimal fractions. However, let's start by reviewing the terminology of common fraction division, and **three important precalculator** steps that may make final manual division easier: **elimination of decimal points, reduction of the fractions,** and **reduction of numbers ending in zero.** The following is a sample of a common fraction division seen in dosages.

**EXAMPLE 1**   $\dfrac{0.25}{0.125} = \dfrac{\text{numerator}}{\text{denominator}}$

You'll recall that the **top number** in a common fraction is called the **numerator**, whereas the **bottom number** is called the **denominator**. If you have trouble remembering which is which, think of **D**, for **down**, for **denominator**. The denominator is on the bottom. With this basic terminology reviewed, we are now ready to look at preliminary math steps that can be used to simplify a fraction or actually solve an equation and eliminate the need for calculator division.

## ELIMINATION OF DECIMAL POINTS

Decimal points can be eliminated from numbers in a decimal fraction without changing its value, if they are moved the same number of places in one numerator and one denominator.

 To eliminate the decimal points from decimal fractions, move them the same number of places to the right in a numerator and a denominator until they are eliminated from both. Zeros may have to be added to accomplish this.

**EXAMPLE 1**   $\dfrac{0.25}{0.125}$   becomes   $\dfrac{250}{125}$

The decimal point must be moved three places to the right in the denominator 0.125 to make it 125. Therefore, it must be moved three places to the right in the numerator 0.25, which requires the addition of one zero to make it 250.

**EXAMPLE 2**   $\dfrac{0.3}{0.15}$   becomes   $\dfrac{30}{15}$

The decimal point must be moved two places in 0.15 to make it 15, so it must be moved two places in 0.3, which requires the addition of one zero to become 30.

**EXAMPLE 3**   $\dfrac{1.5}{2}$   becomes   $\dfrac{15}{20}$

Move the decimal point one place in 1.5 to make it 15; add one zero to 2 to make it 20.

**EXAMPLE 4**   $\dfrac{4.5}{0.95}$   becomes   $\dfrac{450}{95}$

 Eliminating the decimal points from a decimal fraction before final division does not alter the value of the fraction, or the answer obtained in the final division.

## Problems 2.2

Eliminate the decimal points from these common fractions.

1. $\dfrac{17.5}{2}$ = _____

2. $\dfrac{0.5}{25}$ = _____

3. $\dfrac{6.3}{0.6}$ = _____

4. $\dfrac{3.76}{0.4}$ = _____

5. $\dfrac{8.4}{0.7}$ = _____

6. $\dfrac{0.1}{0.05}$ = _____

7. $\dfrac{0.9}{0.03}$ = _____

8. $\dfrac{10.75}{2.5}$ = _____

9. $\dfrac{0.4}{0.04}$ = _____

10. $\dfrac{1.2}{0.4}$ = _____

**Answers** 1. $\dfrac{175}{20}$  2. $\dfrac{5}{250}$  3. $\dfrac{63}{6}$  4. $\dfrac{376}{40}$  5. $\dfrac{84}{7}$  6. $\dfrac{10}{5}$  7. $\dfrac{90}{3}$  8. $\dfrac{1075}{250}$  9. $\dfrac{40}{4}$  10. $\dfrac{12}{4}$

## REDUCTION OF FRACTIONS

Once the decimal points are eliminated, a second simplification step is to reduce the numbers as far as possible using common denominators/divisors, the largest number that will divide both a numerator and a denominator.

 To further reduce fractions, divide numbers by their greatest common denominator (the largest number that will divide into both a numerator and a denominator).

The **greatest common denominator** is usually **2, 3, 4, 5, or multiples of these numbers**, such as 6, 8, 25, and so on.

**EXAMPLE 1**   $\dfrac{175}{20}$    The greatest common denominator is 5

$$\dfrac{\cancel{175}}{\cancel{20}} = \dfrac{35}{4}$$

**EXAMPLE 2**   $\dfrac{63}{6}$    The greatest common denominator is 3

$$\dfrac{\cancel{63}}{\cancel{6}} = \dfrac{21}{2}$$

**EXAMPLE 3**   $\dfrac{1075}{250}$    The greatest common denominator is 25

$$\dfrac{\cancel{1075}}{\cancel{250}} = \dfrac{43}{10}$$

There is a second way you could have reduced the fraction in Example 3, and it is equally as correct. Divide by 5, then by 5 again.

$$\dfrac{\cancel{1075}}{\cancel{250}} = \dfrac{\cancel{215}}{\cancel{50}} = \dfrac{43}{10}$$

 **If the greatest common denominator is difficult to determine, reduce several times by using smaller common denominators.**

**EXAMPLE 4**   $\dfrac{376}{40} = \dfrac{47}{5}$   Divide by 8

Or divide by 4, then 2   $\dfrac{\cancel{376}}{\cancel{40}} = \dfrac{\cancel{94}}{\cancel{10}} = \dfrac{47}{5}$

Or divide by 2, then 2, then 2   $\dfrac{\cancel{376}}{\cancel{40}} = \dfrac{\cancel{188}}{\cancel{20}} = \dfrac{\cancel{94}}{\cancel{10}} = \dfrac{47}{5}$

Remember that **simple numbers are easiest to work with**, and the time spent in extra reductions may be well worth the payoff in safety.

## Problems 2.3

**Reduce the fractions in preparation for final division.**

1. $\dfrac{84}{8}$ = _____

2. $\dfrac{20}{16}$ = _____

3. $\dfrac{250}{325}$ = _____

4. $\dfrac{96}{34}$ = _____

5. $\dfrac{175}{20}$ = _____

6. $\dfrac{40}{14}$ = _____

7. $\frac{82}{28}$ = _____     9. $\frac{50}{75}$ = _____

8. $\frac{100}{75}$ = _____     10. $\frac{60}{88}$ = _____

**Answers** 1. $\frac{21}{2}$ 2. $\frac{5}{4}$ 3. $\frac{10}{13}$ 4. $\frac{48}{17}$ 5. $\frac{35}{4}$ 6. $\frac{20}{7}$ 7. $\frac{41}{14}$ 8. $\frac{4}{3}$ 9. $\frac{2}{3}$ 10. $\frac{15}{22}$

## REDUCTION OF NUMBERS ENDING IN ZERO

The third type of simplification is not solely related to decimal fractions but is best covered at this time. This concerns reductions in a common fraction when both a numerator and a denominator end with zeros.

 Numbers that end in a zero or zeros may be reduced by crossing off the same number of zeros in both a numerator and a denominator.

**EXAMPLE 1**  $\frac{800}{250}$

In this fraction, the numerator, 800, has two zeros, but the denominator, 250, has one zero. The number of zeros crossed off must be the same in both numerator and denominator, so only one zero can be eliminated from each.

$$\frac{80\cancel{0}}{25\cancel{0}} = \frac{80}{25} \qquad \text{Reduce by } 5 = \frac{16}{5}$$

**EXAMPLE 2**  $\frac{24\cancel{00}}{20\cancel{00}} = \frac{24}{20}$  Reduce by $4 = \frac{6}{5}$

Two zeros can be eliminated from the denominator and the numerator in this fraction.

**EXAMPLE 3**  $\frac{15\cancel{000}}{30\cancel{000}} = \frac{15}{30}$  Reduce by $15 = \frac{1}{2}$

In this fraction, three zeros can be eliminated.

## Problems 2.4

**Reduce the fractions to their lowest terms.**

1. $\frac{50}{250}$ = _____       4. $\frac{1,000,000}{750,000}$ = _____

2. $\frac{120}{50}$ = _____       5. $\frac{800}{150}$ = _____

3. $\frac{2500}{1500}$ = _____      6. $\frac{110}{100}$ = _____

7. $\dfrac{200,000}{150,000}$ = _____

9. $\dfrac{60}{40}$ = _____

8. $\dfrac{1000}{800}$ = _____

10. $\dfrac{150}{200}$ = _____

**Answers**  **1.** $\dfrac{1}{5}$  **2.** $\dfrac{12}{5}$  **3.** $\dfrac{5}{3}$  **4.** $\dfrac{4}{3}$  **5.** $\dfrac{16}{3}$  **6.** $\dfrac{11}{10}$  **7.** $\dfrac{4}{3}$  **8.** $\dfrac{5}{4}$  **9.** $\dfrac{3}{2}$  **10.** $\dfrac{3}{4}$

## USING A CALCULATOR

Calculators vary in how addition, subtraction, division, and multiplication must be entered, and in the number of fractional numbers displayed after the decimal point. The first precaution in calculator use is to ensure you **know how to use the one available to you**. If you must do frequent calculations, it would be wise to buy and use your own. The next precaution—and this is critical—is to enter decimal numbers correctly, which includes **entering the decimal points**. This is not as easy to remember as it sounds, and this is a step where dosage calculation errors can occur.

 Calculator entry errors tend to be repetitive, so visually check each entry before entering the next.

## EXPRESSING TO THE NEAREST TENTH

When a fraction is reduced as much as possible, it is ready for final division. If necessary, this is done using a calculator to **divide the numerator by the denominator**. Dosage answers are most frequently rounded off and expressed as decimal fractions to the nearest tenth.

 To express an answer to the nearest tenth, the division is carried to hundredths (two places after the decimal). When the number representing hundredths is 5 or larger, the number representing tenths is increased by one.

**EXAMPLE 1**   $\dfrac{0.35}{0.4} = 0.35 \div 0.4 = 0.87$

Answer = **0.9**

The number representing hundredths is 7, so the number representing tenths is increased by one: 0.87 becomes 0.9.

**EXAMPLE 2**   $\dfrac{0.5}{0.3} = 0.5 \div 0.3 = 1.66 = \mathbf{1.7}$

The number representing hundredths, 6, is larger than 5, so 1.66 becomes 1.7.

**EXAMPLE 3**   $\dfrac{0.16}{0.3} = 0.53 = \mathbf{0.5}$

The number representing hundredths, 3, is less than 5, so the number representing tenths, 5, remains unchanged.

**EXAMPLE 4** $\dfrac{0.2}{0.3} = 0.66 = \mathbf{0.7}$

**EXAMPLE 5** An answer of 1.42 remains **1.4**.

**EXAMPLE 6** An answer of 1.86 becomes **1.9**.

## Problems 2.5

**Use a calculator to divide the common fractions. Express answers to the nearest tenth.**

1. $\dfrac{5.1}{2.3} =$ _____

2. $\dfrac{0.9}{0.7} =$ _____

3. $\dfrac{3.7}{2} =$ _____

4. $\dfrac{6}{1.3} =$ _____

5. $\dfrac{1.5}{2.1} =$ _____

6. $\dfrac{2.7}{1.1} =$ _____

7. $\dfrac{4.2}{5} =$ _____

8. $\dfrac{0.5}{2.5} =$ _____

9. $\dfrac{5.2}{0.91} =$ _____

10. $\dfrac{2.4}{2.7} =$ _____

**Answers 1.** 2.2 **2.** 1.3 **3.** 1.9 **4.** 4.6 **5.** 0.7 **6.** 2.5 **7.** 0.8 **8.** 0.2 **9.** 5.7 **10.** 0.9

## EXPRESSING TO THE NEAREST HUNDREDTH

Some drugs are administered in dosages carried to the nearest hundredth. This is common in pediatric dosages, and in drugs that alter a vital function of the body, for example, heart rate.

To express an answer to the nearest hundredth, the division is carried to thousandths (three places after the decimal point). When the number representing thousandths is 5 or larger, the number representing hundredths is increased by one.

**EXAMPLE 1** 0.736 becomes **0.74**

The number representing thousandths, 6, is larger than 5, so the number representing hundredths, 3, is increased by one to become 4.

**EXAMPLE 2** 0.777 becomes **0.78**

**EXAMPLE 3** 0.373 remains **0.37**

The number representing thousandths, 3, is less than 5, so the number representing hundredths, 7, remains unchanged.

**EXAMPLE 4**    0.934   remains   **0.93**

## Problems 2.6

**Express the numbers to the nearest hundredth.**

1. 0.175 = _____
2. 0.344 = _____
3. 1.853 = _____
4. 0.306 = _____
5. 3.015 = _____
6. 2.154 = _____

7. 1.081 = _____
8. 1.327 = _____
9. 0.739 = _____
10. 0.733 = _____
11. 2.072 = _____
12 0.089 = _____

**Answers  1.** 0.18  **2.** 0.34  **3.** 1.85  **4.** 0.31  **5.** 3.02  **6.** 2.15  **7.** 1.08  **8.** 1.33  **9.** 0.74
**10.** 0.73  **11.** 2.07  **12.** 0.09

## Summary

**This concludes the chapter on multiplication and division of decimals. The important points to remember from this chapter are:**

- When decimal fractions are multiplied manually, the decimal point is placed the same number of places to the left in the product as the total of numbers after the decimal points in the fractions multiplied.

- Zeros must be placed in front of a product if it contains insufficient numbers for the correct placement of the decimal point.

- Excess trailing zeros are eliminated in dosages.

- To simplify fractions for final division, the preliminary steps of eliminating decimal points, reducing the numbers by common denominators, and reducing numbers ending in zeros can be used.

- To express to tenths, increase the answer by one if the number representing the thousandths is 5 or larger.

- To express to hundredths, increase the answer by one if the number representing the thousandths is 5 or larger.

- Practice using a calculator until proficiency is achieved.

- All calculator entries and answers must be double-checked.

- Calculator running totals should be disregarded because they can cause confusion.

- A personal calculator is a must if frequent calculations are necessary.

## Summary Self-Test

**Multiply the decimals. A calculator may be used.**

1. $1.49 \times 0.05$ = _____
2. $0.15 \times 3.04$ = _____
3. $0.025 \times 3.5$ = _____
4. $0.55 \times 2.5$ = _____
5. $1.31 \times 2.07$ = _____

6. $5.3 \times 1.02$ = _____
7. $0.35 \times 1.25$ = _____
8. $4.32 \times 0.05$ = _____
9. $0.2 \times 0.02$ = _____
10. $0.4 \times 1.75$ = _____

11. You are to administer four tablets with a dosage strength of 0.04 mg each. What total dosage are you giving? _____

12. You have given 2½ (2.5) tablets with a strength of 1.25 mg per tablet. What total dosage is this? _____

13. The tablets your patient is to receive are labeled 0.1 mg, and you are to give 3½ (3.5) tablets. What total dosage is this? _____

14. You gave your patient 3 tablets labeled 0.75 mg each, and he was to receive a total of 2.25 mg. Did he receive the correct dosage? _____

15. The tablets available for your patient are labeled 12.5 mg, and you are to give 4½ (4.5) tablets. What total dosage will this be? _____

16. Your patient is to receive a dosage of 4.5 mg. The tablets available are labeled 3.5 mg, and there are 2½ tablets in his medication drawer. Is this a correct dosage? _____

**Divide the fractions. Express answers to the nearest tenth. A calculator may be used.**

17. $\dfrac{1.3}{0.7}$ = _____

18. $\dfrac{1.9}{3.2}$ = _____

19. $\dfrac{32.5}{9}$ = _____

20. $\dfrac{0.04}{0.1}$ = _____

21. $\dfrac{1.45}{1.2}$ = _____

22. $\dfrac{250}{1000}$ = _____

23. $\dfrac{0.8}{0.09}$ = _____

24. $\dfrac{2,000,000}{1,500,000}$ = _____

25. $\dfrac{4.1}{2.05}$ = _____

26. $\dfrac{7.3}{12}$ = _____

27. $\dfrac{150,000}{120,000}$ = _____

28. $\dfrac{0.15}{0.08}$ = _____

29. $\dfrac{2700}{900}$ = _____

30. $\dfrac{0.25}{0.15}$ = _____

**Divide the fractions. Express answers to the nearest hundredth. A calculator may be used.**

31. $\dfrac{900}{1700}$ = _____

32. $\dfrac{0.125}{0.3}$ = _____

33. $\dfrac{1450}{1500}$ = _____

34. $\dfrac{65}{175}$ = _____

35. $\dfrac{0.6}{1.35}$ = _____

36. $\dfrac{0.04}{0.12}$ = _____

37. $\dfrac{750}{10,000}$ = _____

38. $\dfrac{0.65}{0.8}$ = _____

39. $\dfrac{3.01}{4.2}$ = _____

40. $\dfrac{4.5}{6.1}$ = _____

41. $\dfrac{0.13}{0.25}$ = _____

42. $\dfrac{0.25}{0.7}$ = _____

43. $\dfrac{3.3}{5.1}$ = _____

44. $\dfrac{0.19}{0.7}$ = _____

45. $\dfrac{1.1}{1.3}$ = _____

46. $\dfrac{3}{4.1}$ = _____

47. $\dfrac{62}{240}$ = _____

48. $\dfrac{280,000}{300,000}$ = _____

49. $\dfrac{115}{255}$ = _____

50. $\dfrac{10}{14.3}$ = _____

| Answers | | | | |
|---|---|---|---|---|
| **1.** 0.0745 | **11.** 0.16 mg | **22.** 0.3 | **33.** 0.97 | **44.** 0.27 |
| **2.** 0.456 | **12.** 3.125 mg | **23.** 8.9 | **34.** 0.37 | **45.** 0.85 |
| **3.** 0.0875 | **13.** 0.35 mg | **24.** 1.3 | **35.** 0.44 | **46.** 0.73 |
| **4.** 1.375 | **14.** Yes | **25.** 2 | **36.** 0.33 | **47.** 0.26 |
| **5.** 2.7117 | **15.** 56.25 mg | **26.** 0.6 | **37.** 0.08 | **48.** 0.93 |
| **6.** 5.406 | **16.** No | **27.** 1.3 | **38.** 0.81 | **49.** 0.45 |
| **7.** 0.4375 | **17.** 1.9 | **28.** 1.9 | **39.** 0.72 | **50.** 0.7 |
| **8.** 0.216 | **18.** 0.6 | **29.** 3 | **40.** 0.74 | |
| **9.** 0.004 | **19.** 3.6 | **30.** 1.7 | **41.** 0.52 | |
| **10.** 0.7 | **20.** 0.4 | **31.** 0.53 | **42.** 0.36 | |
| | **21.** 1.2 | **32.** 0.42 | **43.** 0.65 | |

# 3

# SOLVING COMMON FRACTION EQUATIONS

## Objectives

The learner will solve equations containing:

1. whole numbers.
2. decimal numbers.
3. multiple numbers.

## Prerequisites

Chapters 1 and 2

The majority of clinical drug dosage calculations involve solving an equation containing one to five common fractions. Two examples are:

$$\frac{2}{5} \times \frac{3}{4} \qquad \text{and} \qquad \frac{20}{1} \times \frac{1000}{60,000} \times \frac{1200}{1} \times \frac{1}{60}$$

Two options are available to solve common fraction equations: calculator use throughout, or initial fraction reduction followed by calculator use for final division. Both options are presented in this chapter, and you may use whichever you wish, or whichever your instructor requires.

 **Common fraction equations are solved by dividing the numerators by the denominators.**

It is important that you do the calculations for each example and then compare them with the math provided. Just reading the examples will not teach you the calculation skills you need. The examples and problems provided incorporate all the content covered in the first two chapters. They represent the full range of calculations you will be doing on a continuing basis.

 **Calculator solution of equations is most safely done by concentrating only on the entries being made, not the numbers that register and change throughout the calculation.**

## WHOLE-NUMBER EQUATIONS

**EXAMPLE 1**  **Option 1: Calculator Use Throughout**

$$\frac{2}{5} \times \frac{3}{4}$$

$2 \times 3 \div 5 \div 4$

Multiply the numerators, 2 and 3, and then divide by the denominators, 5 then 4, in continuous entries

$= 0.3$

Answer $= \mathbf{0.3}$ **(tenth)**

**Option 2:  Initial Reduction of Fractions**

$$\frac{2}{5} \times \frac{3}{4}$$

$\frac{{}^{1}2}{5} \times \frac{3}{4_{2}}$    Divide the numerator, 2, and the denominator, 4, by 2
(to become 1 and 2)

$3 \div 5 \div 2$    Use the calculator to divide the remaining numerator, 3,
by the remaining denominators, 5 and 2

$= 0.3$

Answer $= $ **0.3 (tenth)**

 Initial reduction of fractions in an equation can simplify final calculator entries, especially if the numbers are large, or contain decimal fractions or zeros.

EXAMPLE 2    **Option 1:  Calculator Use Throughout**

$$\frac{250}{175} \times \frac{150}{325}$$

$250 \times 150 \div 175 \div 325$    Multiply the numerators, 250 and 150,
then divide by the denominators, 175
and 325

$= 0.659$

Answer $= $ **0.7 (tenth)** or **0.66 (hundredth)**

**Option 2:  Initial Reduction of Fractions**

$$\frac{250}{175} \times \frac{150}{325}$$

$\frac{\overset{10}{\cancel{250}}}{\underset{7}{\cancel{175}}} \times \frac{\overset{6}{\cancel{150}}}{\underset{13}{\cancel{325}}}$    Divide the numerator, 250, and the denominator,
175, by 25 (to become 10 and 7); divide the
numerator, 150, and denominator, 325, by 25
(to become 6 and 13)

$10 \times 6 \div 7 \div 13$    Use the calculator to multiply the numerators,
10 and 6, then divide by the denominators,
7 and 13

$= 0.659$

Answer $= $ **0.7 (tenth)** or **0.66 (hundredth)**

EXAMPLE 3

**Option 1: Calculator Use Throughout**

$$\frac{7}{50} \times \frac{25}{3} \times \frac{120}{32}$$

$7 \times 25 \times 120 \div 50 \div 3 \div 32$   Multiply the numerators, 7, 25, and 120, then divide by the denominators, 50, 3, and 32

$= 4.375$

Answer $= $ **4.4 (tenth)** or **4.38 (hundredth)**

**Option 2: Initial Reduction of Fractions**

$$\frac{7}{50} \times \frac{25}{3} \times \frac{120}{32}$$

$$\frac{7}{\cancel{50}_2} \times \frac{\cancel{25}^1}{3} \times \frac{\cancel{120}^{15}}{\cancel{32}_4}$$   Divide 25 and 50 by 25, then divide 120 and 32 by 8

$7 \times 15 \div 2 \div 3 \div 4$

$= 4.375$

Answer $= $ **4.4 (tenth)** or **4.38 (hundredth)**

EXAMPLE 4

**Option 1: Calculator Use Throughout**

$$\frac{20}{1} \times \frac{1000}{60,000} \times \frac{1200}{1} \times \frac{1}{60}$$

$20 \times 1000 \times 1200 \div 60,000 \div 60$

$= 6.666$

Answer $= $ **6.7 (tenth)** or **6.67 (hundredth)**

**Option 2: Initial Reduction of Fractions**

$$\frac{20}{1} \times \frac{1000}{60,000} \times \frac{1200}{1} \times \frac{1}{60}$$

$$\frac{\cancel{20}^1}{1} \times \frac{\cancel{1000}^1}{\cancel{60,000}_3} \times \frac{\cancel{1200}^{20}}{1} \times \frac{1}{\cancel{60}_1}$$

$20 \div 3$

$= 6.666$

Answer $= $ **6.7 (tenth)** or **6.67 (hundredth)**

EXAMPLE 5

**Option 1: Calculator Use Throughout**

$$\frac{2000}{1500} \times \frac{2500}{3000}$$

$2000 \times 2500 \div 1500 \div 3000$

$= 1.111$

Answer $= $ **1.1 (tenth)** or **1.11 (hundredth)**

**Option 2:  Initial Reduction of Fractions**

$$\frac{2000}{1500} \times \frac{2500}{3000}$$

$$\frac{\overset{2}{\cancel{2000}}}{\underset{3}{\cancel{1500}}} \times \frac{\overset{5}{\cancel{2500}}}{\underset{3}{\cancel{3000}}}$$

$$2 \times 5 \div 3 \div 3$$

$$= 1.111$$

Answer = **1.1 (tenth)** or **1.11 (hundredth)**

## Problems 3.1

**Solve the equations. Express answers to the nearest tenth and hundredth. A calculator may be used.**

1. $\dfrac{3}{8} \times \dfrac{6}{3}$  = _____ _____

2. $\dfrac{3}{4} \times \dfrac{10}{2}$  = _____ _____

3. $\dfrac{3}{5} \times \dfrac{1050}{40}$  = _____ _____

4. $\dfrac{10}{1} \times \dfrac{750}{40,000} \times \dfrac{1000}{1} \times \dfrac{1}{60}$ = _____ _____

5. $\dfrac{12}{1} \times \dfrac{500}{2700} \times \dfrac{2000}{1} \times \dfrac{1}{60}$ = _____ _____

6. $\dfrac{1500}{750} \times \dfrac{350}{600}$  = _____ _____

7. $\dfrac{1000}{2700} \times \dfrac{1300}{500} \times \dfrac{70}{50}$  = _____ _____

8. $\dfrac{15}{1} \times \dfrac{2500}{20,000} \times \dfrac{1000}{1} \times \dfrac{1}{60}$ = _____ _____

9. $\dfrac{8}{1} \times \dfrac{1000}{5000} \times \dfrac{100}{1} \times \dfrac{1}{60}$ = _____ _____

10. $\dfrac{750}{500} \times \dfrac{250}{300}$  = _____ _____

**Answers  1.** 0.8; 0.75  **2.** 3.8; 3.75  **3.** 15.8; 15.75  **4.** 3.1; 3.13  **5.** 74.1; 74.07  **6.** 1.2; 1.17  **7.** 1.3; 1.35  **8.** 31.3; 31.25  **9.** 2.7; 2.67  **10.** 1.3; 1.25

## DECIMAL FRACTION EQUATIONS

Decimal fraction equations raise an instant warning flag in calculations, because it is here that most dosage errors occur. As with whole-number equations, simplifying the numbers by eliminating decimal points and reducing the numbers is an optional first step. If you elect to do the entire calculation with a calculator, be sure to enter the decimal points carefully. Double-check all calculator entries and answers.

Particular care must be taken with calculator entry of decimal numbers to include the decimal point. Each entry and answer must be routinely double-checked.

**EXAMPLE 1**

**Option 1: Calculator Use Throughout**

$$\frac{0.3}{1.65} \times \frac{2.5}{1}$$

$0.3 \times 2.5 \div 165$     Multiply 0.3 by 2.5, then divide by 1.65

$= 0.454$

Answer $= $ **0.5 (tenth)** or **0.45 (hundredth)**

**Option 2: Initial Elimination of Decimal Points and Reduction of Fractions**

$$\frac{0.3}{1.65} \times \frac{2.5}{1}$$

$$\frac{30}{165} \times \frac{25}{10}$$     Move the decimal point two places in 0.3 and 1.65 (to become 30 and 165) and one place in 2.5 and 1 (to become 25 and 10)

$$\frac{\overset{3}{\cancel{30}}}{\underset{33}{\cancel{165}}} \times \frac{\overset{5}{\cancel{25}}}{\underset{1}{\cancel{10}}}$$     Divide 30 and 10 by 10, then divide 25 and 165 by 5

$$\frac{\overset{1}{\cancel{3}}}{\underset{11}{\cancel{33}}} \times \frac{5}{1}$$     Divide 3 and 33 by 3

$5 \div 11$     Divide the remaining numerator, 5, by the denominator, 11

$= 0.454$

Answer $= $ **0.5 (tenth)** or **0.45 (hundredth)**

**EXAMPLE 2**

**Option 1: Calculator Use Throughout**

$$\frac{0.3}{1.2} \times \frac{2.1}{0.15}$$

$0.3 \times 2.1 \div 1.2 \div 0.15$     Multiply 0.3 by 2.1, then divide by 1.2 and 0.15

$= 3.5$

Answer $= $ **3.5 (tenth)** or **3.5 (hundredth)**

**Option 2: Initial Elimination of Decimal Points and Reduction of Fractions**

$$\frac{0.3}{1.2} \times \frac{2.1}{0.15}$$

$$\frac{3}{12} \times \frac{210}{15}$$     Eliminate the decimal points by moving them one place in 0.3 and 1.2 (to become 3 and 12) and two places in 2.1 and 0.15 (to become 210 and 15)

$$\frac{\overset{1}{\cancel{3}}}{\underset{4}{\cancel{12}}} \times \frac{\overset{42}{\cancel{210}}}{\underset{3}{\cancel{15}}}$$   Divide 3 and 12 by 3, then divide 210 and 15 by 5

$$\frac{1}{\underset{2}{\cancel{4}}} \times \frac{\overset{21}{\cancel{42}}}{3}$$   Divide 42 and 4 by 2

$21 \div 2 \div 3$   Use a calculator to divide the numerator, 21, by 2 and then by 3

$= 3.5$

Answer = **3.5 (tenth)** or **3.5 (hundredth)**

**EXAMPLE 3**

**Option 1:  Calculator Use Throughout**

$$\frac{0.15}{0.17} \times \frac{3.1}{2}$$

$0.15 \times 3.1 \div 0.17 \div 2$   Multiply 0.15 by 3.1, divide by 0.17, and then divide by 2

$= 1.367$

Answer = **1.4 (tenth)** or **1.37 (hundredth)**

**Option 2:  Initial Elimination of Decimal Points and Reduction of Fractions**

$$\frac{0.15}{0.17} \times \frac{3.1}{2}$$

$$\frac{15}{17} \times \frac{31}{20}$$   Move the decimal point two places in 0.15 and 0.17 and one place in 3.1 and 2 (requires adding a zero to 2)

$$\frac{\overset{3}{\cancel{15}}}{17} \times \frac{31}{\underset{4}{\cancel{20}}}$$   Divide 15 and 20 by 5

$3 \times 31 \div 17 \div 4$   Complete this with a calculator

$= 1.367$

Answer = **1.4 (tenth)** or **1.37 (hundredth)**

**EXAMPLE 4**

**Option 1:  Calculator Use Throughout**

$$\frac{2.5}{1.5} \times \frac{1.2}{1.1}$$

$2.5 \times 1.2 \div 1.5 \div 1.1$

$= 1.818$

Answer = **1.8 (tenth)** or **1.82 (hundredth)**

**Option 2: Initial Elimination of Decimal Points and Reduction of Fractions**

$$\frac{2.5}{1.5} \times \frac{1.2}{1.1}$$

$$\frac{25}{15} \times \frac{12}{11}$$

$$\frac{\overset{5}{\cancel{25}}}{\underset{3}{\cancel{15}}} \times \frac{12}{11}$$

$$\frac{5}{\cancel{3}} \times \frac{\overset{4}{\cancel{12}}}{11}$$
$$\underset{1}{}$$

$$5 \times 4 \div 11$$

$$= 1.818$$

Answer = **1.8 (tenth)** or **1.82 (hundredth)**

---

### Problems 3.2

**Solve the equations. Express answers to the nearest tenth and hundredth. A calculator may be used.**

1. $\dfrac{2.1}{1.15} \times \dfrac{0.9}{1.2}$ = _____ _____

2. $\dfrac{3.1}{2.7} \times \dfrac{2.2}{1.4}$ = _____ _____

3. $\dfrac{0.3}{1.2} \times \dfrac{3}{2.1}$ = _____ _____

4. $\dfrac{0.17}{0.3} \times \dfrac{2.5}{1.5}$ = _____ _____

5. $\dfrac{1.75}{0.95} \times \dfrac{1.5}{2}$ = _____ _____

6. $\dfrac{0.75}{1.15} \times \dfrac{3}{1.25}$ = _____ _____

7. $\dfrac{10.2}{1.5} \times \dfrac{2}{5.1}$ = _____ _____

8. $\dfrac{0.125}{0.25} \times \dfrac{2.5}{1.5}$ = _____ _____

9. $\dfrac{0.9}{0.3} \times \dfrac{1.2}{1.4}$ = _____ _____

10. $\dfrac{0.35}{1.7} \times \dfrac{2.5}{0.7}$ = _____ _____

**Answers** **1.** 1.4; 1.37 **2.** 1.8; 1.8 **3.** 0.4; 0.36 **4.** 0.9; 0.94 **5.** 1.4; 1.38 **6.** 1.6; 1.57 **7.** 2.7; 2.67 **8.** 0.8; 0.83 **9.** 2.6; 2.57 **10.** 0.7; 0.74

## MULTIPLE-NUMBER EQUATIONS

The calculation steps just practiced are also used for multiple-number equations, which occur frequently in advanced clinical calculations. **Reduction of numbers may be of particular benefit here because calculations of this type sometimes have numbers that cancel and/or reduce dramatically.** Answers are expressed to the nearest whole number in the examples and problems that follow to replicate actual clinical calculations.

**EXAMPLE 1**

**Option 1:  Calculator Use Throughout**

$$\frac{60}{1} \times \frac{1000}{4} \times \frac{1}{1000} \times \frac{6}{1}$$

$60 \times 1000 \times 6 \div 4 \div 1000$     Multiply 60 by 1000, then by 6; divide by 4 and 1000

$= 90$

Answer $=$ **90**

**Option 2:  Initial Reduction of Fractions**

$$\frac{60}{1} \times \frac{1000}{4} \times \frac{1}{1000} \times \frac{6}{1}$$

$$\frac{60}{1} \times \frac{\overset{1}{\cancel{1000}}}{\underset{2}{\cancel{4}}} \times \frac{1}{\underset{1}{\cancel{1000}}} \times \frac{\overset{3}{\cancel{6}}}{1}$$     Eliminate 1000 from a numerator and denominator, then divide 6 and 4 by 2

$60 \times 3 \div 2$     Multiply 60 by 3, then divide by 2

$= 90$

Answer $=$ **90**     The answer is obtained by cancellation alone

**EXAMPLE 2**

**Option 1:  Calculator Use Throughout**

$$\frac{20}{1} \times \frac{75}{1} \times \frac{1}{60}$$

$20 \times 75 \div 60$     Multiply 20 by 75, then divide by 60

$= 25$

Answer $=$ **25**

**Option 2:  Initial Reduction of Fractions**

$$\frac{20}{1} \times \frac{75}{1} \times \frac{1}{60}$$

$$\frac{\overset{1}{\cancel{20}}}{1} \times \frac{\overset{25}{\cancel{75}}}{1} \times \frac{1}{\underset{3\,\,1}{\cancel{60}}}$$     Divide 20 and 60 by 20 to become 1 and 3, then divide 75 and 3 by 3 to become 25 and 1

$= 25$

Answer $=$ **25**     The answer is obtained by cancellation alone

**EXAMPLE 3**

**Option 1:  Calculator Use Throughout**

$$\frac{2}{0.5} \times \frac{1}{100} \times \frac{275}{1}$$

$2 \times 275 \div 0.5 \div 100$     Multiply 2 by 275, then divide by 0.5 and 100

$= 11$

Answer $=$ **11**

**Option 2: Initial Reduction of Fractions**

$$\frac{2}{0.5} \times \frac{1}{100} \times \frac{275}{1}$$

$$\frac{20}{5} \times \frac{1}{100} \times \frac{275}{1}$$

Eliminate the decimal point by moving it one place in 0.5 and one place in 2, which requires adding a zero to 2 (to become 5 and 20)

$$\frac{\overset{1}{\cancel{20}}}{\underset{1}{\cancel{5}}} \times \frac{1}{\underset{5}{\cancel{100}}} \times \frac{\overset{55}{\cancel{275}}}{1}$$

Divide 20 and 100 by 20, then divide 275 and 5 by 5

$$\frac{1}{\underset{1}{\cancel{5}}} \times \frac{\overset{11}{\cancel{55}}}{1}$$

Divide 5 and 55 by 5

$$= 11$$

Answer = **11**     The answer is obtained by cancellation alone

**EXAMPLE 4**  **Option 1: Calculator Use Throughout**

$$\frac{1}{60} \times \frac{1}{12} \times \frac{10}{1} \times \frac{750}{1}$$

$$10 \times 750 \div 60 \div 12$$

$$= 10.4$$

Answer = **10**

**Option 2: Initial Reduction of Fractions**

$$\frac{1}{60} \times \frac{1}{12} \times \frac{10}{1} \times \frac{750}{1}$$

$$\frac{1}{\underset{6}{\cancel{60}}} \times \frac{1}{\underset{6}{\cancel{12}}} \times \frac{\overset{1}{\cancel{10}}}{1} \times \frac{\overset{375}{\cancel{750}}}{1}$$

$$375 \div 6 \div 6$$

$$= 10.4$$

Answer = **10**

---

### Problems 3.3

Solve the equations. Express answers to the nearest whole number.

1. $\dfrac{15}{1} \times \dfrac{350}{5} \times \dfrac{1}{60}$ = _____

2. $\dfrac{1}{32} \times \dfrac{60}{1} \times \dfrac{7.5}{3.1}$ = _____

3. $\dfrac{10}{1} \times \dfrac{2500}{24} \times \dfrac{1}{60}$ = _____

4. $\dfrac{1.7}{2.3} \times \dfrac{15.3}{12.1} \times \dfrac{6.2}{0.3}$ = _____

5. $\dfrac{20}{1} \times \dfrac{1200}{16} \times \dfrac{1}{60}$ = _____

6. $\dfrac{5}{1} \times \dfrac{320}{1.5} \times \dfrac{1}{60}$ = _____

7. $\dfrac{100}{1} \times \dfrac{1750}{200} \times \dfrac{1}{60}$ = _____

8. $\dfrac{60}{1} \times \dfrac{1150}{200} \times \dfrac{1}{100}$ = _____

9. $\dfrac{25}{4} \times \dfrac{1000}{8} \times \dfrac{1}{60}$ = _____    10. $\dfrac{18}{10} \times \dfrac{120}{7} \times \dfrac{9}{17}$ = _____

**Answers   1.** 18   **2.** 5   **3.** 17   **4.** 19   **5.** 25   **6.** 18   **7.** 15   **8.** 3   **9.** 13   **10.** 16

## Summary

**This concludes the chapter on solving common fraction equations. The important points to remember from this chapter are:**

- Most clinical calculations consist of an equation containing one to five common fractions.

- In solving equations, all the numerators are multiplied, then divided by the denominators.

- Numbers in an equation may initially be reduced using common denominators/divisors to simplify final multiplication and division.

- Zeros may be eliminated from the same number of numerators and denominators without altering the value.

- Double-check all calculator entries and answers.

- Answers may be expressed as whole numbers, or to the nearest tenth or hundredth, depending on the calculation being done.

## Summary Self-Test

**Solve the equations. Express answers to the nearest tenth and hundredth.
A calculator may be used.**

1. $\dfrac{0.8}{0.65} \times \dfrac{1.2}{1}$ = _____  _____

2. $\dfrac{350}{1000} \times \dfrac{4.4}{1}$ = _____  _____

3. $\dfrac{0.35}{1.3} \times \dfrac{4.5}{1}$ = _____  _____

4. $\dfrac{0.4}{1.5} \times \dfrac{2.3}{1}$ = _____  _____

5. $\dfrac{1}{75} \times \dfrac{500}{1}$ = _____  _____

6. $\dfrac{0.15}{0.12} \times \dfrac{1.45}{1}$ = _____  _____

7. $\dfrac{100,000}{80,000} \times \dfrac{1.7}{1}$ = _____  _____

8. $\dfrac{1.45}{2.1} \times \dfrac{1.5}{1}$ = _____  _____

9. $\dfrac{1550}{500} \times \dfrac{0.5}{1}$ = _____  _____

10. $\dfrac{4}{0.375} \times \dfrac{0.25}{1}$ = _____  _____

11. $\dfrac{0.08}{0.1} \times \dfrac{2.1}{1}$ = _____  _____

12. $\dfrac{1.5}{1.25} \times \dfrac{1.45}{1}$     = _____ _____

13. $\dfrac{0.5}{0.15} \times \dfrac{0.35}{1}$     = _____ _____

14. $\dfrac{300,000}{200,000} \times \dfrac{1.7}{1}$     = _____ _____

15. $\dfrac{13.5}{10} \times \dfrac{1.8}{1}$     = _____ _____

16. $\dfrac{1,000,000}{800,000} \times \dfrac{1.4}{1}$     = _____ _____

17. $\dfrac{1.3}{0.2} \times \dfrac{0.25}{1}$     = _____ _____

18. $\dfrac{1.5}{0.1} \times \dfrac{0.25}{1}$     = _____ _____

19. $\dfrac{1.9}{3.5} \times \dfrac{3.2}{1.4}$     = _____ _____

20. $\dfrac{15,000}{7500} \times \dfrac{3.5}{1.2}$     = _____ _____

21. $\dfrac{4.7}{1.3} \times \dfrac{50}{20} \times \dfrac{4}{25} \times \dfrac{8.2}{2.1}$     = _____ _____

22. $\dfrac{40}{24} \times \dfrac{250}{5} \times \dfrac{0.375}{7.5}$     = _____ _____

23. $\dfrac{6.9}{21.6} \times \dfrac{250}{5} \times \dfrac{0.75}{2.1}$     = _____ _____

24. $\dfrac{1}{60} \times \dfrac{1}{25} \times \dfrac{10}{1} \times \dfrac{1000}{1}$     = _____ _____

25. $\dfrac{50.5}{22.75} \times \dfrac{4.7}{6.3} \times \dfrac{31.7}{10.2}$     = _____ _____

**Solve the equations. Express answers to the nearest whole number. A calculator may be used.**

26. $\dfrac{104}{95} \times \dfrac{20}{15} \times \dfrac{63}{1.6}$     = _____

27. $\dfrac{40,000}{10,000} \times \dfrac{30}{1} \times \dfrac{3.7}{12.5}$     = _____

28. $\dfrac{60}{1} \times \dfrac{500}{50} \times \dfrac{1}{1000} \times \dfrac{116}{1}$ = _____

29. $\dfrac{1.5}{0.6} \times \dfrac{10}{14} \times \dfrac{3.2}{5.3} \times \dfrac{100}{2}$     = _____

30. $\dfrac{60}{1} \times \dfrac{50}{250} \times \dfrac{1}{100} \times \dfrac{455}{1}$     = _____

31. $\dfrac{33.7}{15.9} \times \dfrac{19.2}{2.6} \times \dfrac{2.9}{3.85}$     = _____

32. $\dfrac{20}{4} \times \dfrac{100}{88} \times \dfrac{1200}{250} \times \dfrac{10}{30}$     = _____

33. $\dfrac{14}{7.9} \times \dfrac{88}{8}$     = _____

34. $\dfrac{10}{1} \times \dfrac{325}{1.5} \times \dfrac{1}{60}$ = _____

35. $\dfrac{60}{1} \times \dfrac{300}{400} \times \dfrac{1}{800} \times \dfrac{400}{1}$ = _____

36. $\dfrac{3.7}{1.3} \times \dfrac{12}{8} \times \dfrac{3.1}{7.4} \times \dfrac{5}{1}$ = _____

37. $\dfrac{20}{2} \times \dfrac{125}{25} \times \dfrac{2}{750} \times \dfrac{216}{1}$ = _____

38. $\dfrac{4}{3} \times \dfrac{45}{1} \times \dfrac{22.5}{37.8}$ = _____

39. $\dfrac{7.5}{12.3} \times \dfrac{55}{5} \times \dfrac{23.2}{1.2}$ = _____

40. $\dfrac{1000}{1} \times \dfrac{50}{250} \times \dfrac{20}{1} \times \dfrac{1}{60}$ = _____

41. $\dfrac{15}{1} \times \dfrac{1000}{4000} \times \dfrac{800}{1} \times \dfrac{1}{60}$ = _____

42. $\dfrac{15}{1} \times \dfrac{500}{3} \times \dfrac{1}{60}$ = _____

43. $\dfrac{25}{3} \times \dfrac{750}{8} \times \dfrac{0.1}{1}$ = _____

44. $\dfrac{40}{2} \times \dfrac{250}{50} \times \dfrac{1}{800} \times \dfrac{154}{1}$ = _____

45. $\dfrac{33}{4} \times \dfrac{75}{40} \times \dfrac{2}{150} \times \dfrac{432}{1}$ = _____

46. $\dfrac{22.5}{7} \times \dfrac{100}{5} \times \dfrac{1}{700} \times \dfrac{3}{80} \times \dfrac{3150}{1}$ = _____

47. $\dfrac{100}{250} \times \dfrac{50}{1} \times \dfrac{27.5}{1.375}$ = _____

48. $\dfrac{2.2}{0.25} \times \dfrac{3.6}{1} \times \dfrac{3.7}{7.1}$ = _____

49. $\dfrac{1.3}{0.21} \times \dfrac{0.3}{2} \times \dfrac{10.1}{0.75}$ = _____

50. $\dfrac{27.5}{10} \times \dfrac{40}{7} \times \dfrac{8.5}{1.9}$ = _____

**Answers**

| | | | |
|---|---|---|---|
| **1.** 1.5; 1.48 | **13.** 1.2; 1.17 | **26.** 57 | **39.** 130 |
| **2.** 1.5; 1.54 | **14.** 2.6; 2.55 | **27.** 36 | **40.** 67 |
| **3.** 1.2; 1.21 | **15.** 2.4; 2.43 | **28.** 70 | **41.** 50 |
| **4.** 0.6; 0.61 | **16.** 1.8; 1.75 | **29.** 54 | **42.** 42 |
| **5.** 6.7; 6.67 | **17.** 1.6; 1.63 | **30.** 55 | **43.** 78 |
| **6.** 1.8; 1.81 | **18.** 3.8; 3.75 | **31.** 12 | **44.** 19 |
| **7.** 2.1; 2.13 | **19.** 1.2; 1.24 | **32.** 9 | **45.** 89 |
| **8.** 1; 1.04 | **20.** 5.8; 5.83 | **33.** 19 | **46.** 11 |
| **9.** 1.6; 1.55 | **21.** 5.6; 5.65 | **34.** 36 | **47.** 400 |
| **10.** 2.7; 2.67 | **22.** 4.2; 4.17 | **35.** 23 | **48.** 17 |
| **11.** 1.7; 1.68 | **23.** 5.7; 5.7 | **36.** 9 | **49.** 13 |
| **12.** 1.7; 1.74 | **24.** 6.7; 6.67 | **37.** 29 | **50.** 70 |
| | **25.** 5.1; 5.15 | **38.** 36 | |

# SECTION 2

# Introduction to Drug Measures

**CHAPTER 4**
Metric/International (SI)
System / 36

**CHAPTER 5**
Unit, Percentage,
Milliequivalent, Ratio,
Household, and Apothecary
Measures / 46

# 4

# METRIC/ INTERNATIONAL (SI) SYSTEM

You are probably already familiar with the metric system, which is the major system of weights and measures used in medicine. The metric/international/SI (from the French Système International) system was invented in France in 1875, and takes its name from the meter, a length roughly equivalent to a yard, from which all other units of measure in the system are derived. The strength of the metric system lies in its simplicity, because all units of measure differ from each other in powers of ten (10). Conversions between units in the system are accomplished by simply moving a decimal point.

> A major strength of the metric system is that all its units of measure differ from each other in powers of ten (10), and conversions between the units can be made by simply moving the decimal point.

This is also one of the metric system's greatest hazards. This is because a misplaced decimal point alters the value of a number by a multiple of at least 10. It is not necessary for you to know the entire metric system to administer medications safely, but you must understand its basic structure and become familiar with the units of measure you will be using in the clinical setting.

> The greatest hazard of the metric system in drug dosages is that a misplaced decimal point will alter a dosage by a multiple of at least 10.

## BASIC UNITS OF THE METRIC/SI SYSTEM

Three types of metric measures are in common clinical use: those for **length**, **volume** (or capacity), and **weight**. The basic units of these measures are:

> length — meter
> volume — liter
> weight — gram

Memorize the basic units if you do not already know them. In addition to the basic units, **there are both larger and smaller units of measure** for length, volume, and weight. Let's compare this concept with something familiar. The pound is a unit of weight that we use every day. A smaller unit of measure is the ounce; a larger, the ton. **However, all are units measuring weight.**

In the same way, there are smaller and larger units than the basic meter, liter, and gram. In the metric system, however, there is one very important advantage: **all other units, whether larger or smaller than the basic units, have the name of the basic unit incorporated in them.** So when you see a unit of metric measure, there is no doubt what it is measuring: **meter—length**, **liter—volume**, and **gram—weight**.

## Problems 4.1

**Identify the metric measures with their appropriate category of weight, length, or volume.**

1. milligram  _____
2. centimeter  _____
3. milliliter  _____
4. millimeter  _____

5. kilogram  _____
6. microgram  _____
7. kilometer  _____
8. kiloliter  _____

**Answers**   **1.** weight   **2.** length   **3.** volume   **4.** length   **5.** weight   **6.** weight   **7.** length   **8.** volume

## METRIC/SI PREFIXES

Prefixes are used in combination with the names of the basic units to identify larger and smaller units of measure. The same prefixes are used with all three measures. Therefore, there is a kilo**meter**, kilo**gram**, and a kilo**liter**.

 **Identical prefixes are used to identify units that are larger or smaller than the basic metric measures.**

Prefixes also change the value of each of the basic units by the same amount. For example, the prefix "kilo" identifies a unit of measure that is larger than (or multiplies) the basic unit by 1000.

$$1 \text{ kilometer} = 1000 \text{ meters}$$
$$1 \text{ kilogram} = 1000 \text{ grams}$$
$$1 \text{ kiloliter} = 1000 \text{ liters}$$

**Kilo** is the only prefix you will be using in the clinical setting that identifies a measure **larger** than the basic unit. Kilograms are frequently used as a measure for body weight, especially for infants and children.

You will see only three measures **smaller** than the basic unit in common clinical use. The prefixes for these are:

**milli**—as in milligram—for weight
**micro**—as in microgram—for weight
**centi**—as in centimeter—for length

Therefore, you will actually be working with only four prefixes: **kilo**, which identifies a larger unit of measure than the basic; and **milli**, **micro**, and **centi**, which identify smaller units than the basic.

## METRIC/SI ABBREVIATIONS

In clinical use, units of metric measure are abbreviated.

 The basic units are abbreviated to their first initial and printed in small (lowercase) letters, with the exception of liter, which is capitalized (uppercase).

meter is abbreviated **m**

gram is abbreviated **g**

liter is abbreviated **L**

 The abbreviations for the prefixes used in combination with the basic units are all printed using small letters.

kilo is **k** (as in kilogram—kg)

milli is **m** (as in milligram—mg)

micro is **mc** (as in microgram—mcg)

centi is **c** (as in centimeter—cm)

Micro has an additional abbreviation, the symbol $\mu$, but its use has been discontinued in medication dosages. This became necessary because medication errors were made when handwritten $\mu$g was misread as mg, a dosage 1000 times the mcg dosage ordered.

 Micro is always abbreviated using the prefix mc rather than the symbol $\mu$, which has an inherent safety risk.

**In combination, liter remains capitalized.** Therefore, milliliter is **mL** and kiloliter is **kL**.

### Problems 4.2

**Abbreviate the following metric units.**

1. microgram _____
2. liter _____
3. kilogram _____
4. milliliter _____
5. centimeter _____
6. milligram _____
7. meter _____
8. kiloliter _____
9. millimeter _____
10. gram _____

**Answers 1.** mcg **2.** L **3.** kg **4.** mL **5.** cm **6.** mg **7.** m **8.** kL **9.** mm **10.** g

## METRIC/SI NOTATION RULES

To remember the rules of metric **notations**, in which **a unit of measure is expressed with a quantity**, it is helpful to memorize some prototypes (examples) that incorporate all the rules. For the metric system, the notations for one-half, one, and one and one-half milliliters incorporate all the official notation rules.

Prototype notations:   **0.5 mL    1 mL    1.5 mL**

**RULE 1**   **The quantity is written in Arabic numerals: 1, 2, 3, 4, and so forth.**
*Example:*    0.5        1        1.5

**RULE 2**   **The numerals representing the quantity are placed in front of the abbreviations.**
*Example:*    0.5 mL    1 mL    1.5 mL    (**not** mL 0.5, mL 1, mL 1.5)

**RULE 3**   **A full space is used between the numeral and the abbreviation.**
*Example:*    0.5 mL    1 mL    1.5 mL    (**not** 0.5mL, 1mL, 1.5mL)

**RULE 4**   **Fractional parts of a unit are expressed as decimal fractions.**
*Example:*    0.5 mL    1.5 mL    (**not** ½ mL, 1½ mL)

**RULE 5**   **A zero is placed in front of the decimal when it is not preceded by a whole number to emphasize the decimal point.**
*Example:*    0.5 mL    (**not** .5 mL)

**RULE 6**   **Excess zeros following a decimal fraction are eliminated.**
*Example:*    0.5 mL    1 mL    1.5 mL    (**not** 0.50 mL, 1.0 mL, 1.50 mL)

## Problems 4.3

Write the metric measures using official abbreviations and notation rules.

1. two grams                              _____
2. five hundred milliliters               _____
3. five-tenths of a liter                 _____
4. two-tenths of a milligram              _____
5. five-hundredths of a gram              _____
6. two and five-tenths kilograms          _____
7. one hundred micrograms                 _____
8. two and three-tenths milliliters       _____
9. seven-tenths of a milliliter           _____
10. three-tenths of a milligram           _____
11. two and four-tenths liters            _____
12. seventeen and five-tenths kilograms   _____

13. nine-hundredths of a milligram  _____

14. ten and two-tenths micrograms  _____

15. four-hundredths of a gram  _____

---

**Answers** **1.** 2 g  **2.** 500 mL  **3.** 0.5 L  **4.** 0.2 mg  **5.** 0.05 g  **6.** 2.5 kg  **7.** 100 mcg  **8.** 2.3 mL
**9.** 0.7 mL  **10.** 0.3 mg  **11.** 2.4 L  **12.** 17.5 kg  **13.** 0.09 mg  **14.** 10.2 mcg  **15.** 0.04 g

---

## CONVERSION BETWEEN METRIC/SI UNITS

When you administer medications, you will be routinely **converting units of measure within the metric system;** for example, g to mg and mg to mcg. Learning the relative value of the units with which you will be working is the first prerequisite for accurate conversions.

There are only four metric **weights** commonly used in medicine. From **greater** to **lesser** value, these are:

| | | |
|---|---|---|
| kg | = | kilogram |
| g | = | gram |
| mg | = | milligram |
| mcg | = | microgram |

Only two units of **volume** are frequently used. From **greater** to **lesser** value, these are:

| | | |
|---|---|---|
| L | = | liter |
| mL | = | milliliter |

**Each of these clinical metric measures differs from the next by 1000.**

| | | |
|---|---|---|
| 1 kg | = | 1000 g |
| 1 g | = | 1000 mg |
| 1 mg | = | 1000 mcg |
| 1 L | = | 1000 mL |

1000 L = 1 kL.

Once again, from greater to lesser value, the units are, for weight: kg—g—mg—mcg; for volume: L—mL. Each unit differs in value from the next by 1000, and **all conversions will be between touching units of measure;** for example, g to mg, mg to mcg, and L to mL.

---

Problems 4.4

**Choose true (T) or false (F) for each conversion.**

1. T  F    1000 mL  = 1000 L             6. T  F    1 kg      = 1000 g
2. T  F    1000 mg  = 1 g                7. T  F    1 mg      = 1000 g
3. T  F    1000 g    = 1 kg              8. T  F    1000 mcg = 1 mg
4. T  F    1000 mg  = 1 mcg             9. T  F    1 g        = 100 mcg
5. T  F    1000 mcg = 1 g              10. T  F    1000 L    = 1 kL

---

**Answers** **1.** F  **2.** T  **3.** T  **4.** F  **5.** F  **6.** T  **7.** F  **8.** T  **9.** F  **10.** T

Because the metric system is a decimal system, **conversions between the units are accomplished by moving the decimal point.** Also, because each unit of measure in clinical use differs from the next by 1000, if you know one conversion, you know them all.

How far do you move the decimal point? There is an unforgettable memory cue that can be used with **all** metric conversions. There are **three zeros in 1000.** The decimal point moves **three places,** the **same number of places as the zeros** in the conversion.

> In metric conversions between touching units of clinical measures differing by 1000, the decimal point is moved three places, the same as the number of zeros in 1000.

This rule holds true for **all** decimal conversions in the metric system. If the difference in value was **10,** which has **one zero,** it would move **one place.** If the difference was **100,** which has **two zeros,** it would move **two places.** When the difference is **1000,** as in clinical conversions, which has **three zeros,** the decimal point moves **three places.**

Which way do you move the decimal point? If you are converting to a **smaller** unit of measure—for example, g to mg or L to mL—the **quantity must get larger.** The decimal point must move three places to the **right.**

**EXAMPLE 1**    0.5 g = _____ mg

You are converting to smaller units of measure, from **g to mg,** so the quantity will be **larger.** Move the decimal point **three places to the right.** To do this, you must **add two zeros** to the end of the quantity, and **eliminate the zero in front** of it. The larger 500 mg quantity indicates that you have moved the decimal point in the correct direction.

Answer    **0.5 g = .500. mg**    Move the decimal three places to the right

**EXAMPLE 2**    2.5 L = _____ mL

You are converting to smaller units of measure, so the quantity will be **larger.** Move the decimal point **three places to the right.** To do this, you must **add two zeros.** The larger 2500 mL quantity indicates that you have moved the decimal point in the correct direction.

Answer    **2.5 L = 2.500. mL**

## Problems 4.5

**Convert the metric measures.**

1. 7 mg    = _____ mcg
2. 1.7 L    = _____ mL
3. 3.2 g    = _____ mg
4. 0.03 kg  = _____ g
5. 0.4 mg   = _____ mcg

6. 1.5 mg    = _____ mcg
7. 0.7 g     = _____ mg
8. 0.3 L     = _____ mL
9. 7 kg      = _____ g
10. 0.01 mg  = _____ mcg

**Answers  1.** 7000 mcg  **2.** 1700 mL  **3.** 3200 mg  **4.** 30 g  **5.** 400 mcg  **6.** 1500 mcg
**7.** 700 mg  **8.** 300 mL  **9.** 7000 g  **10.** 10 mcg

In metric conversions from **smaller to larger units** of measurement, such as mL to L and mcg to mg, the quantity will be **smaller**. The decimal point is moved **three places to the left**.

> **EXAMPLE 1**        200 mL = _____ L

You are converting to a larger unit of measure, **mL** to **L**, so the quantity will be **smaller**. Move the decimal point **three places to the left**.

$$.200. \text{ mL} = .200 \text{ L}$$

Eliminate the two unnecessary zeros at the end of the quantity (to make it .2), then add a zero in front of the decimal point to correctly write the dosage as 0.2 L.

$$\text{Answer} = .200. \text{ mL} = 0.2 \text{ L}$$

> **EXAMPLE 2**        1500 mcg = _____ mg

You are converting to a larger unit of measure, so the quantity will be smaller. Move the decimal point **three places to the left**. **Place a decimal point in front of** the 5, and **eliminate the two zeros** after the 5.

$$\text{Answer} = 1.500. \text{ mcg} = 1.5 \text{ mg}$$

> **EXAMPLE 3**        300 mcg = _____ mg

You are converting to a larger unit of measure, **mcg** to **mg**, so the quantity will be **smaller**. Move the decimal point **three places to the left**.

$$.300. \text{ mcg} = .300 \text{ mg}$$

Two zeros will need to be eliminated from the end of this decimal fraction (to make it .3), and a zero must be placed in front of the decimal point to complete the decimal fraction.

$$\text{Answer} = 300 \text{ mcg} = 0.3 \text{ mg}$$

## Problems 4.6

**Convert the metric measures.**

1. 3500 mL  = _____ L
2. 520 mg  = _____ g
3. 1800 mcg = _____ mg
4. 750 mL  = _____ L
5. 150 mg  = _____ g
6. 250 mcg  = _____ mg
7. 1200 mg  = _____ g
8. 600 mL  = _____ L
9. 100 mg  = _____ g
10. 950 mcg  = _____ mg

**Answers**  **1.** 3.5 L  **2.** 0.52 g  **3.** 1.8 mg  **4.** 0.75 L  **5.** 0.15 g  **6.** 0.25 mg  **7.** 1.2 g  **8.** 0.6 L
**9.** 0.1 g  **10.** 0.95 mg

## COMMON ERRORS IN METRIC/SI DOSAGES

Most errors in the metric system occur because orders are not written using correct notation rules, or they are not transcribed correctly. **Errors usually involve decimal fractions.** Even though you have just finished learning metric notation rules, let's review the most common errors.

One error is the **failure to enter a zero in front of a decimal point**; for example, .2 mg instead of **0.**2 mg. Regardless of the presence of a zero in front of the decimal in a written order, one must be added when the order is transcribed to a medication administration record.

 Fractional dosages in the metric system are transcribed with a zero in front of the decimal point.

Another common error is to **include zeros where they should not be**; for example, 2.**0** mg instead of 2 mg or .**20** mg instead of 0.2 mg. Each error can be misread as 20 mg, a dosage greatly in excess of the intended dosage.

 Unnecessary zeros are eliminated when metric dosages are transcribed.

Errors are also more likely to occur in **calculations that include decimal fractions**. The presence of a decimal fraction in a calculation raises a warning flag to slow down and double-check all math. **Use your reasoning powers.** If a decimal is misplaced, the answer will be a minimum of 10 times too large or 10 times too small. **Question quantities that seem unreasonable.** A 1.5 mL IM injection dosage makes sense, but a 0.15 mL or 15 mL does not, and this is the type of error you might see.

 Question orders and calculations that seem unreasonably large or small.

Additional errors to be aware of are in **conversions within the metric system.** Errors in conversions can be eliminated by thinking **three.** All conversions between the g, mg, mcg, mL, and L measures are accomplished by moving the decimal point **three** places. Always and forever. There are not many things for which you can use the words "always" and "forever," but converting between these units of measure in the metric system is one of those rare instances.

 Conversions between g, mg, mcg, mL, and L units of measure in metric measures require moving the decimal point three places.

Be constantly mindful of these problem areas to become a safe clinical practitioner.

## Summary

**This concludes the refresher on the metric system. The important points to remember from this chapter are:**

☑ The meter-m, liter-L, and gram-g are the basic units of metric measure.

☑ Only liter is capitalized, L.

☑ Larger and smaller units than the basics are identified by the use of prefixes.

☑ The prefixes are printed using small (lowercase) letters.

☑ The one larger unit you will be seeing is the kilo, whose prefix is k.

☑ The smaller units you will be seeing are milli—m, micro—mc, and centi—c.

☑ Each prefix changes the value of a basic unit by the same amount.

☑ Converting from one unit to another within the system is accomplished by moving a decimal point.

☑ When you convert from larger to smaller units of measurement, the quantity will increase.

☑ To convert from larger to smaller units, the decimal point is moved to the right.

☑ When you convert from smaller to larger units of measurement, the quantity will get smaller.

☑ To convert from smaller to larger units, the decimal point is moved to the left.

☑ Conversions between g to mg, mg to mcg, and mL to L all require moving the decimal point three places.

☑ Fractional dosages are transcribed with a zero in front of the decimal point.

☑ Unnecessary zeros are eliminated from dosages.

## Summary Self-Test

**List the basic units of measure of the metric system and the measure they are used for.**

1. _____    _____

   _____    _____

   _____    _____

**Identify the official metric/SI abbreviations.**

2. a) L          e) mg
   b) g          f) kg
   c) kL         g) ml
   d) mgm        h) G

   _____

**Use official metric abbreviations and notation rules to express these as numerals.**

3. six-hundredths of a milligram    _____

4. three hundred and ten milliliters    _____

5. three-tenths of a kilogram _____

6. four-tenths of a milliliter _____

7. one and five-tenths grams _____

8. one-hundredths of a gram _____

9. four thousand milliliters _____

10. one and two-tenths milligrams _____

**List the four commonly used clinical units of weight and the two of volume from greater to lesser value.**

11. Weight _____  _____  _____  _____

    Volume _____  _____

**Convert the metric measures.**

12. 160 mg    = _____ g

13. 10 kg     = _____ g

14. 1500 mcg  = _____ mg

15. 750 mg    = _____ g

16. 200 mL    = _____ L

17. 0.3 g     = _____ mg

18. 0.05 g    = _____ mg

19. 0.15 g    = _____ mg

20. 1.2 L     = _____ mL

21. 1800 mL   = _____ L

22. 2 mg      = _____ mcg

23. 900 mcg   = _____ mg

24. 2.1 L     = _____ mL

25. 475 mL    = _____ L

26. 0.9 L     = _____ mL

27. 300 mg    = _____ g

28. 2.5 mg    = _____ mcg

29. 1 kL      = _____ L

30. 3 L       = _____ mL

31. 2 L       = _____ mL

32. 0.7 mg    = _____ mcg

33. 4 g       = _____ mg

34. 1000 mL   = _____ L

35. 2500 mL   = _____ L

36. 1000 mg   = _____ g

37. 0.2 mg    = _____ mcg

38. 2000 g    = _____ kg

39. 1.4 g     = _____ mg

40. 2.5 L     = _____ mL

**Answers**

1. gram-weight; liter-volume; meter-length
2. a, b, c, e, f
3. 0.06 mg
4. 310 mL
5. 0.3 kg
6. 0.4 mL
7. 1.5 g
8. 0.01 g
9. 4000 mL
10. 1.2 mg
11. kg, g, mg, mcg, L, mL
12. 0.16 g
13. 10,000 g
14. 1.5 mg
15. 0.75 g
16. 0.2 L
17. 300 mg
18. 50 mg
19. 150 mg
20. 1200 mL
21. 1.8 L
22. 2000 mcg
23. 0.9 mg
24. 2100 mL
25. 0.475 L
26. 900 mL
27. 0.3 g
28. 2500 mcg
29. 1000 L
30. 3000 mL
31. 2000 mL
32. 700 mcg
33. 4000 mg
34. 1 L
35. 2.5 L
36. 1 g
37. 200 mcg
38. 2 kg
39. 1400 mg
40. 2500 mL

# UNIT, PERCENTAGE, MILLIEQUIVALENT, RATIO, HOUSEHOLD, AND APOTHECARY MEASURES

## Objectives

The learner will recognize dosages:

1. measured in units.

2. measured as percentages.

3. using ratio strengths.

4. in milliequivalents.

5. in household measures.

6. in the apothecary system as obsolete.

Although metric measures predominate in medications, there are several other measures frequently used, particularly in parenteral (injectable) solutions, that are important for you to know. In addition, you must be familiar with several measures in the household system because you may occasionally see these.

## INTERNATIONAL UNITS (units)

A number of drugs are measured in International Units. Insulin, penicillin, and heparin are commonly seen examples. Antibiotics, such as penicillin, have dosages in the hundredths of thousands and millions, and heparin has dosages in the thousandths. A unit **measures a drug in terms of its action**, not its physical weight. The word "units" is **not abbreviated; it is written in lower case using Arabic numerals in front of the measure**, with a space between; for example, 2000 units or 1,000,000 units. **Commas are not usually used in a quantity unless it has at least five numbers;** for example, 45,000 units.

### Problems 5.1

**Express the unit dosages in numerals.**

1. two hundred and fifty thousand units  _____

2. ten units  _____

3. five thousand units  _____

4. forty-four units  _____

5. forty thousand units  _____

6.  one million units          _____

7.  one thousand units        _____

8.  twenty-five hundred units _____

9.  thirty-four units         _____

10.  one hundred units         _____

---

**Answers   1.** 250,000 units   **2.** 10 units   **3.** 5000 units   **4.** 44 units   **5.** 40,000 units
**6.** 1,000,000 units   **7.** 1000 units   **8.** 2500 units   **9.** 34 units   **10.** 100 units

---

## PERCENTAGE (%) MEASURES

Percentage strengths are used extensively in intravenous solutions, and somewhat less commonly for a variety of other medications, including eye and topical (for external use) ointments. **Percentage (%) means parts per hundred. The greater the percentage strength, the stronger the solution or ointment**; for example, 3% is stronger than 1%. Fractional percentages are expressed as decimal fractions; for example, 0.45%. Notice that, unlike other written dosages, percentages are generally written with **no space between the quantity and percentage sign**.

 In solutions, percent represents the number of grams of drug per 100 mL of solution.

| EXAMPLE 1 | 100 mL of a 1% solution will contain 1 g of drug. |
| EXAMPLE 2 | 100 mL of a 2.5% solution will contain 2.5 g of drug. |
| EXAMPLE 3 | 100 mL of a 10% solution will contain 10 g of drug. |
| EXAMPLE 4 | 100 mL of a 0.9% solution will contain 0.9 g of drug. |

 These examples are included to point out that percentage solutions contain a significant amount of drug or other solute, and that reading percentage labels requires the same care as that used with other drug dosages.

## MILLIEQUIVALENT (mEq) MEASURES

Milliequivalents (**mEq**) is **an expression of the number of grams of a drug contained in 1 mL of a normal solution**. This is a definition that is quite understandable to a pharmacist or chemist, but you need not memorize it. Milliequivalent dosages are also written using **Arabic numerals**, with a space between the **abbreviation that follows**, for example, 30 mEq. You will see milliequivalents used in a variety of oral and parenteral solutions, potassium chloride being a common intravenous example.

## Problems 5.2

**Express the milliequivalent dosages in numerals.**

1. sixty milliequivalents _____
2. fifteen milliequivalents _____
3. forty milliequivalents _____
4. one milliequivalent _____
5. fifty milliequivalents _____
6. eighty milliequivalents _____
7. fifty-five milliequivalents _____
8. seventy milliequivalents _____
9. thirty milliequivalents _____
10. twenty milliequivalents _____

Answers **1.** 60 mEq **2.** 15 mEq **3.** 40 mEq **4.** 1 mEq **5.** 50 mEq **6.** 80 mEq **7.** 55 mEq
**8.** 70 mEq **9.** 30 mEq **10.** 20 mEq

## RATIO MEASURES

Ratio strengths are used primarily in solutions. They represent **parts of drug per parts of solution**; for example, 1 : 1000 (one part drug to 1000 parts solution).

**EXAMPLE 1** A 1 : 100 strength solution has 1 part drug in 100 parts solution.

**EXAMPLE 2** A 1 : 5 solution contains 1 part drug in 5 parts solution.

**EXAMPLE 3** A solution that is 1 part drug in 2 parts solution would be written 1 : 2

 The less solution a drug is dissolved in, the stronger the solution.

For example, a ratio strength of 1 : 10 (1 part drug to 10 parts solution) is much stronger than a 1 : 100 (1 part drug in 100 parts solution).

Ratio strengths are always expressed in their **simplest terms**. For example, 2 : 10 would be incorrect because it can be reduced to 1 : 5. Notice that ratio dosages are written separated by a colon, with a space between both numbers and the colon. Dosages using ratio strengths are not common, but you do need to know what they represent.

## Problems 5.3

**Express as ratios.**

1. 1 part drug to 200 parts solution _____
2. 1 part drug to 4 parts solution _____
3. 1 part drug to 7 parts solution _____

Identify the strongest solution.

4. a) 1 : 20        b) 1 : 200        c) 1 : 2        _____

5. a) 1 : 50        b) 1 : 20        c) 1 : 100        _____

6. a) 1 : 1000        b) 1 : 5000        c) 1 : 2000        _____

**Answers    1.** 1 : 200    **2.** 1 : 4    **3.** 1 : 7    **4.** c    **5.** b    **6.** a

## HOUSEHOLD AND APOTHECARY MEASURES

Household and apothecary measures are most often used in the home care setting, and their clinical use is becoming less frequent. The measures you may occasionally see include the **ounce, tablespoon, teaspoon, dram, and drop.** Abbreviations and/or names for all of these measures, except the drop, **still appear on many disposable medication cups,** and care must be taken not to confuse them with metric dosages. It is quite possible that these measures will be eliminated in the future because the health care industry has been moving rapidly to improve dosage labeling and medication abbreviation guidelines to reduce the possibility of errors.

The various abbreviations for household dosages and their metric equivalents are as follows:

| Household Measure | Abbreviation | Metric Equivalent |
| --- | --- | --- |
| ounce | oz | 30 mL |
| tablespoon | T, TBS, tbs | 15 mL |
| teaspoon | t, TSP, tsp | 5 mL |
| dram | dr | 4 mL |
| drop | gtt | 1 mL |

 The volume of a drop depends on the size of the dropper being used.

A drop is so inaccurate a measure that medication droppers are now an integral part of small-volume liquid medication preparations. The use of drops is largely restricted to eye and ear drop use. One exception is in small-volume pediatric liquid medications, which are prepared with **integral medicine droppers that are calibrated by volume, or by actual dosage.**

## APOTHECARY MEASURES

Apothecary measures are mentioned here only to point out that they are no longer used. However, in the event your instructor thinks that you must be familiar with these measures, please refer to Appendix 1 for a brief discussion of this system.

## Summary

This concludes your introduction to the additional measures you will see used in dosages and in solutions. The important points to remember from this chapter are:

- International units measure a drug by its action rather than its weight.

- There is no abbreviation for units, which is written in full, units, in lower case letters.

- Percentage (%) strengths are frequently used in solutions and ointments.

▣ Percent represents grams of drug per 100 mL of solution.

▣ The greater the percentage strength, the stronger the solution.

▣ Milliequivalent is abbreviated mEq and is frequently used in solution measurements.

▣ Ratio strengths represent parts of drug per parts of solution.

▣ The smaller the volume of solution, the greater the ratio strength.

▣ T or tbs is the abbreviation for tablespoon (15 mL), and t or tsp for teaspoon (5 mL).

▣ The abbreviation gtt is used for drop, and oz for ounce.

▣ Apothecary measures are now obsolete and should not be used.

## Summary Self-Test

**Express the dosages using the official symbols/abbreviations.**

1. three hundred thousand units      _____

2. forty-five units      _____

3. ten percent      _____

4. two and a half percent      _____

5. forty milliequivalents      _____

6. a one in two thousand ratio      _____

7. a one in ten ratio      _____

8. one percent      _____

9. one drop      _____

10. two thousand units      _____

11. five milliequivalents      _____

12. nine-tenths percent      _____

13. ten units      _____

14. a one in two ratio      _____

15. five percent      _____

16. twenty milliequivalents      _____

17. fourteen units      _____

18. twenty percent      _____

19. two million units      _____

20. one hundred thousand units      _____

| **Answers** | **6.** 1 : 2000 | **12.** 0.9% | **18.** 20% |
| --- | --- | --- | --- |
| **1.** 300,000 units | **7.** 1 : 10 | **13.** 10 units | **19.** 2,000,000 units |
| **2.** 45 units | **8.** 1% | **14.** 1 : 2 | **20.** 100,000 units |
| **3.** 10% | **9.** 1 gtt | **15.** 5% | |
| **4.** 2.5% | **10.** 2000 units | **16.** 20 mEq | |
| **5.** 40 mEq | **11.** 5 mEq | **17.** 14 units | |

# SECTION 3

# Reading Medication Labels and Syringe Calibrations

**CHAPTER 6**
Oral Medication
Labels and Dosage
Calculation / 52

**CHAPTER 7**
Safe Medication
Administration / 75

**CHAPTER 8**
Hypodermic Syringe
Measurement / 85

**CHAPTER 9**
Parenteral Medication
Labels and Dosage
Calculation / 100

**CHAPTER 10**
Reconstitution of
Powdered Drugs / 122

**CHAPTER 11**
Measuring Insulin
Dosages / 138

# 6

# ORAL MEDICATION LABELS AND DOSAGE CALCULATION

## Objectives

**The learner will:**

1. identify scored tablets, unscored tablets, and capsules.

2. read drug labels to identify trade and generic names.

3. locate dosage strengths and calculate average dosages.

4. measure oral solutions using a medicine cup.

In this chapter, you will be introduced to labels of oral medications for both solid (tablet and capsule) and liquid (mL) medications. Medication label information includes trade and generic drug names, metric dosage strengths, manufacturer's name, and other details you need to be aware of, primarily so that you can quickly locate the correct dosage strength to calculate ordered dosages. You will then use actual drug labels to calculate a full range of oral medication dosages. **Average dosage calculations require only the information you have already learned on the metric system and in the Refresher Math Section on addition and subtraction**. They are routinely done mentally. Advanced calculations are needed primarily in clinical specialty areas, and they will be covered in later chapters.

 **Most oral dosages consist of one-half to three tablets or capsules, or one-half to double the mL volume of liquid medications, and are done mentally.**

We will begin with labels for solid drug preparations. These include tablets, scored tablets (which contain an indented marking to make breakage for partial dosages possible), enteric-coated tablets (which delay absorption until the drug reaches the small intestine), capsules (powdered or oily drugs in a gelatin cover), and sustained or controlled–release capsules (action spread over a prolonged period of time; for example, 12 hours). See illustrations in Figure 6-1.

Tablets          Scored Tablets          Enteric-Coated Tablets

Capsules          Gelatin Capsules          Controlled-Release Capsules

**Figure 6-1**

## TABLET AND CAPSULE LABELS

The most common type of label you will see in the clinical setting is the **unit dosage label**, in which each tablet or capsule is packaged separately. However, the dosage information on both unit and multiple dose labels is identical.

**EXAMPLE 1**

Look at the Synthroid® label in Figure 6-2. The first thing to notice is that this drug has two names. The first, **Synthroid**, is its **trade name**, which is identified by the ® registration symbol. Trade names are usually **capitalized** and **printed first** on the label. The name in smaller print, **levothyroxine sodium**, is the **generic** or

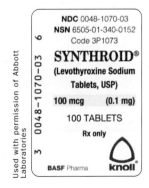

**Figure 6-2**

**official name** of the drug. Each drug has only **one** official name but may have **several trade names**, each for the exclusive use of the company that manufactures it. It is important to remember, however, that most labels do contain **both** names. Drugs may be ordered by either name depending on hospital policy or prescriber preference. You will frequently need to cross-check trade and generic names for accurate drug identification.

Next on the label is the **dosage strength**, 100 mcg or 0.1 mg. The prepared dosage is often representative of the **average dosage strength; the dosage given to the average patient at one time**. This label also identifies the **manufacturer** of this drug, Knoll Pharmaceuticals.

Notice that **100 TABLETS** is printed near the **bottom** of the label. This is the **total number** of tablets in the bottle. Be careful not to confuse the quantity of tablets or capsules with the dosage strength. **The dosage strength always has a unit of measure associated with it**; in this case, mcg and mg. Because label designs vary widely, this is an important point to remember.

**EXAMPLE 2**

The **Percocet®** label in Figure 6-3 is an example of a medication that contains not one but **two drugs**: 5 mg of the narcotic oxycodone and 325 mg of acetaminophen, an analgesic. The dosages in multiple drug products are routinely written in the same order as the drugs listed in the product. Oxycodone and acetaminophen are generic names, and Percocet is the manufacturer's trade name for this product. Medications that contain more than one drug are usually **ordered by trade name and number of tablets or capsules** to be given rather than by dosage.

The balance of the label information includes the total number of tablets near the bottom, 100; average dosage considerations; a bar code; and a space where the manufacturer would enter the drug lot number and expiration date. Expiration dates are carefully monitored by clinical pharmacies, but you must also make checking them a habit.

 Tablets and capsules that contain more than one drug are usually ordered by trade name and number of tablets or capsules to be given, rather than by dosage.

**Figure 6-3**

**EXAMPLE 3**

The small unit dosage label in Figure 6-4 bears only one name, **phenobarbital**, which is actually the **generic** name of the drug. Generic labeling is common with drugs that have been in use for generations. The official (generic) name was so well established that drug manufacturers did not try to promote their own trade names. Also notice that following the drug name are the initials **U.S.P.** This is the abbreviation for **U**nited **S**tates **P**harmacopeia, one of the two official national listings of drugs. The other is the **N**ational **F**ormulary, **NF**. You will see U.S.P. and NF on drug labels and must not confuse them with other initials that identify additional drugs or specific action of drugs in a preparation. Also notice that the label contains the dosage strength in both the metric, **15 mg**, and apothecaries, **1/4 gr**, measures. Finally, on the right of the label, printed sideways, is Exp 6-6-16, which identifies the last date when the drug should be used.

Next, refer to Figure 6-5. Notice that this label also contains the dosage strength of nitroglycerin in both the **0.3 mg metric** and the **1/200 gr (grains)** of the obsolete **apothecaries** system units of measure. As with phenobarbital, the inclusion of apothecaries dosages on this label relates to the age and historic use of this drug. Relabeling is already well under way by manufacturers to remove apothecaries dosages completely from their products.

For safety in medication administration, focus on the drug name and its dosage strength.

**Figure 6-4**

**Figure 6-5**

## Problems 6.1

**Refer to the label in Figure 6-5 and answer the questions about this drug.**

1. What is the generic name?                                     _____

2. What is the trade name?                                       _____

3. What is the dosage strength in metric units?                 _____

4. What is the dosage strength in the obsolete apothecary measure?   _____

5. If nitroglycerine 0.3 mg is ordered, how many tablets will be required?   _____

6. Read the information above the Nitrostat name.
   What kind of tablets are these?                              _____

7. How must the drug be administered?   _____

8. Who is the manufacturer of this drug?   _____

9. How many tablets will be needed to give a 0.6 mg dosage of nitroglycerin?   _____

**Answers   1.** nitroglycerin   **2.** Nitrostat®   **3.** 0.3 mg   **4.** 1/200 gr   **5.** 1 tab   **6.** sublingual
**7.** under the tongue   **8.** Parke Davis, a division of Pfizer Pharmaceuticals LLC   **9.** 2 tab

## Problems 6.2

Refer to the label in Figure 6-6 and answer the questions about this drug.

1. What is the generic name?   _____
2. What is the trade name?   _____
3. What is the dosage strength?   _____
4. What company manufactured this drug?   _____
5. How many tablets are in this container?   _____
6. If Prinivil 5 mg is ordered, how many tablets will you give?   _____
7. If lisinopril 10 mg is ordered, how many tablets will you give?   _____

Figure 6-6

**Answers   1.** lisinopril   **2.** Prinivil®   **3.** 5 mg   **4.** Merck & Co., Inc.   **5.** 100 tablets   **6.** 1 tab   **7.** 2 tab

Refer to the Sinemet® label in Figure 6-7. Sinemet is another example of a combined drug tablet. The **generic** names of the drugs it contains are **carbidopa** and **levodopa**. These are listed on the label in several places: directly under the trade name and with the **amount** of each drug in the fine print near the bottom of the label. Also, notice the box to the right of the trade name, which contains the numbers 25-100. This again is the amount of carbidopa—25 mg—and levodopa—100 mg. Contrast this label with the Sinemet labels in Figures 6-8 and 6-9.

In Figure 6-8, the dosage strengths are different. A blue box to the right of the Sinemet trade name identifies the strengths of carbidopa and levodopa as **10 mg** and **100 mg**, respectively, which are actually lower dosages. And, finally, Figure 6-9 is a label for Sinemet® **CR**, a **c**ontrolled-**r**elease or sustained-release tablet, with yet another dosage strength of 50-200: **carbidopa 50 mg** and **levodopa 200 mg**. Unlike the previous combined drug tablet discussed, an order for Sinemet **must** include the dosage because it is available in several strengths.

 Extra numbers after a drug name may be used to identify the dosage strengths of more than one drug in a preparation, and extra initials may be used to identify a special drug action.

Figure 6-7

Figure 6-8

Figure 6-9

## TABLET/CAPSULE DOSAGE CALCULATION

When the time comes for you to administer medications, you will have to read a **M**edication **A**dministration **R**ecord, abbreviated MAR, to prepare the dosage. This will tell you the name and amount of drug to be given, but it will not tell you how many tablets or capsules contain this dosage. This you must calculate yourself. However, remember that most tablets/capsules are prepared in average dosage strengths, and most orders will involve giving one-half to three tablets (or one to three capsules, since capsules cannot be broken in half). **Learn to question orders for more than three tablets or capsules.** Although some drugs require multiple tablets, most do not. Some clinical pharmacies do carry a limited quantity of a particular medication as a cost-saving factor, so if a drug came in 25 mg, 50 mg, 100 mg, and 200 mg dosages and that facility's pharmacy only carried 25 mg tablets, an order for 200 mg would translate into 8 tablets, which would seem unreasonable. In the 100 or 200 mg supply, the order results in 1 or 2 tablets, which is reasonable. Always question an order of more than 3 tablets, and double-check your calculations.

**An unusual number of tablets or capsules could be a warning of an error in prescribing, transcribing, or calculation.**

Let's now look at some sample orders and do some actual dosage calculations. **Assume that tablets are scored and can be broken in half.**

## Problems 6.3

**Refer to the Inderal®LA label in Figure 6-10 to answer these questions.**

1. What is the dosage strength?  _____
2. If you have an order for 120 mg, give  _____
3. If you have an order for 60 mg, give  _____
4. What is the generic name of this drug?  _____
5. What is the total number of capsules in this package?  _____

**Figure 6-10**

**Answers** **1.** 60 mg  **2.** 2 cap  **3.** 1 cap  **4.** propranolol hydrochloride  **5.** 100 capsules

## Problems 6.4

**Refer to the Aricept® label in Figure 6-11 to answer these questions.**

1. What is the dosage strength?  _____
2. If 10 mg is ordered, give  _____
3. If 2.5 mg is ordered, give  _____
4. If 5 mg is ordered, give  _____
5. What is the generic name of this drug?  _____
6. What is the total number of tablets in this package?  _____

**Figure 6-11**

**Answers   1.** 5 mg   **2.** 2 tab   **3.** ½ tab   **4.** 1 tab   **5.** donepezil HCl   **6.** 30 tablets

It is not uncommon to have a drug **ordered** in one unit of metric measure—**for example, mg**—and discover that it is **labeled** in another measure—**for example, g**. It will then be necessary to **convert the metric units to calculate the dosage**. Conversions will always be between touching units of measure: g and mg or mg and mcg. **Converting involves moving the decimal point three places**.

**EXAMPLE 1**

Refer to the Halcion® label in Figure 6-12. A dosage of 250 mcg has been ordered. The label reads 0.25 mg. Convert the mg to mcg by moving the decimal point three places to the right, and you can mentally verify that these dosages are identical. Give 1 tablet.

**Figure 6-12**

**EXAMPLE 2**

Refer to the Klonopin® label in Figure 6-13. A dosage of 1000 mcg is ordered. The label reads 0.5 mg, so you must give 2 tablets (1 tab = 500 mcg, so 1000 mcg requires 2 tab). The decimal moves three places to the right in this conversion from mg to mcg.

**Figure 6-13**

## Problems 6.5

Locate the appropriate labels for the following dosages, and indicate how many tablets or capsules are needed to give them. Assume all tablets are scored and can be broken in half. Labels may be used in more than one problem.

1. verapamil HCl 0.12 g _____ cap

2. Terbutaline® 10 mg _____ tab

3. Ritalin® HCl 7.5 mg _____ tab

4. methyphenidate HCl 2500 mcg _____ tab

**Answers   1.** 1 cap   **2.** 2 tab   **3.** 1½ tab   **4.** ½ tab

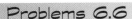

## Problems 6.6

Locate the appropriate labels for the following drug orders, and indicate the number of tablets/capsules that will be required to administer the dosages ordered. Assume that all tablets are scored and can be broken in half. Notice that both generic and trade names are used for the orders and that a label may be used in more than one problem.

1. isosorbide dinitrate 80 mg          _____ cap

2. sulfasalazine 0.5 g                 _____ tab

3. Azulfidine® 1 g                     _____ tab

4. terbutaline sulfate 2500 mcg        _____ tab

5. chlordiazepoxide HCl 50 mg          _____ cap

6. Librium® 25 mg                      _____ cap

7. Dilatrate®–SR 80 mg                 _____ cap

8. Synthroid® 0.2 mg                   _____ tab

9. levothyroxine Na 0.2 mg             _____ tab

10. terbutaline sulfate 3.75 mg        _____ tab

**Answers   1.** 2 cap   **2.** 1 tab   **3.** 2 tab   **4.** 1 tab   **5.** 2 cap   **6.** 1 cap   **7.** 2 cap   **8.** 2 tab
**9.** 2 tab   **10.** 1½ tab

## ORAL SOLUTION LABELS

In liquid drug preparations, the dosage is contained in a certain mL **volume of solution**. Let's review dosages in some solid and liquid drug preparations to illustrate the difference.

**EXAMPLE 1**    **Solid** 250 mg in **1 tablet**        **Liquid:** 250 mg in **5 mL**

**EXAMPLE 2**    **Solid:** 100 mg in **1 capsule**      **Liquid:** 100 mg in **10 mL**

**EXAMPLE 3**

Refer to the Lomotil® label in Figure 6-14. The information it contains will be familiar. **Lomotil** is the **trade** name and **diphenoxylate** is the **generic** or official name. The dosage strength is **2.5 mg per 5 mL**. As with solid drugs, the medication administration record, MAR, will tell you the **dosage of the drug** to be administered, but it **will not specify the volume that contains this dosage**.

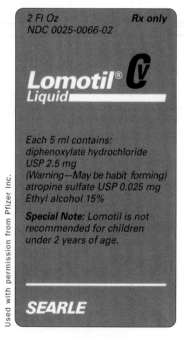

Used with permission from Pfizer Inc.

**Figure 6-14**

---

Problems 6.7

Refer to the Lomotil® label in Figure 6-14 to calculate these dosages.

1. The order is for diphenoxylate 2.5 mg. Give _____
2. The order is for Lomotil 5 mg. Give _____

## Problems 6.8

Refer to the Penicillin® V label in Figure 6-15 to calculate these dosages.

1. The order is for Penicillin V 400,000 units.   _____
2. Penicillin V 125 mg has been ordered.   _____
3. Penicillin V 375 mg has been ordered.   _____

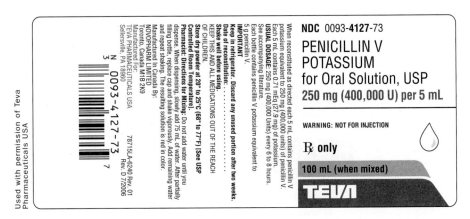

**Figure 6-15**

## Problems 6.9

Refer to the solution labels in Figures 6-16 and 6-17 to calculate these dosages.

1. Prozac® soln. 10 mg   _____
2. cefaclor susp. 187 mg   _____
3. cefaclor susp. 374 mg   _____
4. fluoxetine HCl soln. 30 mg   _____

5. Prozac® soln. 40 mg          _____

6. fluoxetine HCl soln. 20 mg   _____

**Figure 6-16**

**Figure 6-17**

## MEASUREMENT OF ORAL SOLUTIONS

Oral solutions are most commonly measured using a disposable **calibrated medication cup**. Take a close look at the schematic drawing of the medication cup calibrations in Figure 6-18. Many disposable medication cups, like this one, still contain the TSP (teaspoon), TBS (tablespoon), and OZ (ounce) calibrations of the household system and the obsolete DR (for dram) of the apothecaries system. Some also contain the increasingly disused cc (cubic centimeter) calibration, which is identical to a mL. Oral solutions are **most safely poured at eye level**. Because of the number of units of measure on these cups, **always read calibrations very carefully**.

**Figure 6-18**

Small-volume solution dosages can also be measured using specially calibrated **oral syringes** such as those illustrated in Figures 6-19 and 6-20. Oral syringes have safety features built into their design to prevent their being mistaken for hypodermic syringes. One of these features is **color**, as illustrated in Figure 6-19. Hypodermic syringes are not colored, although their packaging and needle covers are colored to aid in identification. A second feature is the syringe tip, which is a **different size and shape** and is often **off center** (**termed eccentric**). Figure 6-20 illustrates an eccentric oral syringe tip. Hypodermic syringes **without a needle** can also be used to measure and administer oral dosages.

**Figure 6-19**

**Figure 6-20**

The main concern with correct syringe identification is that **oral syringes, which are not sterile**, should not be confused and used for **hypodermic medications, which are sterile.** This mistake **has** been made in spite of the fact that hypodermic needles do not fit correctly on oral syringes. The precaution, therefore, does need to be stressed.

Oral solutions may also be ordered as drops (gtt), and when this is the case, the dropper is attached to the bottle stopper. Medicine droppers are often calibrated in mL or by actual dosage, such as 125 mg, and so forth. (Refer to Chapter 20 for more information on droppers.)

## Summary

**This concludes the chapter on reading oral medication labels. The important points to remember from this chapter are:**

- Most labels contain both generic and trade names.

- Dosages are clearly printed on the label, including preparations containing multiple drugs.

- Combined dosage tablets and capsules may be ordered by trade name and number of tablets/capsules to be given and may include dosages.

- The letters U.S.P. (United States Pharmacopeia) and NF (National Formulary) on drug labels identify their official generic listings.

- Additional letters that follow a drug name are used to identify additional drugs in the preparation or a special action of the drug.

- Most dosages of tablets or capsules consist of one-half to three tablets (1–3 capsules, which cannot be broken in half). An unusual number of tablets or capsules may indicate an error.

- Check expiration dates on labels before use.

- For accurate measurement, solutions are poured at eye level when a medicine cup is used.

- Liquid oral medications may be measured and administered using an oral medication syringe or a hypodermic syringe without a needle.

- Care must be taken not to use oral syringes for hypodermic medication preparation because these are not sterile.

## Summary Self-Test

**Locate the appropriate label for each of the following drug orders, and indicate the number of tablets, capsules, or mL that will be required to administer them. Assume that all tablets are scored and can be broken in half. Labels may be used more than once in each problem set.**

PART I

1. Glucotrol® 15 mg          *3 tabs*

2. dexamethasone 4 mg        *2 tabs*

3. Dilatrate®-SR 80 mg       *2 capsules*

4. morphine sulfate 20 mg    *2 capsules*

NDC 0091-0920-01

Store at controlled room temperature 15°-30°C (59°-86°F) in a dry place.

Dispense in tight containers as described in USP-NF.

100 Capsules

**Dilatrate®-SR**
*(isosorbide dinitrate)*
Sustained Release Capsules

℞ Only

40 mg

**SCHWARZ**
P H A R M A

6505-01-244-9942

*Distributed by*
**ROERIG** *Pfizer*
A division of Pfizer Inc. N.Y., N.Y. 10017

NDC 0662-4110-73

500 Tablets

**Glucotrol®**
glipizide

**5 mg**

CAUTION: Federal law prohibits dispensing without prescription.

*Distributed by*
**ROERIG** *Pfizer*
A division of Pfizer Inc. N.Y., N.Y. 10017

NDC 0054-8176-25

10 x 10 Tablets

**2 mg**

**DEXAMETHASONE**
**Tablets USP**

LOT

EXP.

4238501

**Roxane**
Laboratories, Inc.
Columbus, Ohio 43216

108
© RLI, 1998

NDC 63857-410-11

**KADIAN®**
Morphine Sulfate
Extended-Release Capsules

**10 mg**

℞ only        100 Capsules

**ALPHARMA.**
Pharmaceuticals

**Each capsule contains:** 10 mg morphine sulfate as extended-release pellets.
**Usual Dosage:** See accompanying prescribing information.
The pellets from KADIAN® capsules should NOT be chewed, crushed or dissolved.
**Warning:** As with all medication, keep out of the reach of children.
Dispense in a sealed, tamper-evident, childproof, light-resistant container.
Store at 25°C (77°F); excursions permitted to 15°-30°C (59°-86°F). Protect from light and moisture.

Manufactured for:
Alpharma Pharmaceuticals LLC
One New England Avenue
Piscataway, NJ 08854
by Actavis Elizabeth LLC, 200 Elmora Avenue
Elizabeth, NJ 07207 USA        Rev. 04/07

Lot No.:

63857-410-11

## PART II

5. piroxicam 20 mg          *1 capsule*

6. cefaclor susp. 250 mg    _____

7. Lortab® 5/500 2 tab      _____

8. Halcion® 250 mcg         _____

9. alprazolam 750 mcg       _____

10. gabapentin 0.2 g        _____

11. Biaxin® 1 g             _____

12. Xanax® 500 mcg          _____

13. clarithromycin 0.5 g    _____

14. triazolam 500 mcg       _____

---

Used with permission from Pfizer Inc.

**Store below 86°F (30°C)**

Dispense in tight, light-resistant containers (USP).

**DOSAGE AND USE**
See accompanying prescribing information.
One capsule per day.

Each capsule contains 20 mg piroxicam.

**IMPORTANT:** This closure is not child-resistant.

**CAUTION:** Federal law prohibits dispensing without prescription.

NDC 0069-3230-66

**100 Capsules**

**Feldene®**
(piroxicam) 20

**20 mg**

**Pfizer** Pfizer Labs
Division of Pfizer Inc, NY, NY 10017

6505-01-137-4628
0069-3230-66 2
3
05-4300-00-5
MADE IN USA
1292

---

Used with permission of Abbott Laboratories.

**SPECIMEN** ©Abbott

Exp.
Lot
03-2126-2/R4

0074258660

Store tablets at 15° to 30°C (59° to 86°F).

NDC 0074-2586-60
**60 Tablets**

**BIAXIN®**
**FILMTAB®**
clarithromycin
tablets

**500 mg**

abbott Caution: Federal (U.S.A.) law prohibits dispensing without prescription.

**6505-01-354-8581**
Do not accept if break-away ring on cap is broken or missing.
Dispense in a USP tight, light-resistant container.
Each tablet contains:
500 mg clarithromycin.
Each yellow tablet bears the Ⓐ and Abbo-Code KL for product identification.
Usual Adult Dose: One tablet every twelve hours. See enclosure for full prescribing information.
Filmtab—Film-sealed tablets, Abbott.
Abbott Laboratories
North Chicago, IL 60064, U.S.A.

---

Used with permission of UCB Pharma, Inc.

**ucb Pharma**

**PHARMACIST:** Dispense in a tight, light-resistant container with a child-resistant closure.

Store at controlled room temperature, 15°-30°C (59°-86°F).

Lot No.:
Exp. Date:

Manufactured for
**UCB Pharma, Inc.**
Smyrna, GA 30080
**by Mallinckrodt Inc.**
Hobart, NY 13788

NDC 50474-902-01    **100 TABLETS**

**LORTAB® 5/500**

**HYDROCODONE BITARTRATE AND ACETAMINOPHEN TABLETS, USP**
**5 mg/500 mg**

Each scored, white with blue specks tablet contains:

Hydrocodone Bitartrate . . . . . . . . . . 5 mg
Acetaminophen . . . . . . . . . . . . . . . 500 mg

**℞ only**

**USUAL DOSAGE:** See package insert for complete dosage recommendations.

N 3 50474-902-01 1

Rev. 6/01
P/N 1003723

**R** RANBAXY

NDC 63304-**954**-01

# CEFACLOR

For Oral Suspension USP

**125 mg/5 mL**

**75 mL** (when mixed)

SHAKE WELL BEFORE USE

Rx only

Manufactured for:
Ranbaxy Pharmaceuticals Inc.
Jacksonville, FL 32216 USA
by: Ranbaxy Laboratories Ltd.
New Delhi - 110 019, India

0903

**Usual Dosage:** Children, 20 mg/kg a day (40 mg/kg in otitis media) in three divided doses.
Adults, 250 mg three times a day. See literature for complete dosage information.
Contains Cefaclor monohydrate equivalent to 1.875 g cefaclor in a dry, pleasantly flavored mixture.
**Prior to Mixing,** store at 20 - 25° C (68 - 77° F). (See USP Controlled Room Temperature). Protect from moisture.
**Directions for Mixing: Add 53 mL** of water in two portions to dry mixture in the bottle. Shake well after each addition.
Each 5 mL (Approx. one teaspoonful) will then contain Cefaclor USP monohydrate equivalent to 125 mg anhydrous cefaclor.
Over size bottle provides extra space for shaking.
**Store in a refrigerator.** May be kept for 14 days without significant loss of potency. Keep tightly closed. Discard unused portion in 14 days.

50308460

non varnish area

LOT:
EXP:

N 3 63304 95401 2

---

NDC 0054-
8176-25

10 x 10
Tablets

**2 mg**

## DEXAMETHASONE
Tablets USP

LOT
EXP.

**Roxane**
Laboratories, Inc.
Columbus, Ohio 43216

4238501

108

© RLI, 1998

---

# Halcion® C IV

triazolam tablets, USP

**0.25 mg**

*Distributed by*
**Pharmacia & Upjohn Co**
Div of Pfizer Inc,
NY, NY 10017

← 2

EXP 00/0000  LOT 0000

N0009001755

---

Store at controlled room temperature 15°-30°C (59°-86°F).

NDC 0071-0803-24

**100 Capsules**    Rx only

**DOSAGE AND USE**
See package insert for full prescribing information.

Each capsule contains 100 mg of gabapentin.

Manufactured by:
Pfizer Pharmaceuticals Ltd.
Vega Baja, PR 00694

**Neurontin®** 100

(gabapentin) capsules

**100 mg**

*Distributed by*
**Pfizer** **Parke-Davis**
Division of Pfizer Inc, NY, NY 10017

---

©Abbott

0074336860

Exp.

Lot 03-2127-3/R4

Store tablets at 15° to 30°C (59° to 86°F).

NDC 0074-3368-60
60 Tablets

## BIAXIN®
FILMTAB®

clarithromycin tablets

**250 mg**

Caution: Federal (U.S.A.) law prohibits dispensing without prescription.

6505-01-354-8582
Do not accept if break-away ring on cap is broken or missing.
Dispense in a USP tight, light-resistant container.
Each tablet contains:
250 mg clarithromycin.
Each yellow tablet bears the ◨ and Abbo-Code KT for product identification.
Usual Adult Dose: One or two tablets every twelve hours. See enclosure for full prescribing information.
Filmtab – Film-sealed tablets, Abbott.
Abbott Laboratories
North Chicago, IL 60064, U.S.A.

---

**R** only
See package insert for complete product information.

Keep container tightly closed.

Dispense in tight, light-resistant container.

Store at controlled room temperature 20° to 25° C (68° to 77° F) [see USP].

Pharmacia & Upjohn
Company
Kalamazoo, MI 49001, USA

NDC 0009-0029-01
6505-01-143-9269

## Xanax®  C IV

alprazolam tablets, USP

**0.25 mg**

812 004 712

100 Tablets

LOT
EXP

N 3 0009-0029-01 2

## PART III

15. acetaminophen 650 mg  _____

16. Aldactone® 75 mg  _____

17. meclizine HCl 50 mg  _____

18. Kadian® 20 mg  _____

19. ciprofloxacin HCl 0.375 g  _____

20. metoprolol tartrate 0.15 g  _____

21. nifedipine 10 mg  _____

22. piroxicam 20 mg  _____

23. Feldene® 40 mg  _____

24. Lomotil® 2.5 mg  _____

25. Librium® 75 mg  _____

26. codeine 45 mg  _____

27. Aldactone® 50 mg  _____

28. Synthroid® 225 mcg  _____

29. nitroglycerin 600 mcg  _____

Used with permission of McNeil Consumer and Specialty Pharmaceuticals

**Regular Strength**
**TYLENOL®**
Pain Reliever - Fever Reducer  ACETAMINOPHEN
**Tablets**
**100 TABLETS—325 mg each**  THIS PACKAGE FOR HOUSEHOLDS WITHOUT YOUNG CHILDREN

Used with permission of Valeant Pharmaceuticals

NDC 0187-3758-10
**Librium®** C IV
(chlordiazepoxide HCl)
**25 mg**
Each capsule contains
25 mg chlordiazepoxide HCl
℞ only
**100 Capsules**
ICN

Used with permission from Pfizer Inc.

**1000 Tablets**
**Antivert®** 25
(meclizine HCl)
**25 mg**
Distributed by
**Pfizer  Roerig**
Division of Pfizer Inc, NY, NY 10017

Used with permission from Pfizer Inc.

Store below 86°F (30°C)
Dispense in tight, light-resistant containers (USP).
**DOSAGE AND USE**
See accompanying prescribing information. One capsule per day.
Each capsule contains 20 mg piroxicam.
**IMPORTANT:** This closure is not child-resistant.
CAUTION: Federal law prohibits dispensing without prescription.

NDC 0069-3230-66
**100 Capsules**
**Feldene®**
(piroxicam) 20
**20 mg**
**Pfizer  Pfizer Labs**
Division of Pfizer Inc, NY, NY 10017

6505-01-137-4628
0069-3230-66  2
05-4300-00-5
MADE IN USA
1292

Used with permission from Pfizer Inc.

Store below 25°C (77°F).
**Protect from light.**
Dispense in tight, light-resistant, child-resistant containers (USP).
**DOSAGE AND USE:**
See accompanying prescribing information.
Each tablet contains 25 mg spironolactone.

NDC 0025-1001-31
**Rx only**
**100 Tablets**
**Aldactone®**
spironolactone tablets, USP  25
**25 mg**
Distributed by
**Pfizer  G.D. Searle LLC**
Division of Pfizer Inc, NY, NY 10017

Used with permission of ALPHARMA LLC

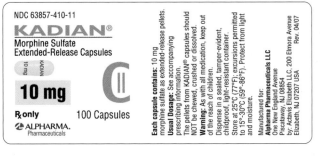

NDC 63857-410-11

**KADIAN®**

Morphine Sulfate
Extended-Release Capsules

**10 mg**

R̠ only          100 Capsules

**ALPHARMA.**
Pharmaceuticals

**C II**

**Each capsule contains:** 10 mg
morphine sulfate as extended-release pellets.
**Usual Dosage:** See accompanying
prescribing information.
The pellets from KADIAN® capsules should
NOT be chewed, crushed or dissolved.
**Warning:** As with all medication, keep out
of the reach of children.
Dispense in a sealed, tamper-evident,
childproof, light-resistant container.
Store at 25°C (77°F); excursions permitted
to 15°-30°C (59°-86°F). Protect from light
and moisture.

Manufactured for:
**Alpharma Pharmaceuticals LLC**
One New England Avenue
Piscataway, NJ 08854
by: Actavis Elizabeth LLC, 200 Elmora Avenue
Elizabeth, NJ 07207 USA          Rev. 04/07

Used with permission of Novartis AG

NDC 0028-0051-10
6505-01-071-6557

**Lopressor® 50 mg**

metoprolol tartrate USP

1000 tablets

Rx only

**♦ NOVARTIS**

Used with permission of Roxane Laboratories Inc.

See Package Insert for
Complete Prescribing Information.

Store at Controlled Room Temperature
15°-30°C (59°-86°F).

PROTECT FROM MOISTURE.

Dispense in a well-closed container
as defined in the USP/NF.

TABLETS IDENTIFIED  54 783
(Side One)  ⊖  54 783  (Side Two)
DO NOT USE UNLESS TABLETS
CARRY THIS IDENTIFICATION

NDC 0054-
4156-25          100 Tablets          EXP. LOT

**30 mg**          **C II**

**CODEINE**
Sulfate
Tablets USP

Each tablet contains
Codeine Sulfate 30 mg
R̠ only.

**Roxane**
Laboratories, Inc.
Columbus, Ohio 43216

4151001
039
© RLI, 1999

3  0054-4156-25  7

Used with permission of Abbott Laboratories

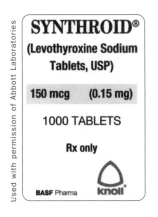

**SYNTHROID®**

**(Levothyroxine Sodium
Tablets, USP)**

**150 mcg      (0.15 mg)**

**1000 TABLETS**

**Rx only**

**BASF** Pharma          **knoll®**

Used with permission from Pfizer Inc.

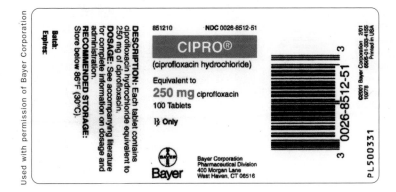

Store at Controlled Room Temperature
20°-25°C (68°-77°F) [see USP].

Dispense in original, unopened container.

**DOSAGE AND USE**
See accompanying prescribing information.

Each tablet contains 0.3 mg nitroglycerin.

**Keep this and all drugs out
of the reach of children.**

**Warning**—To prevent loss of potency, keep
these tablets in the original container or in a
supplemental Nitroglycerin container
specifically labeled as being suitable for
Nitroglycerin Tablets. Close tightly
immediately after each use.

Manufactured by:
**Pfizer Pharmaceuticals LLC**
Vega Baja, PR 00694          8210

NDC 0071-0417-24
Rx only

**100 Sublingual Tablets**

**Nitrostat®**
(Nitroglycerin
Tablets, USP)          0.3

**0.3 mg (1/200 gr)**

05-5930-32-2

**Pfizer** Distributed by
**Parke-Davis**
Division of Pfizer Inc, NY, NY 10017

Used with permission from Pfizer Inc.

Store below 25°C (77°F).

**Pharmacist:** Caution patient
not to exceed recommended
dose and to keep out of reach
of children. Dispense only in
a well-closed, light-resistant,
child-resistant container.

**DOSAGE AND USE:**
See accompanying
prescribing information.

*Each tablet contains: 2.5 mg
diphenoxylate hydrochloride
(Warning—May be habit
forming) and 0.025 mg
atropine sulfate USP.

**Special Note:**
Lomotil is not recommended for
children under 2 years of age.

NDC 0025-0061-31
100 Tablets          Rx only

**Lomotil®  C V**
(diphenoxylate
hydrochloride and
atropine sulfate tablets USP)

**2.5 mg/0.025 mg***

**Pfizer** Distributed by
**G.D. Searle LLC**
Division of Pfizer Inc, NY, NY 10017

Used with permission of Bayer Corporation

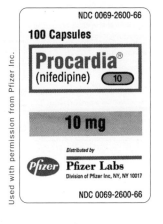

Batch:
Expires:

**DESCRIPTION:** Each tablet contains
ciprofloxacin hydrochloride equivalent to
250 mg of ciprofloxacin.
**DOSAGE:** See accompanying literature
for complete information on dosage and
administration.
**RECOMMENDED STORAGE:**
Store below 86°F (30°C).

851210          NDC 0026-8512-51

**CIPRO®**
(ciprofloxacin hydrochloride)

Equivalent to
**250 mg** ciprofloxacin
100 Tablets

R̠ Only

**Bayer**
Bayer Corporation
Pharmaceutical Division
400 Morgan Lane
West Haven, CT 06516

©2001 Bayer Corporation  2/01
6505-01-333-4195
Printed in USA
10278

3  0026-8512-51  3

PL500331

Used with permission from Pfizer Inc.

NDC 0069-2600-66

**100 Capsules**

**Procardia®**
(nifedipine)          10

**10 mg**

**Pfizer** Distributed by
**Pfizer Labs**
Division of Pfizer Inc, NY, NY 10017

NDC 0069-2600-66

PART IV

30. cefaclor susp. 0.25 g         _____

31. propanolol hydrocloride 120 mg    _____

32. metronidazole 0.75 g         _____

33. piroxicam 40 mg         _____

34. Lopid® 300 mg         _____

**6**

## PART V

35. Vantin® 150 mg _____

36. spironolactone 0.1 g _____

37. cefpodoxime proxetil 0.2 g _____

38. Azulfidine® 0.75 g _____

39. potassium chloride 40 mEq _____

40. Cipro® 250 mg _____

Used with permission of Pharmaceutical Associates, Inc.

Delivers **15 mL**
NDC 0121-0465-15
**POTASSIUM CHLORIDE**
**ORAL SOLUTION** USP 10%
**20 mEq per 15 mL**
Sugar Free        Alcohol 5%
**DILUTE BEFORE USING**

(01) 0 03 01210 465154

**Rx ONLY**
FOR INSTITUTIONAL USE ONLY
PHARMACEUTICAL ASSOCIATES, INC.
GREENVILLE, SC 29605
SEE INSERT

Used with permission from Pfizer Inc.

Store below 25°C (77°F).
**Protect from light.**
Dispense in tight, light-resistant, child-resistant containers (USP).
**DOSAGE AND USE:**
See accompanying prescribing information.
Each tablet contains 100 mg spironolactone.

**100 Tablets**          NDC 0025-1031-31          **Rx only**

**Aldactone®**
spironolactone
tablets, USP          (100)

**100 mg**

*Distributed by*
**Pfizer** **G.D. Searle LLC**
Division of Pfizer Inc, NY, NY 10017

2137

N3 0025-1031-31 1
05-6589-32-1

Used with permission of Pfizer Inc.

**Azulfidine®**
sulfasalazine tablets, USP

**500 mg**
Rx only

MADE IN SWEDEN
Mfd. for: Pharmacia & Upjohn Co.
        Kalamazoo, MI 49001, USA
by:   Pharmacia & Upjohn AB
        Stockholm, Sweden

300 Tablets          **Pharmacia & Upjohn**

NDC 0009-3615-03
50 mL (when mixed)

**Vantin®** For Oral Suspension
cefpodoxime proxetil
for oral suspension

**100 mg** per 5 mL

Equivalent to 100 mg per 5 mL
cefpodoxime when constituted

**Pharmacia & Upjohn**

Used with permission of Pfizer Inc.

Used with permission of Bayer Corporation

Batch:
Expires:

851210          NDC 0026-8512-51

**CIPRO®**
(ciprofloxacin hydrochloride)

Equivalent to
**250 mg** ciprofloxacin
100 Tablets

Rx Only

**DESCRIPTION:** Each tablet contains ciprofloxacin hydrochloride equivalent to 250 mg of ciprofloxacin.
**DOSAGE:** See accompanying literature for complete information on dosage and administration.
**RECOMMENDED STORAGE:**
Store below 86°F (30°C).

**Bayer**
Bayer Corporation
Pharmaceutical Division
400 Morgan Lane
West Haven, CT 06516

©2001 Bayer Corporation  2/01
6505-01-333-4155
10276          Printed in USA

3 0026-8512-51 3

PL500331

**Answers**

| | | | | |
|---|---|---|---|---|
| **1.** 3 tab | **9.** 3 tab | **18.** 2 cap | **27.** 2 tab | **36.** 1 tab |
| **2.** 2 tab | **10.** 2 cap | **19.** 1½ tab | **28.** 1½ tab | **37.** 10 mL |
| **3.** 2 cap | **11.** 2 tab | **20.** 3 tab | **29.** 2 tab | **38.** 1½ tab |
| **4.** 2 cap | **12.** 2 tab | **21.** 1 cap | **30.** 10 mL | **39.** 30 mL |
| **5.** 1 cap | **13.** 2 tab | **22.** 1 cap | **31.** 2 cap | **40.** 1 tab |
| **6.** 10 mL | **14.** 2 tab | **23.** 2 cap | **32.** 1½ tab | |
| **7.** 2 tab | **15.** 2 tab | **24.** 1 tab | **33.** 2 cap | |
| **8.** 1 tab | **16.** 3 tab | **25.** 3 cap | **34.** ½ tab | |
| | **17.** 2 tab | **26.** 1½ tab | **35.** 7.5 mL | |

# SAFE MEDICATION ADMINISTRATION

In this chapter you will be introduced to a sample **Medication Administration Record (MAR)** that may be used to prepare, administer, and chart medications. Additional instruction will include the **Six Rights of Medication Administration:** the basic guidelines for all medication administration; information on the most common sources of **medication errors;** and the **actions that you must take when errors occur**. You'll also be introduced to new transcription rules for medication dosages and abbreviations that have been addressed by the major watchdog organizations for medication safety: **The Joint Commission** and **The Institute for Safe Medication Practices (ISMP)**.

## MEDICATION ADMINISTRATION RECORDS

The focus of this section is to familiarize you with a sample MAR so that you will understand the many columns and features it contains. Your instructors will orient you to the actual MARs you will use in your clinical experiences, and you will quickly discover that there is **no one universal form** in use. Each clinical facility using MARs makes its own determination on the particular format that suits its needs. What you will notice, however, is that **all MARs are more similar than different**. A MAR is, simply stated, **a paper record of all medications a patient is receiving and has received**.

    The most prominent MAR feature is a **large column** where medications **given on a continuing basis** are listed. This column will contain a **drug name** (or names, if trade and generic listing is appropriate), **dosage, frequency, actual times of administration, and precautions related to administration, such as checking blood pressure, pulse, or body weight**. Other columns provide the following: an area that the person who transcribed the dosages initials; the start date of the medication; columns where dosages administered are recorded; an area for the initials of the nurse who gives the dosage; and an additional area where all staff initials are identified with a full name. A MAR may consist of a single sheet of paper printed on both sides, or two sheets, to allow separate space for p.r.n. (pro re nata or "as needed") medications (given on an as needed basis), for parenteral medications and site identification, and IV medications and/or fluids.

## Objectives

The learner will:

1. read a MAR to identify medications to be administered.

2. record medications administered.

3. list and discuss the six rights of medication administration.

4. explain "partnering with the patient" in medication administration.

5. list common causes of dosage errors.

6. list the five steps to take when a dosage error occurs.

7. list the two major safety concerns addressed by The Joint Commission and ISMP.

Refer now to the sample MAR in Figure 7-1, and locate the following column headings and entries.

**Column 1**  Labeled "Start" and "Stop." The three drugs listed are being given on a continuing basis. They were started on "5–1." None has been discontinued.

**Column 2**  Labeled "Medication and Dose." The first drug listed is Lanoxin® including its generic name, digoxin. The dosage, "0.25 mg," and frequency, "daily," is next. There is a precautionary designation to "Check pulse" (ck pulse).

**Column 3**  Labeled "Schedule." Gives the actual times of each medication's administration. For Lanoxin, this is 8 am.

**Column 4**  This column has two designations: "Route," which is oral or "PO" for all three medications. The "Nurse" space, which "GJ" has initialed, identifies the transcriber of these medication orders.

**Column 5**  There are three designations here: "Time," the actual hour the drug is to be given (i.e., "8 am"); "Site" if the drug is parenteral; and "Initials," where the nurse who gave the drug, "BPP," verified administration. The pulse, "64," is recorded next to the 8 am dosage.

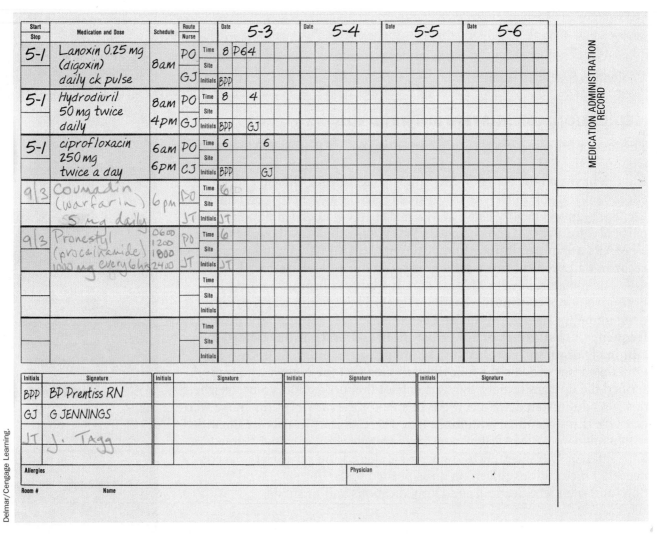

**Figure 7-1** | Medication administration record.

This particular MAR covers only four days of medications, "5–3" through "5–6." However, most MARs provide for longer periods of up to a month. At the bottom of this MAR is an area for identification of staff initials, where "GJ" is clearly identified as "G Jennings" and "BPP" as "BP Prentiss."

## Problems 7.1

**Refer to the MAR provided to answer the following questions.**

1. List the second and third listed drugs and dosages on this sample record.

   _Hydrodiurll 50 mg_    _ciprofloxacin 250 mg_

2. Who administered the 4 pm dosage for the second drug listed?

   _G. Jennings_

3. Drug number 3 is administered twice a day. Identify the hours these dosages are to be given. _6 am_    _6 pm_

**Answers   1.** Hydrodiuril 50 mg, ciprofloxacin 250 mg   **2.** G. Jennings   **3.** 6 am and 6 pm

## Problems 7.2

**Use the drug entries on the MAR provided as a guide to enter the following two additional drugs and dosages. Use today's date as the start date. Have your instructor or a fellow student check your entries.**

1. Coumadin® (warfarin) 5 mg PO daily 6 pm.
2. Pronestyl® (procainamide) 1000 mg PO every 6 hours: 6 am, noon, 6 pm, and midnight.
3. Identify your initials as the transcriber of these dosages.
4. Sign for the initial 6 pm dosage administration for each drug.

Information needs to be filled in on the MAR.

Computer-controlled records, usually keyed to drug label bar codes, are making a strong appearance in the health care field. The Veterans Administration System in the United States is already completely computerized, and this has resulted in increased safety and lower costs in medication services. It is wise to remember, however, that errors can occur anywhere, and the newer systems of administration will have identified their own safety precautions for error-prone areas.

## THE SIX RIGHTS OF MEDICATION ADMINISTRATION

The **Six Rights** of administration consist of the right **drug**, the right **dosage**, the right **route**, the right **time**, to the right **person**, and the right **recording** of a dosage when it is administered. These rights will be covered in more detail in your fundamentals text, but it is appropriate to discuss them briefly here.

## RIGHT DRUG

When preparing dosages, the **drug order and drug label are routinely checked against each other three times: when you locate the drug, just before you open or pour it, and immediately before you administer it**. There are three specific safety reminders related to reading labels that need to be revisited. The first is that **a drug may be ordered by trade name but available only in a generic** so make sure you have the drug ordered. The second concern is that **many drug names, particularly generic, are very similar**, and must be identified carefully. And, finally, because it is easy to miss the **special initials that follow a drug name**—a familiar example is CR, for controlled release—look for and identify these. When doing the three required order and label cross checks, all these precautions to locate the correct drug apply.

## RIGHT DOSAGE

Dosage is **a particular concern in metric dosages containing a decimal**. Think back to your instruction in conversions between the different units of metric measure containing decimals. You know that in conversions in metric dosages, **the decimal point will always move three places**. If you are **converting from a greater to a lesser unit**: g to mg or mg to mcg, **the number will become larger**; if you are **converting from a lesser to a greater unit**: mcg to mg or mg to g, **the number will become smaller**. If you inadvertently **convert in the wrong direction, the numbers often don't make sense**: 0.25 mg **cannot** be 250 g; and 2 mg **cannot** be 0.002 mcg. Remember that medications are **prepared in average dosages** and usually consist of **one-half to three times the average dose (tablet or capsule) available**. Ask yourself if the conversion makes sense, and recognize when it doesn't.

## RIGHT ROUTE

**Oral medications** are swallowed. This is not always easy for patients to do, and this is why many children's medications are prepared as liquids. This means you must **watch the patient actually take oral medications**. If you have any doubt that the medications have been swallowed, check the patient's mouth.

An additional oral route is the **sublingual: under the tongue**. There has been a considerable increase in the number of sublingual drugs in use, so this route designation is one to carefully identify. A sublingual drug swallowed will not have the desired effect, if it has any at all, because the acid of the stomach will destroy it.

**Drops** are another administration route, and eye, nose, and ear drops are quite common. Eye medications are also prepared as **ointments**, and, understandably, they are clearly labeled for their intended **ophthalmic** use. **Locating the ophthalmic designation** is mandatory before the use of any preparation on the eyes.

An increasing number of **topical** drugs is in use. These are **ointments** or, less commonly, **liquids** that are applied to the skin. The amount of ointment or liquid to be used is specific, as is the cleansing of a site for repeated ointment applications, and covering or not covering the site after application.

Now in very wide use are **transdermal patches**. The precautions in their use relate to where the patch must be applied, how long it is to stay on, and examination for local skin reaction to the adhesive that secures the patch. Unfortunately, many people are sensitive to transdermal patch adhesives. A rash may appear when a patch is used for the first time, or even after repeated use. Inflamed skin will not absorb well, and inflammation can cause acute discomfort.

A large number of **inhalation** medications is in common use. One of the newest is Exubera®, a form of inhalation insulin. These medications are usually self-administered, and your responsibility will be to make sure that the patient understands how to use the inhalation device, how many activations each dosage requires, how many times a day to use the medication, and precautions in use, such as for temporary dizziness.

The **creams and suppositories** used for the genitorectal systems provide another method of direct medication application. These are very clearly labeled and recognizable.

Finally, there are the **parenterals: medications administered under the skin.** The **intravenous** is the primary parenteral route, with **intramuscular (IM)** and **subcutaneous** coming in second, and **intradermal** a distant third. Most injectable drugs are **site-specific,** and are labeled for either IV, IM, or subcutaneous use. You'll be reading many drug labels that identify specific parenteral site routes in the balance of this text.

## RIGHT TIME

The time each drug is to be given is **often critical**, such as insulin immediately before a meal or, more correctly, a meal as soon as insulin is injected. Drugs may be ordered at **specific hours during the day or only at bedtime**. Some drugs must be given **before or after specific blood tests**. Pain medications are given **p.r.n.,** which means **as needed.** Pain medications are extremely **time-sensitive,** and must be given before pain becomes severe in postoperative situations, and at least half an hour before a painful procedure, including postoperative ambulation.

Each clinical facility designates routine administration times; however, twice a day may mean 9 am and 5 pm or 9 am and 9 pm, depending on the action of the drug being given. Each MAR identifies **two time-related specifics: frequency**—for example, "twice a day"—then **specific hours**—for example, 9 (am) and 5 (pm) or, in International military time, 09 and 17, representing 0900 and 1700.

A final consideration, just illustrated, is **standard versus international/ military time**. A clinical facility will use **either one time or the other, but not both**. International/military time uses a 24-hour clock, starting with 0001 for one minute after midnight, to 2400 for midnight of the same (next date) day. To convert from standard to international/military time, add 12 hours to each hour beginning with 1 pm standard time. For example, 2 pm plus 12 hours is 1400; 4 pm plus 12 (hours) is 1600. Using international time, if you are unfamiliar with it, will initially require careful thought. Refer to Figure 7-2 for a complete time conversion chart.

| Standard am | International/Military am | Standard pm | International/Military pm |
|---|---|---|---|
| 1:00 | 0100 | 1:00 | 1300 |
| 2:00 | 0200 | 2:00 | 1400 |
| 3:00 | 0300 | 3:00 | 1500 |
| 4:00 | 0400 | 4:00 | 1600 |
| 5:00 | 0500 | 5:00 | 1700 |
| 6:00 | 0600 | 6:00 | 1800 |
| 7:00 | 0700 | 7:00 | 1900 |
| 8:00 | 0800 | 8:00 | 2000 |
| 9:00 | 0900 | 9:00 | 2100 |
| 10:00 | 1000 | 10:00 | 2200 |
| 11:00 | 1100 | 11:00 | 2300 |
| 12:00 noon | 1200 | 12:00 midnight | 2400 |

Delmar/Cengage Learning.

**Figure 7-2 |** Comparison of standard and international/military time.

## RIGHT PERSON

Administering medications to the **right person** should be foolproof, but it isn't. All MARs identify patients by the **room number and bed** they occupy. But sometimes patients are moved, so room and bed number cannot be relied on for identification. The current identification procedure is to **ask an individual her or his name**, then check the response against the wrist **Identa-Band®**. Obviously, some people will not be able to state their name. But if they can, they must be asked.

Of considerable concern is the possibility of having two people with the same surname on the same floor or even, though more rarely, in the same room. **Duplicate names** are a source of errors, so **read both surname and first name** on each Identa-Band. **Do this every time you give a medication. No exceptions. Once a drug is administered, there is no way to get it back.**

## RIGHT RECORDING

If an administered drug **is not charted, it can be given again in error**. There is an **absolute rule that a drug given must be recorded immediately**. It is also necessary to **record and report unusual reactions to a medication**, such as nausea or dizziness, or a patient's **refusal to take a medication**. In such an occurrence, **record and report the incident immediately**.

If you give a **parenteral** medication other than by IV, **the injection site used is usually recorded**, so that a different site can be used next time. Diabetic or other patients receiving frequent injections may tell you which site they prefer, which they have a perfect right to do. Or, ask them if they have a preference. In actual practice, **sites are chosen by the condition of the tissues at acceptable sites**, because previous injection sites are generally easy to see and must be avoided.

## THE SEVENTH RIGHT: PARTNERING WITH THE PATIENT

Partnering with the patient/recipient is so important a concern that it should be a Seventh Right. You are only half of a medication administration twosome. **The medication recipient is one of your best assists in preventing errors.** Consider the following, not uncommon, verbal reports: "I just had my medication." Or, "My doctor told me he was stopping this drug." Or, "The doctor said I needed a bigger dose." Or, "This pill doesn't look the same as the one I had before." Or, "Where is my . . . pill?" Or, "This pill made me sick the last time I took it." Learn to listen very carefully, and **consider the patient correct until proven otherwise**.

You will also be responsible for **helping the patient learn what drugs and dosages he or she is taking, what they are for, what time they must be taken, and how they must be taken**. Most individuals will be discharged with medications, so the sooner they—or, if they are not deemed responsible, their caretaker—can learn what they are taking, the better. They must also learn about common side effects and, if particularly relevant, what untoward effects they should watch for. Patients taking medications are essentially under chemical assistance, or assault, and they or their caretakers must be full partners in their medication administration.

An important safety precaution is recognition of the patient/recipient as a full partner in medication administration.

## COMMON MEDICATION ERRORS

Prescription drugs are estimated to kill close to 100,000 people a year in the United States, although not all these deaths are hospital-based. Medication errors happen, and they will continue to happen in **all three of the modalities** related to drug orders: the **prescribing** (done by a licensed practitioner), the **transcribing** (done by a person who specializes in this responsibility, frequently the pharmacy staff), or in the **administration** (primarily a nursing responsibility). The vast majority of errors is in the prescribing and transcribing areas, but those attributable to administration still represent a very large number of incidents.

There has been a concerted **international** effort in recent years to identify the source of, and take active steps to reduce, the incidence of medication errors caused by the use of administration abbreviations. The primary and an ongoing leader in this project is **The Joint Commission**, formerly known as the **Joint Commission on Accreditation of Healthcare Organizations (JCAHO)**.

Most safety recommendations fall into **two major categories: abbreviations for administration and drug names, and in metric dosages containing decimals**.

## ERRORS IN ABBREVIATIONS AND DRUG NAMES

A number of abbreviations designating **the frequency and routes of medication administration** have been eliminated. For example: the abbreviations Q.D., QD, q.d., and qd used for a **single daily dose** and Q.O.D., QOD, q.o.d., and qod used for a dosage given **every other day**. These are no longer used but are now clearly written as **"daily"** or **"every other day."** Similarly, q.d. and QD for "every day" has been eliminated and is now designated "daily"; qhs, formerly used for "nightly" and misread as "every hour," is now written "nightly"; SC or sub q used for "subcutaneous" has been changed to "subcut" or "subcutaneous"; the use of "per os" for "by mouth" has been eliminated in favor of "PO," "by mouth," or "orally." An additional abbreviation, q2 h or q2hr (or **any** specific hour) is now clearly written "every 2 hours." Another deletion is the use of a lowercase "u" or uppercase "U" or "IU" for "units." As you have already learned, units is not abbreviated, but written as "units." A current list of acceptable administration abbreviations is available on the inside front cover of this text, but do keep in mind that there may be future changes in this evolving area of concern.

Common examples of confusing **drug name abbreviations** are MS for morphine sulfate and $MSO_4$ or $MgSO_4$ for magnesium sulfate. These drugs are now identified using their complete names. Figure 7–3, Official "Do Not Use" List, identifies these changes.

## ERRORS IN WRITING METRIC DOSAGES

All the correct rules for writing metric dosages have been covered earlier in this text. But let's revisit the culprit areas, which are also identified in Figure 7-3. The first error is in **placing a decimal and a zero (0) following a whole number dosage** (called a **trailing zero**); for example, 4.**0** g instead of 4 g. The decimal could easily be missed and 10 times the ordered dosage, 40 g, administered. The second error is **failing to place a zero in front of a decimal fraction** (referred to as lack of a **leading zero**); for example, .5 mg instead of **0**.5 mg. Once again, the decimal could be missed and 5 mg administered. Unfortunately, you may still see an occasional commercial drug label that has not yet been standardized to reflect the new recommended notation rules. But at least on a drug label you will not have the problem of trying to **interpret indecipherable handwriting**, which is often the direct cause of many of the errors just discussed. Commercial drug labels are being redesigned to reflect these new guidelines.

Additional changes have since been recommended by **ISMP**, the **Institute for Safe Medication Practices**. Those of you re-entering the health care field after a significant absence may want to review the ISMP lists, in Appendix B. These tables are for reference only and need not be memorized.

## ACTION STEPS WHEN ERRORS OCCUR

You will almost certainly meet with an error in one way or another during your career. So, let's look at the routine steps you must take when one occurs.

**STEP 1**   Errors must be reported as soon as they are discovered.

**STEP 2**   Necessary remedial measures must be instituted immediately.

**STEP 3**   The reason for the error must be determined.

**STEP 4**   An incident/accident report must be prepared.

**STEP 5**   Corrective policies/procedures must be instituted, if possible, to prevent the error from recurring.

### Official "Do Not Use" List[1]

| Do Not Use | Potential Problem | Use Instead |
|---|---|---|
| U (unit) | Mistaken for "0" (zero), the number "4" (four), or "cc" | Write "unit" |
| IU (International Unit) | Mistaken for IV (intravenous) or the number 10 (ten) | Write "International Unit" |
| Q.D., QD, q.d., qd (daily) | Mistaken for each other | Write "daily" |
| Q.O.D., QOD, q.o.d, qod (every other day) | Period after the Q mistaken for "I" and the "O" mistaken for "I" | Write "every other day" |
| Trailing zero (X.0 mg)* Lack of leading zero (.X mg) | Decimal point is missed | Write X mg Write 0.X mg |
| MS | Can mean morphine sulfate or magnesium sulfate | Write "morphine sulfate" Write "magnesium sulfate" |
| $MSO_4$ and $MgSO_4$ | Confused for one another | |

[1] Applies to all orders and all medication-related documentation that is handwritten (including free-text computer entry) or on preprinted forms.

*Exception:  A "trailing zero" may be used only where required to demonstrate the level of precision of the value being reported, such as for laboratory results, imaging studies that report size of lesions, or catheter/tube sizes. It may not be used in medication orders or other medication-related documentation.

**Figure 7-3** | Official "Do Not Use" list of medical abbreviations. © The Joint Commission, 2008. Reprinted with permission.

**The most important step after ensuring the safety of the patient is reporting the error.** If an error isn't reported, no action can be taken. Keep in mind that **an error is an accident, and it is not necessarily a reflection on competency, nor will reporting an error terminate your career. Distraction and fatigue play a significant role in medication errors**, and when in stressful situations, you must be particularly aware and vigilant that **you** do not become the person making an error.

 The major factors in nursing medication administration errors are distraction and fatigue, and particular vigilance is necessary in these stressful situations.

In time, and with repeat practice, administering medications will become familiar and comfortable. The irony is that when it does, you must **exercise more caution than ever. Routine medication administration must never be routine.**

 Regardless of the source of an error, if you give a wrong drug or dosage, you are legally responsible for it.

## Summary

**This completes your introduction to safe medication administration. The important points to remember from this chapter are:**

- When identifying a drug, pay particular attention to generic names and any initials that identify additional drug components or action.

- When identifying dosages, take special precautions with metric dosages containing a decimal.

- The route of administration is critical to medication safety and effectiveness.

- Parenteral medications are site-specific: IV, IM, subcutaneous, and intradermal.

- Time of administration is especially important for p.r.n. medications for pain, and for drugs with a rapid action such as insulin.

- Identification of the right person begins with asking the patient his or her name, followed by checking the Identa-Band.

- Making the patient or caretaker a full partner in medication administration is a major safety consideration

- Recent changes in abbreviations for drug names and administration are creating increased safety in the clinical setting.

- Dosage errors must be reported as soon as discovered to set in motion the four additional steps you must take.

- Administering medications must never become routine.

- Fatigue and/or clinical distractions are major factors in medication errors.

- MARs are the immediate reference for medication administration, and keeping them up-to-the-minute is of prime importance.

## Summary Self-Test

**Answer the questions as succinctly as possible.**

1. List the six rights of medication administration. _right drug, right dosage, right recording, right person, right time, right route of drug_

2. What consideration was stressed regarding reading generic names? _generic drug names are often very similar_

3. What might extra initials following a drug name identify? _a specific drug action or additional information._

4. List the two major transcribing considerations for metric dosages containing a decimal. _Don't use a decimal and zero after a whole #. DO use a zero before a decimal if # < 1_

5. What use will you make of the fact that medications are prepared in average dosages? _Recognize when a dose is excessively high or low._

6. Name and discuss the two time-sensitive medications that were identified in this chapter. _Insulin - give a meal as soon as insulin is injected. Pain Meds - must be given before pain is severe._

7. What two patient identification steps follow arrival at the room and bed number indicated on a MAR? _Ask the patient his/her name & cross check with the ID band._

8. What will you do if a patient refuses a medication? _Ask them why, document in their chart, & report it_

9. List the steps you must take when a medication error occurs. _Report it, institute remedial measures, determine why error occurred, prepare incident report, institute corrective policies._

10. List your medication responsibilities in preparing a patient for discharge. _Have the patient list all drugs and their dosages, frequency, when they take them, & how they must be taken. Also any side effects they may experience._

**Answers 1.** Drug, dosage, route, person, time, and recording **2.** Read carefully; they are often similar **3.** Additional medications in a preparation or special action **4.** Use a zero in front of a decimal to draw attention to it; no decimal or zero following a whole number dosage **5.** An unusual number of oral tablets or capsules or excessively large mL volumes must be questioned **6.** Pain medications—give before pain becomes severe or half an hour before a painful procedure; insulin—make sure a meal is available shortly after administration **7.** Ask the patient for his or her name; check the Identa-Band **8.** Ask why, record it, report it **9.** Report the error, take remedial measures as necessary, determine the cause, and institute a policy to prevent a repeat **10.** Review all the discharge drugs by asking the patient to explain the dosage, frequency, time, and route of administration for each. Review these again as necessary, including side effects and precautions

# HYPODERMIC SYRINGE MEASUREMENT

A variety of hypodermic syringes is in clinical use. This chapter focuses most heavily on the frequently used 3 mL syringe. However, larger volume syringes are used on occasion, so it is necessary that you learn the **differences** as well as the **similarities** of all syringes in use.

Regardless of a syringe's volume or capacity—0.5, 1, 3, 5, 10, or 20 mL—all except specialized insulin syringes **are calibrated in mL**. Because some syringe manufacturers have not yet replaced the labeling on their syringes with the official mL volume measurement, you may still see cc on syringes. Keep in mind, however, that these two measures, mL and cc, are essentially identical. They will be correctly referred to throughout this text as mL. The various capacity syringes contain **calibrations that differ from each other**. Recognizing the difference in syringe calibrations is the chief safety concern of this chapter.

 The calibrations on different volume syringes differ from each other, requiring particular care in dosage measurement.

## Objectives

The learner will measure parenteral solutions using:

1. a standard 3 mL syringe.
2. a tuberculin syringe.
3. 5 and 10 mL syringes.
4. a 20 mL syringe.

## STANDARD 3 mL SYRINGE

The most commonly used hypodermic syringe is the 3 mL size illustrated in Figure 8-1. Notice the calibrations for the metric mL scale, and that **longer calibrations** identify zero (0) and each ½ and full mL measure. These longer calibrations are numbered: ½, 1, 1½, 2, 2½, and 3.

Next, notice the **number of calibrations in each mL**, which is 10, indicating that on this syringe, each mL is **calibrated in tenths**. Tenths of a mL are written as **decimal fractions**; for example 1.2 mL, 2.5 mL, or 0.4 mL. Also, notice the arrow on this syringe, which identifies a 0.8 mL dosage.

**Figure 8-1** | A 3 mL syringe.

## Problems 8.1

**Use decimal numbers—for example, 2.2 mL—to identify the measurements indicated by the arrows on the standard 3 mL syringes that follow.**

1. _0.2 mL_

2. _1.4 mL_

3. _1.9 mL_

**Answers** **1.** 0.2 mL **2.** 1.4 mL **3.** 1.9 mL

Did you have difficulty with the 0.2 mL calibration in Problem 1? Remember that **the first long calibration on all syringes is zero**. It is slightly longer than the 0.1 mL and subsequent one-tenth calibrations. Be careful not to mistakenly count it as 0.1 mL.

You have just been looking at photos of syringe barrels only. In assembled syringes, the colored suction tip of the plunger has two widened areas in contact with the barrel that look like two distinct rings. **Calibrations are read from the front, or top, ring.** Do not become confused by the second, or bottom, ring or by the raised middle section of the suction tip.

## Problems 8.2

What dosages are measured by the following three assembled syringes?

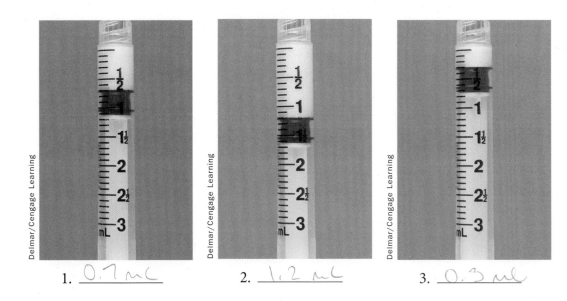

1. _0.7 mL_   2. _1.2 mL_   3. _0.3 mL_

**Answers**  **1.** 0.7 mL  **2.** 1.2 mL  **3.** 0.3 mL

## Problems 8.3

Draw an arrow or shade in the following syringe barrels to indicate the required dosages. Have your instructor check your accuracy.

1. 1.3 mL          2. 2.4 mL          3. 0.9 mL

4. 2.5 mL        5. 1.7 mL        6. 2.1 mL

Verify your answers with your instructor.

## Problems 8.4

Identify the dosages measured on the following 3 mL syringes.

1. _____    2. _____    3. _____

4. _____       5. _____       6. _____

**Answers**   **1.** 1.5 mL   **2.** 2.3 mL   **3.** 0.8 mL   **4.** 2.6 mL   **5.** 1.9 mL   **6.** 1.4 mL

## SAFETY SYRINGES

A number of safety syringes has been developed in recent years to reduce the danger of accidental contaminated needle sticks. Several of these syringes are illustrated in the following photos. Take a few minutes to become familiar with them, as you will in all probability be using them in the clinical setting.

Refer first to the photos in Figure 8-2, which show two B-D SafetyGlide™ syringes. Each of these syringes contains a protective needle guard that can be activated by a single finger to cover and seal the needle after injection.

A

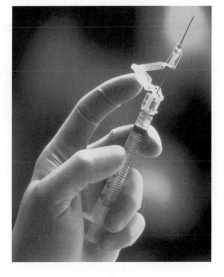

B

**Figure 8-2A and B** | SafetyGlide™ syringes. Courtesy and © Becton, Dickinson and Company.

The syringe shown in Figure 8-3, the VanishPoint®, has a needle that automatically retracts into the barrel after injection.

**Figure 8-3** | VanishPoint®. Courtesy of Retractable Technologies.

A third type of safety needle commonly used is the Magellan Safety Needle by Covidien™, as shown in Figure 8-4. This design also offers one-handed activation. It can be activated one of three ways: by thumb, forefinger, or on a flat surface. As with the other safety syringes, once activated, its safety shield covers the entire needle, providing protection during and after disposal.

A B

**Figure 8-4A and B** | Magellan Safety Needle. Courtesy of Covidien.

## TUBERCULIN (TB) SYRINGE

When very small dosages are required, they are measured in special tuberculin (TB) **0.5 or 1 mL syringes calibrated in hundredths**. Originally designed for the small dosages required for tuberculin skin testing, these syringes are also widely used in a variety of sensitivity and allergy tests. Pediatric dosages frequently require measurement in hundredths, as does heparin, an anticoagulant drug.

Refer to the 0.5 mL TB syringe in Figure 8-5, and take a careful look at its metric calibrated hundredth scale. Notice that slightly longer calibrations identify zero, 0.05, 0.1, 0.15, 0.2, and so on through the 0.5 mL measure. Shorter calibrations lie between these to measure the hundredths. Each tenth mL, .1, .2, .3, .4, and .5, is numbered on this particular TB syringe. Take a moment to study the dosage measured by the arrow in Figure 8-5, which is 0.43 mL.

The closeness and small size of TB syringe calibrations mandate particular care and an unhurried approach in TB syringe dosage measurement.

**Figure 8-5** | A tuberculin (TB) syringe.

## Problems 8.5

**Identify the measurements on the six TB syringes provided.**

1. _____     2. _____     3. _____

4. <u>0.06 mL</u>    5. <u>0.27 mL</u>    6. <u>0.41 mL</u>

**Answers**    **1.** 0.24 mL    **2.** 0.46 mL    **3.** 0.15 mL    **4.** 0.06 mL    **5.** 0.27 mL    **6.** 0.41 mL

## Problems 8.6

Draw an arrow on the barrel to identify the dosages indicated on these TB syringes. Have your instructor check your answers.

1. 0.28 mL                    2. 0.32 mL                    3. 0.45 mL

4.  0.12 mL          5.  0.27 mL          6.  0.35 mL

Verify your answers with your instructor.

## 5 AND 10 mL SYRINGES

When volumes larger than 3 mL are required, a 5 or 10 mL syringe is typically used. Refer to Figure 8-6, and examine the calibrations between the numbered mLs to determine how these syringes are calibrated.

**Figure 8-6** | A 5 mL and a 10 mL syringe.

As you may have discovered, the calibrations divide each mL of these syringes into **five** so that **each shorter calibration actually measures 0.2 mL**. The 5 mL syringe on the left measures 4.6 mL, and the 10 mL syringe on the right measures 7.4 mL. These syringes are most often used to measure whole rather than fractional dosages, but in your practice readings, we will include a full range of measurements.

## Problems 8.7

What dosages are measured on the following syringes?

1. _____

2. _____

3. _____

4. _____

5. _____

**Answers**  **1.** 3.4 mL  **2.** 5 mL  **3.** 4.6 mL  **4.** 1.8 mL  **5.** 9.4 mL

## Problems 8.8

**Measure the dosages indicated on the syringes provided. Have an instructor check your accuracy.**

1.  1.4 mL

2.  3.2 mL

3.  6.8 mL

4.  9.4 mL

5.  4.4 mL

6.  5.6 mL

Verify your answers with your instructor.

## 20 mL AND LARGER SYRINGES

Examine the 20 mL syringe in Figure 8-7, and determine how it is calibrated.

**Figure 8-7** | A 20 mL syringe.

As you can see, this syringe is calibrated in **1 mL increments**, with longer calibrations identifying the 0, 5, 10, 15, and 20 mL volumes. Syringes with a capacity larger than 20 mL are also calibrated in full mL measures. These syringes are used only for measurement of very large volumes.

### Problems 8.9

**What dosages are measured on these syringes?**

1. _____          2. _____          3. _____

**Answers   1.** 7 mL  **2.** 12 mL  **3.** 16 mL

## Problems 8.10

Shade in or draw arrows on the three syringe barrels provided to identify the volumes listed. Have your answers checked by your instructor.

1. 11 mL          2. 18 mL          3. 9 mL

Verify your answers with your instructor.

## Summary

This concludes your introduction to syringe calibrations. The important points to remember from this chapter are:

- 3 mL syringes are calibrated in tenths.

- TB syringes are calibrated in hundredths.

- 5 and 10 mL syringes are calibrated in fifths (two-tenths).

- Syringes larger than 10 mL are calibrated in full mL measures.

- The first long calibration on all syringes indicates zero.

- All syringe calibrations must be read from the top, or front, ring of the plunger's suction tip.

## Summary Self-Test

**Identify the dosages measured on the following syringes**

1. _____

2. _____

3. _____

4. _____

5. _____

6. _____

7. _____

8. _____

9. _____

Draw arrows or shade the barrels on the following syringes/cartridges to measure the indicated dosages. Have your answers checked by your instructor.

10. 0.42 mL

11. 0.31 mL

12. 0.44 mL

13. 13 mL

14. 1.2 mL

15. 7.6 mL

16. 1.7 mL

17. 2.2 mL

18. 0.9 mL

**Answers  1.** 0.5 mL  **2.** 2.5 mL  **3.** 1.6 mL  **4.** 0.18 mL  **5.** 0.25 mL  **6.** 0.08 mL  **7.** 6.4 mL
**8.** 4.8 mL  **9.** 17 mL  **10–18.** Verify your answers with your instructor.

# CHAPTER

# 9

## Objectives

**The learner will:**

1. read parenteral solution labels and identify dosage strengths.

2. calculate average parenteral dosages from the labels provided.

3. measure parenteral dosages in metric, milliequivalent, unit, percentage, and ratio strengths using 3 mL, TB, 5, 10, and 20 mL syringes.

# PARENTERAL MEDICATION LABELS AND DOSAGE CALCULATION

Parenteral medications are administered by injection, with intravenous (IV), intramuscular (IM), and subcutaneous (subcut) being the most frequently used routes. The labels of oral and parenteral solutions are very similar, but the size of the average parenteral dosage label is much smaller. Intramuscular solutions are manufactured so that the **average adult dosage will be contained in a volume of between 0.5 mL and 3 mL**, with subcutaneous injections being smaller, and seldom exceeding 1 mL. Excessively larger or smaller volumes would need to be questioned and calculations rechecked.

 Volumes larger than 3 mL are difficult for a single IM injection site to absorb, and the 0.5 to 3 mL volume can be used as a guideline for accuracy of calculations in IM and subcutaneous dosages

Intravenous medication administration is usually a two-step procedure. The dosage is prepared first, then may be further diluted in IV fluids before administration. In this chapter, we will be concerned only with the **first step of IV drug preparation, which is accurate measurement of the prescribed dosage**.

Parenteral medications are packaged in a variety of single-use glass ampules, single- and multiple-use rubber-stoppered vials, and premeasured syringes and cartridges. See Figure 9-1.

## READING METRIC/SI SOLUTION LABELS

Let's begin by looking at parenteral solution labels on which the dosages are expressed in metric units of measure.

Delmar/Cengage Learning

**Figure 9-1** | Ampules, vials, and a pre-filled cartridge.

### EXAMPLE 1

Refer to the Vistaril® label in Figure 9-2. The immediate difference you will notice between this and oral solution labels is the **size**. Ampules and vials are small and their labels are small, which requires that they be **read with particular care**. The information, however, is similar to oral labels. Vistaril is the trade name of the drug; hydroxyzine hydrochloride is the generic name. The dosage strength is 50 mg per mL (in the red rectangular area). The total vial contents are 10 mL (in black, center). Keep in mind that average intramuscular and subcutaneous dosages usually consist of one-half to double the average dosage strength, which for this IM Vistaril is 50 mg per mL.

> For 50 mg, you would give 1 mL
> For 25 mg, you would give 0.5 mL
> For 100 mg, you would give 2 mL
> For 75 mg, you would give 1.5 mL

These average dosages are within the usual 0.5 to 3 mL IM volume.

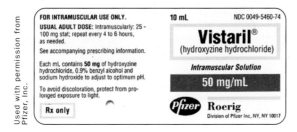

Used with permission from Pfizer, Inc.

FOR INTRAMUSCULAR USE ONLY.

USUAL ADULT DOSE: Intramuscularly: 25 - 100 mg stat; repeat every 4 to 6 hours, as needed.

See accompanying prescribing information.

Each mL contains **50 mg** of hydroxyzine hydrochloride, 0.9% benzyl alcohol and sodium hydroxide to adjust to optimum pH.

To avoid discoloration, protect from prolonged exposure to light.

Rx only

10 mL          NDC 0049-5460-74

**Vistaril®**
(hydroxyzine hydrochloride)

*Intramuscular Solution*

**50 mg/mL**

*Pfizer* **Roerig**
Division of Pfizer Inc, NY, NY 10017

**Figure 9-2**

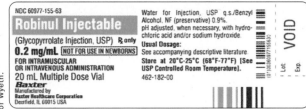

**Figure 9-3**

**EXAMPLE 2**

The Robinul® (glycopyrrolate) medication in Figure 9-3 has a dosage strength of 0.2 mg/mL.

For a 0.2 mg dosage, you would give 1 mL
For a 0.1 mg dosage, you would give 0.5 mL
For a 200 mcg dosage, you would give 1 mL
For a 100 mcg dosage, you would give 0.5 mL
For a 0.4 mg dosage, you would give 2 mL
For a 400 mcg dosage, you would give 2 mL

## Problems 9.1

**Refer to the Celestone® label in Figure 9-4 to answer the following questions.**

1. What is the dosage strength of this solution? _6 mg/mL_
2. How many mL are required for a dosage of 3 mg? _0.5 mL_
3. How many mL for a 6 mg dosage? _1 mL_
4. How many mL for a 9 mg dosage? _1.5 mL_
5. How many mL for a 12 mg dosage? _2 mL_

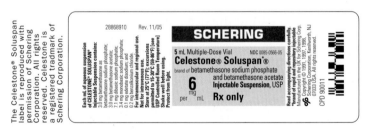

**Figure 9-4**

**Answers  1.** 6 mg/mL  **2.** 0.5 mL  **3.** 1 mL  **4.** 1.5 mL  **5.** 2 mL

## Problems 9.2

Refer to the gentamicin label in Figure 9-5 to answer the following questions.

1. What is the total volume of this vial? _____ 20 mL
2. What is the dosage strength? _____ 40 mg/mL
3. If 80 mg were ordered, how many mL would this be? _____ 2 mL
4. If 60 mg were ordered, how many mL would this be? _____ 1.5 mL
5. How many mL would you need to prepare a 20 mg dosage? _____ 0.5 mL

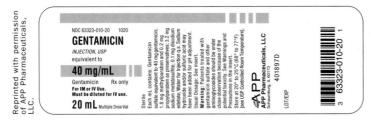

**Figure 9-5**

**Answers** **1.** 20 mL  **2.** 40 mg/mL  **3.** 2 mL  **4.** 1.5 mL  **5.** 0.5 mL

## PERCENT (%) AND RATIO SOLUTION LABELS

Drugs labeled as **percentage solutions** often express the dosage strength in **metric measures in addition to percentage strength**. The lidocaine label in Figure 9-6, a 2% solution, is an example.

But directly underneath this is a "20 mg/mL" designation. Lidocaine HCl is most often ordered in mg, but it is also used as a local anesthetic, and when it is, a physician may ask you to prepare a volume dosage specifying % strength.

## Problems 9.3

Refer to the lidocaine label in Figure 9-6 to answer the following questions.

1. How many mL are needed for a 10 mg dosage? _____ 0.5 mL
2. How many mL for a 20 mg dosage? _____ 1 mL
3. If you are asked to prepare 5 mL of a 2% solution? _____ 5 mL
4. If you are asked to prepare 15 mg? _____ 0.75 mL

**Figure 9-6**

## Problems 9.4

Refer to the lidocaine label in Figure 9-7 to answer the following questions.

1. What is the percentage strength of this lidocaine solution? _____

2. How many mL does the vial contain? _____

3. If you are asked to prepare 20 mL of a 1% lidocaine solution, how many mL will you draw up in the syringe? _____

4. What is the metric dosage strength of this solution? _____

5. If you are asked to prepare 25 mg from this vial, what volume will you draw up? _____

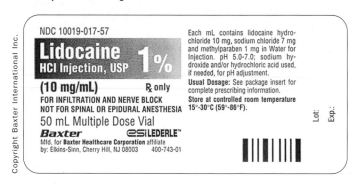

**Figure 9-7**

Refer to the calcium gluconate label in Figure 9-8 to answer the following questions.

6. What is the percentage strength of this solution? _____

7. How many mL does this preparation contain? _____

8. What is the per mL mEq dosage strength of this solution? _____

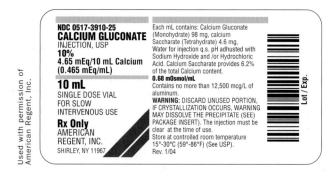

**Figure 9-8**

Parenteral medications expressed in **ratio strengths** are not common, and **when they are ordered, it will be by number of mL**. Ratio labels may also contain dosages in metric weights.

## Problems 9.5

Refer to the epinephrine label in Figure 9-9 to answer the following questions.

1. What is the ratio strength of this solution?　　　＿＿＿＿＿＿
2. What volume is this contained in?　　　＿＿＿＿＿＿
3. What is the metric dosage strength of this solution?　　　＿＿＿＿＿＿

**NDC 0517-1071-25**
**EPINEPHRINE**
INJECTION, USP **1:1000** (1 mg/mL)

**1 mL** AMPULE
FOR SC AND IM USE. FOR IV
AND IC USE AFTER DILUTION.
**Rx Only**
**CONTAINS NO SULFITES.**
**PRESERVATIVE FREE.**
Store at controlled room temperature
up to 25°C (77°F) (See USP).   Rev. 1/04
**AMERICAN REGENT, INC.**
SHIRLEY, NY 11967

Used with permission from American Regent, Inc.

**Figure 9-9**

**Answers   1.** 1 : 1000   **2.** 1 mL   **3.** 1 mg/mL

## SOLUTIONS MEASURED IN INTERNATIONAL UNITS

A number of drugs are measured in **International Units**. The following labels will introduce you to several examples.

## Problems 9.6

Refer to the heparin label in Figure 9-10 to answer the following questions.

1. What is the total volume of this vial?　　　＿＿＿＿＿＿
2. What is the dosage strength?　　　＿＿＿＿＿＿
3. If a volume of 1.5 mL is prepared, how many units will this be?　　　＿＿＿＿＿＿
4. How many mL will you need to prepare a dosage of 5500 units?　　　＿＿＿＿＿＿
5. If 0.25 mL of this medication is prepared, what dosage will this be?　　　＿＿＿＿＿＿

**Figure 9-10**

**Refer to the Bicillin® C-R label in Figure 9-11 to answer the following questions.**

6. What is the dosage strength of this medication?   _____

7. If 600,000 units are ordered, how many mL would this require?   _____

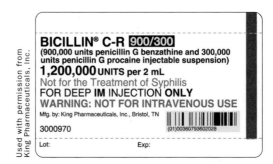

**Figure 9-11**

---

**Answers**   **1.** 10 mL   **2.** 1000 units/mL   **3.** 1500 units   **4.** 5.5 mL   **5.** 250 units
**6.** 1,200,000 units/2 mL   **7.** 1 mL

---

## SOLUTIONS MEASURED AS MILLIEQUIVALENTS (mEq)

The next four labels will introduce you to milliequivalent (mEq) dosages. Refer to the calcium gluconate label in Figure 9-12 and notice that in addition to its 10% strength, this vial has a dosage of 0.465 mEq/mL. If a dosage of 0.465 mEq were ordered, you would draw up 1 mL in the syringe.

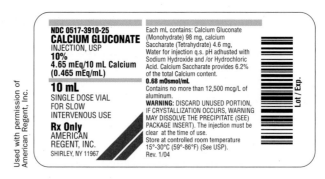

**Figure 9-12**

### Problems 9.7

Refer to the potassium chloride label in Figure 9-13 to answer the following questions.

1. What are the total dosage and volume of this vial?   _____

2. What is the dosage in mEq per mL?   _____

3. If you were asked to prepare 15 mEq for addition to an IV, what volume would you draw up?   _____

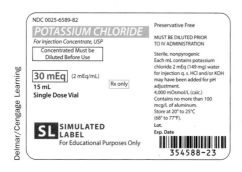

**Figure 9-13**

Refer to the potassium acetate label in Figure 9-14 to answer the following dosage questions.

4.  What is the strength of this solution in mEq per mL?          _____

5.  If you were asked to prepare 40 mEq for addition to an IV solution, what volume would you draw up in the syringe?          _____

6.  What volume would you need for a dosage of 20 mEq?          _____

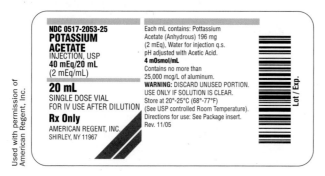

**Figure 9-14**

Refer to the sodium bicarbonate label in Figure 9-15. Notice that this solution lists the drug strength in mEq, percentage, and g. Read the label very carefully to answer the following questions.

7.  What is the dosage strength expressed in mEq/mL?          _____

8.  What is the total volume of the vial, and how many mEq does this volume contain?          _____

9.  What is the strength per mL expressed as g?          _____

10. If you were asked to prepare 10 mL of an 8.4% sodium bicarbonate solution, what volume would you draw up in a syringe?          _____

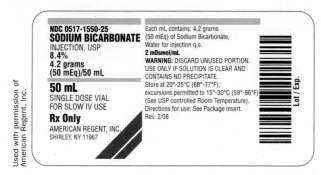

**Figure 9-15**

**Answers**  **1.** 30 mEq; 15 mL  **2.** 2 mEq/mL  **3.** 7.5 mL  **4.** 2 mEq/mL  **5.** 20 mL  **6.** 10 mL  **7.** 1 mEq/mL  **8.** 50 mL/50 mEq; 1 mEq/mL  **9.** 4.2 g/mL  **10.** 10 mL

## Summary

**This concludes the introduction to parenteral solution labels. The important points to remember from this chapter are:**

- The most commonly used parenteral administration routes are IV, IM, and subcutaneous.

- The labels of most parenteral solutions are quite small and must be read with particular care.

- The average IM dosage will be contained in a volume of between 0.5 mL and 3 mL.

- These 0.5 to 3 mL volumes can be used as a guideline to accuracy of calculations.

- The average subcutaneous dosage volume is between 0.5 and 1 mL.

- IV medication preparation is usually a two-step procedure: measurement of the dosage, then dilution according to manufacturers' recommendations or a physician's or prescriber's order.

- Parenteral drugs may be measured in metric, ratio, percentage, unit, or mEq dosages.

- If dosages are ordered by percentage or ratio strength, they are usually specified in mL to be administered.

- Most IM dosages are prepared using a 3 mL syringe.

- Most subcutaneous dosages are prepared using a 3 mL or tuberculin syringe.

## Summary Self-Test

**Read the parenteral drug labels provided to measure the following dosages. Then, indicate on the syringe provided exactly how much solution you will draw up to obtain these dosages. Have your answers checked by your instructor to be sure you have measured the dosages correctly.**

**Dosage Ordered**                                                    **mL Needed**

1. terbutaline sulfate 500 mcg                                    _____

## Dosage Ordered

## mL Needed

2. furosemide 10 mg

_____

3. heparin 2500 units

_____

4. acyclovir Na 100 mg

_____

| **Dosage Ordered** | **mL Needed** |
|---|---|

5. atropine 0.2 mg                _____

6. hydroxyzine HCl 25 mg           _____

7. Robinul® 100 mcg              _____

## Dosage Ordered

## mL Needed

8. nitroglycerine 25 mg

_____

9. methotrexate 0.25 g

_____

10. cyanocobalamin 1 mg

_____

**Dosage Ordered**                                               **mL Needed**

11. hydralazine hydrochloride 10 mg                              _____

NDC 0517-0901-25
**HYDRALAZINE HYDROCHLORIDE**
INJECTION, USP
**20 mg/mL**

**1 mL** SINGLE DOSE VIAL
FOR IM OR IV USE

**Rx Only**
AMERICAN REGENT, INC
SHIRLEY, NY 11967

**WARNING:** DISCARD UNUSED PORTION. Store at 20°-25°C (68°-77°F) (See USP Controlled Room Temperature). Directions for Use: See Package Insert. Rev. 11/05

Used with permission from American Regent, Inc.

Delmar/Cengage Learning

12. epinephrine 2 mg                                             _____

NDC 0517-1071-25
**EPINEPHRINE**
INJECTION, USP **1:1000** (1 mg/mL)

**1 mL** AMPULE
FOR SC AND IM USE. FOR IV AND IC USE AFTER DILUTION.
**Rx Only**
**CONTAINS NO SULFITES.**
**PRESERVATIVE FREE.**
Store at controlled room temperature up to 25°C (77°F) (See USP).   Rev. 1/04

**AMERICAN REGENT, INC.**
SHIRLEY, NY 11967

Used with permission from American Regent, Inc.

Delmar/Cengage Learning

13. Fentanyl® 125 mcg                                            _____

NDC 10019-033-72
**Fentanyl**
Citrate Injection, USP

**250 mcg/5 mL**
**50 mcg/mL (0.05 mg/mL)**
**10 x 5 mL** DOSETTE® Ampuls
**FOR INTRAVENOUS OR INTRAMUSCULAR USE**

*Baxter*
Mtd. for an affiliate of
**Baxter Healthcare Corporation**
Deerfield, IL 60015 USA
by: Elkins-Sinn, Inc., Cherry Hill, NJ 08003

℞ only

Each mL contains fentanyl citrate equivalent to 50 mcg (0.05 mg) fentanyl base in Water for Injection. pH 4.0-7.5; sodium hydroxide and/or hydrochloric acid added, if needed, for pH adjustment. Contains no preservative. **Usual Dosage:** See package insert for complete prescribing information.
**PROTECT FROM LIGHT:** Keep covered in carton until time of use.
**Store at controlled room temperature 15°-30°C (59°-86°F).**
To open ampuls, ignore color line; break at constriction.

DOSETTE® is a registered trademark of A.H. Robins Company

⊜SiLEDERLE™

460-120-00

Copyright Baxter International Inc.

Delmar/Cengage Learning

## Dosage Ordered                                                                          ## mL Needed

### 14. calcium gluconate 0.93 mEq

_____

### 15. Ceftriaxone 0.7 g

_____

### 16. heparin 500 units

_____

### 17. ondansetron 3 mg

_____

**Dosage Ordered**                                                          **mL Needed**

18.  epinephrine 0.5 mg                                        _____

NDC 0517-1071-25
**EPINEPHRINE**
INJECTION, USP **1:1000** (1 mg/mL)

**1 mL** AMPULE
FOR SC AND IM USE. FOR IV
AND IC USE AFTER DILUTION.
**Rx Only**
**CONTAINS NO SULFITES.
PRESERVATIVE FREE.**
Store at controlled room temperature
up to 25°C (77°F) (See USP).   Rev. 1/04
**AMERICAN REGENT, INC.**
SHIRLEY, NY 11967

Used with permission from American Regent, Inc.

19.  Ketorolac tromethamine 30 mg                      _____

Used with permission of Bedford Laboratories, A Division of Ben Venue Laboratories Inc. A Boehringer-Ingelheim Company

**KETOROLAC**
TROMETHAMINE
INJECTION USP

**15 mg/mL**
**1 mL Vial**

FOR IM OR IV USE ONLY

NDC 55390-480-01
1 mL Single-dose Vial
**Protect from light.**
**Rx ONLY**

Manufactured for:
Bedford Laboratories™
Bedford, OH 44146

KC-KRLV01

20.  gentamicin 60 mg                                           _____

Reprinted with permisson of APP Pharmaceuticals, LLC

NDC 63323-010-20    1020
**GENTAMICIN**
INJECTION, USP
equivalent to
**40 mg/mL**
Gentamicin        Rx only
**For IM or IV Use.**
**Must be diluted for IV use.**
**20 mL** Multiple Dose Vial

Sterile
Each mL contains: Gentamicin
sulfate equivalent to 40 mg gentamicin;
1.8 mg methylparaben and 0.2 mg
propylparaben as preservatives; 3.2 mg
sodium metabisulfite; 0.1 mg disodium
edetate; Water for Injection q.s. Sodium
hydroxide and/or sulfuric acid may
have been added for pH adjustment.
Usual Dosage: See insert.
**Warning:** Patients treated with
gentamicin sulfate and other
aminoglycosides should be under
close observation because of the
potential toxicity. See Warnings and
Precautions in the insert.
Store at 20° to 25°C (68° to 77°F)
[see USP Controlled Room Temperature].

**APP**
**APP Pharmaceuticals, LLC**
Schaumburg, IL 60173

401897D
LOT/EXP

3  63323-010-20  1

**Dosage Ordered**                                                                                           **mL Needed**

21.  lidocaine HCl 50 mg                                                            _____

NDC 10019-017-56

**Lidocaine** **1%**
HCl Injection, USP

**(10 mg/mL)**          ℞ only
FOR INFILTRATION AND NERVE BLOCK
NOT FOR SPINAL OR EPIDURAL ANESTHESIA
30 mL Multiple Dose Vial

**Baxter**        **℮Sī LEDERLE™**
Mfd. for **Baxter Healthcare Corporation** affiliate
by: Elkins-Sinn, Cherry Hill, NJ 08003      400-741-01

Copyright Baxter International Inc.

Each mL contains lidocaine hydrochloride 10 mg, sodium chloride 7 mg
and methylparaben 1 mg in Water for
Injection.  pH 5.0-7.0; sodium hydroxide and/or hydrochloric acid used,
if needed, for pH adjustment.
**Usual Dosage:** See package insert for
complete prescribing information.
Store at controlled room temperature
15°-30°C (59°-86°F).

Lot.:
Exp.:

22.  sodium chloride 40 mEq                                                         _____

NDC 0025-6589-82

**SODIUM CHLORIDE**
INJECTION, USP

**CONCENTRATED**
PHARMACY BULK PACKAGE–
Not for direct infusion

**23.4%  4 mEq/mL**
FOR IV USE ONLY
AFTER DILUTION

100 mL          Rx only

**SL  SIMULATED**
**LABEL**
For Educational Purposes Only

Delmar/Cengage Learning

**Preservative Free**
Each mL contains: sodium chloride 234 mg;
water for injection q.s. pH may have been
adjusted with hydrochloric acid.

8008 mOsmol/L  4,000 mEq/L
Directions for pharmacy bulk package: Swab
stopper with an antiseptic solution. Withdraw
contents of the vial using a sterile dispensing
set. If prompt fluid transfer is not possible, a
maximum time of 4 hours from the time of
initial entry is allowed to complete the
transferring operations. Discard the container
no later than 4 hours after initial closure.

Use only if solution is clear and seal intact.
Store at controlled room temperature 15° to
30°C (59° to 86°F). Do not freeze.

Lot.
Exp. Date

354588-23

23.  atropine 200 mcg                                                              _____

**Dosage Ordered**                                              **mL Needed**

24. meperidine 50 mg                                    _____

25. clindamycin 0.3 g                                    _____

26. morphine sulfate 15 mg                         _____

## Dosage Ordered

## mL Needed

27. acyclovir Na 150 mg _____

28. cisplatin 20 mg _____

29. sodium chloride 20 mEq _____

**Dosage Ordered**

**mL Needed**

30. meperidine 50 mg

31. furosemide 30 mg

32. gentamicin 60 mg

**Dosage Ordered**                                                **mL Needed**

33. meperidine 50 mg                                                  _____

34. dexamethasone 2 mg                                              _____

35. Vistaril® 50 mg                                                    _____

| **Dosage Ordered** | **mL Needed** |
|---|---|
| 36. fentanyl 0.05 mg | _____ |

37. morphine 15 mg _____

38. cyanocobalamin 1 mg _____

## Dosage Ordered

## mL Needed

39. ketorolac tromethamine 15 mg

_____

KETOROLAC
TROMETHAMINE
INJECTION USP

30 mg/mL
1 mL Vial

FOR IM OR IV USE ONLY

NDC 55390-481-01
1 mL Single-dose Vial
Protect from light.
Rx ONLY

Manufactured for:
Bedford Laboratories™
Bedford, OH 44146

KC-KRLVA02

Used with permission of Bedford Laboratories, A Division of Ben Venue Laboratories Inc. A Boehringer-Ingelheim Company

40. Robinul 200 mcg

_____

NDC 10019-016-81

**Robinul**
**Injectable**
(glycopyrrolate
injection, USP)

**0.2 mg/mL**
FOR IM OR IV USE
1 mL
Single Dose Vial
Mfd. for an affiliate of
**Baxter Healthcare Corp.**
by: A.H. Robins Co.
Richmond, VA 23220
400-938-01

Lot:

Exp.:

Used with permission of Baxter International Inc. Robinul is a trademark of Wyeth Pharmaceuticals Division of Wyeth

| Answers | | | | |
|---|---|---|---|---|
| | **9.** 10 mL | **18.** 0.5 mL | **27.** 3 mL | **36.** 1 mL |
| **1.** 0.5 mL | **10.** 1 mL | **19.** 2 mL | **28.** 20 mL | **37.** 1.5 mL |
| **2.** 1 mL | **11.** 0.5 mL | **20.** 1.5 mL | **29.** 5 mL | **38.** 1 mL |
| **3.** 0.5 mL | **12.** 2 mL | **21.** 5 mL | **30.** 2 mL | **39.** 0.5 mL |
| **4.** 2 mL | **13.** 2.5 mL | **22.** 10 mL | **31.** 3 mL | **40.** 1 mL |
| **5.** 2 mL | **14.** 2 mL | **23.** 2 mL | **32.** 1.5 mL | |
| **6.** 1 mL | **15.** 2 mL | **24.** 0.5 mL | **33.** 2 mL | |
| **7.** 0.5 mL | **16.** 0.5 mL | **25.** 2 mL | **34.** 0.5 mL | |
| **8.** 5 mL | **17.** 1.5 mL | **26.** 1 mL | **35.** 2 mL | |

# 10

# RECONSTITUTION OF POWDERED DRUGS

## Objectives

The learner will:

1. prepare solutions from powdered drugs using directions printed on vial labels.

2. prepare solutions from powdered drugs using drug literature or inserts.

3. determine the expiration date and time for reconstituted drugs.

4. calculate dosages for reconstituted drugs.

Many drugs are shipped in powdered form because they **retain their potency only a short time in solution**. Reconstitution of these drugs is often the responsibility of clinical pharmacies, but you will need to know how to read and follow reconstitution directions and how to label drugs with an expiration date and time once they have been reconstituted. The drug label, or instructional package insert, will give specific directions for reconstitution of the drug. Reading these requires care, and this chapter will take you step by step through the entire process.

### RECONSTITUTION OF A SINGLE STRENGTH SOLUTION

Let's start with the simplest type of reconstitution instructions, for a single strength solution. Examine the label for the Solu-Medrol® 500 mg vial in Figure 10-1.

Rx only

See package insert for complete product information. Store at controlled room temperature 20° to 25°C (68° to 77°F) [see USP]. Protect from light. Reconstitute with 8 mL Bacteriostatic Water for Injection with Benzyl Alcohol. **When reconstituted as directed each 8 mL contains:** Methylprednisolone sodium succinate equivalent to 500 mg methylprednisolone (62.5 mg per mL). Store solution at controlled room temperature 20° to 25°C (68° to 77°F) [see USP] and use within 48 hours after mixing. Lyophilized in container. Protect from light.
Reconstituted: _____

Pharmacia & Upjohn Co., Kalamazoo, MI 49001, USA

8123365909

NDC 0009-0758-01
4—125 mg doses

**Solu-Medrol®**
methylprednisolone sodium succinate for injection, USP

**500 mg***

For intramuscular or intravenous use
Diluent Contains Benzyl Alcohol as a Preservative

**Figure 10-1**

Reconstitution directions on vial labels may be small and difficult to read, and extreme care in reading them is essential.

The first step in reconstitution is to locate the directions. They are on the left side of this label.

Locate the **Reconstitute with 8 mL Bacteriostatic Water for injection with Benzyl Alcohol** instructions. Water, or any other solution specified for reconstitution, is called the **diluent**. The **type of diluent** specified will be **different for different drugs**. The **volume of diluent will also vary**. Therefore, reading the label carefully to identify both the type and the volume of diluent to be used is mandatory.

Once the type of diluent is identified, the next step is to use a **sterile syringe and aseptic technique** to draw up the 8 mL volume required. Inject it slowly into the vial **above the medication level, because air bubbles can distort drug dosages**. If the diluent volume is large, as in this case, be aware that **the syringe plunger will be forced out to expel air to reequalize the internal vial pressure as you inject**. Very large volumes of diluent will have to be injected in divided amounts to keep the internal vial pressure equalized. When all the diluent has been injected, the vial is rotated and upended until all the medication has been dissolved. **Do not shake** unless directed to do so, because this also can add air bubbles to some medications and distort dosages.

After reconstitution locate the information that relates to the **length of time the reconstituted solution may be stored**, and **how it must be stored**. Look again at the Solu-Medrol directions and locate this information. You will find that this solution can be stored at room temperature and that it must be used within 48 hours of reconstitution.

The next step is to **print your initials on the label as the person who reconstituted the drug**, in case any questions subsequently arise concerning the preparation. Next, **add the expiration date and time to the label**. Let's assume you reconstituted this Solu-Medrol solution at **2 pm on January 3**. What expiration (EXP) date and time will you print on the label? The reconstituted drug lasts only 48 hours at room temperature, so you would print **Exp. Jan. 5, 2 pm**, which is 48 hours (2 days) from the time you reconstituted it.

The person who reconstitutes a drug is responsible for labeling it with the date and time of expiration, and with his or her initials.

Next, identify the total dosage strength of this vial, which is **500 mg**. Near the top of the label, you can locate the individual dosage strength: **4–125 mg doses**. Because you have injected 8 mL of diluent, this will be approximately **2 mL for each 125 mg** dose, but if you read the small print on the label, you will see that the individual dosage is clearly identified as **62.5 mg per mL**.

**Reconstituted volumes do not always exactly equal the amount of diluent added**; in fact, most do not. This is because the medication itself has a volume, and it usually makes the total volume somewhat larger than the amount of diluent injected. Our next examples of a single-strength reconstitution will illustrate this increased volume concept.

If a 62.5 mg dosage is ordered, you will need 1 mL.

If a 125 mg dosage is needed, you will need 2 mL (125 mg = 62.5 mg × 2).

If a 250 mg dosage is needed, you will need 4 mL; and if 500 mg is ordered, the total is 8 mL.

Reconstituted volumes may exceed the volume of the diluent added, because the drug itself has a volume.

## Problems 10.1

Other drugs shipped in powdered form are antibiotics. Read the label in Figure 10-2 to answer the following questions about reconstituting this drug. All the information you need is printed sideways on the right of the label.

1. How should this drug be stored before reconstitution?   *← 85°*

2. How is this drug administered?   *IV | IM*

3. How long will this solution retain its potency at room temperature after reconstitution?   *2-8 hrs*

4. How long if refrigerated?   *24-72 hrs*

5. If you reconstitute this drug at 10:10 am on October 3 and it is refrigerated, what expiration time will you print on the label?   *Exp. 10:10 Oct 4*  *10:10 Oct 6*

6. What else will you print on the label?   *initials*

7. What is the total dosage of this reconstituted IV solution?   *1.5 g*

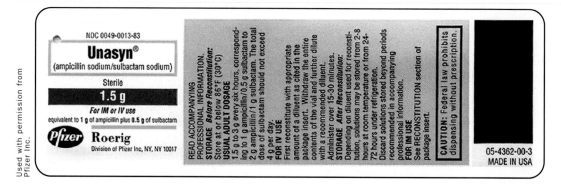

**Figure 10-2**

Used with permission from Pfizer Inc.

Answers  **1.** at or below 86°F (30°C)  **2.** IM or IV  **3.** 2–8 hours  **4.** 24–72 hours  **5.** Exp. Oct. 4 10:10 am to Oct. 6 10:10 am (your answer must include "Exp." to be correct)  **6.** Your initials  **7.** 1.5 g

## Problems 10.2

Refer to the penicillin V potassium oral suspension label in Figure 10-3 to answer the following questions.

1. How much diluent is needed to reconstitute this large-volume oral suspension preparation?   *75 ul*

2. What kind of diluent will you use?   *water*

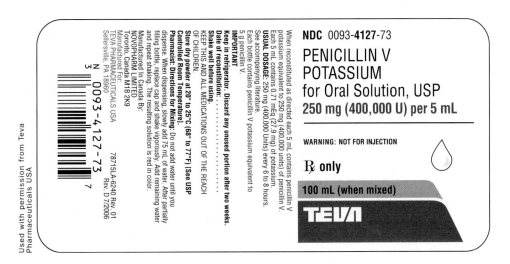

**Figure 10-3**

3. The label is specific about how to add this diluent. What does it tell you?

   *Add half, shake, add rest, shake again*

4. This is an oral suspension. Does the diluent need to be sterile?

   *No*

5. What is the mg dosage strength of the prepared solution?

   *250 mg/5 ml*

6. Determine the expiration date if you reconstitute this drug on March 15 at 4:40 pm.

   *March 29 4:40 pm*

7. How must the reconstituted solution be stored?

   *refrigerator*

8. If the dosage ordered is 125 mg, how many mL are needed?

   *2.5 ml*

9. For a 500 mg dosage, how many mL are needed?

   *10 ml*

10. How many units of medication will there be in a 5 mL dose?

    *400,000 units*

11. What should you do to this medication before administering it?

    *Check expiration, shake well.*

12. What must the person who reconstitutes the medication print on the label?

    *initials*

---

**Answers**  **1.** 75 mL  **2.** Water  **3.** Slowly add water, partially fill bottle and shake vigorously. Add remaning water and shake  **4.** No, this is an oral medication  **5.** 250 mg/5 mL  **6.** Exp. March 29 4:40 pm  **7.** In a refrigerator  **8.** 2.5 mL  **9.** 10 mL  **10.** 400,000 units  **11.** Shake well  **12.** Her initials

**Figure 10-4**

## Problems 10.3

**Refer to the Rocephin® label in Figure 10-4 to answer the following questions.**

1. What is the total dosage of this vial?  *500 mg*

2. How much diluent is used for IM reconstitution?  *1 mL*

3. What kind of diluent is specified for IM reconstitution?  *1% lidocaine hydro*

4. What dosage will 1 mL of IM reconstituted solution contain?  _____

5. What is the generic name of this drug?  _____

6. How many mL must be added for IV reconstitution?  _____

7. Where does it tell you to look for information on the kind of diluent to use for IV reconstitution?  _____

8. What dosage will 1 mL of reconstituted IV solution contain?  _____

9. Where will you find storage and expiration details?  _____

10. What will you print on the label in addition to the expiration date?  _____

**Answers  1.** 500 mg  **2.** 1 mL  **3.** 1% lidocaine hydrochloride injection or sterile water for injection  **4.** 350 mg  **5.** ceftriaxone  **6.** 4.8 mL  **7.** Package insert  **8.** 100 mg  **9.** Package insert  **10.** Your initials

## Problems 10.4

**Refer to the clindamycin label provided in Figure 10-5 to answer the following questions.**

1. What is the total dosage in this vial?  *9 gms*

2. Where will you locate reconstitution instructions?  _____

3. How long may the reconstituted solution be used?  _____

4. How much clindamycin will a 6 mL IV volume contain?  _____

5. How many mL will be needed for a 1500 mg IV dosage?  _____

6. What is the mL strength of the reconstituted solution?  _____

7. How is this drug administered?  _____

**Figure 10-5**

## Problems 10.5

Refer to the cytarabine label in Figure 10-6 to answer the following questions.

1. What is the total dosage strength of this vial? _____
2. How much diluent is required for reconstitution? _____
3. What will be the dosage strength per mL of the
   reconstituted solution? _____
4. What type of diluent is to be used? _____
5. How long can the reconstituted solution be retained? _____
6. How is this medication administered? _____

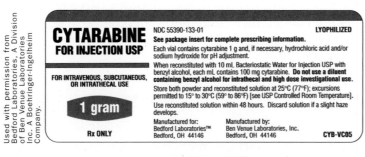

**Figure 10-6**

## Problems 10.6

Refer to the cytarabine label in Figure 10-7 to answer the following questions.

1. What is the total dosage strength of this vial? _____
2. How much diluent is required for reconstitution? _____
3. What will be the dosage per mL of the reconstituted
   solution? _____
4. What is the expiration time of the reconstituted solution? _____
5. What diluent must be used for subcutaneous injection? _____

**Figure 10-7**

**Answers** **1.** 500 mg **2.** 10 mL **3.** 50 mg per mL **4.** 48 hours **5.** Bacteriostatic water USP with benzyl alcohol

# RECONSTITUTION FROM PACKAGE INSERT DIRECTIONS

The package insert directions provided represent just a small portion of the information that drug package inserts contain. Additional information includes specific use of the drug for diagnosed conditions, such as bacterial meningitis, infections of the gastrointestinal or genitourinary tracts, and so forth; dosage recommendations if the vial label does not contain them; and untoward or adverse reactions, to name just a sample of the topics covered.

## Problems 10.7

Refer to the selected package insert information in Figure 10-8 to answer the following questions.

1. Identify the types of diluent that may be used for reconstitution under the section labeled **For Intramuscular Use**. _____

2. Look next at the four-column table for reconstitution, and notice that information is provided for the four different strengths of vials available: 250 mg, 500 mg, 1 g, and 2 g. What volume of diluent is specified for a 250 mg vial? _____

3. How much diluent is required for a 500 mg vial? _____

4. How much diluent is required for a 1 g vial? _____

5. How much diluent is required for a 2 g vial? _____

6. The mL dosage strength of all four reconstituted solutions is the same. What is it? _____

7. Refer to the information under **For Direct Intravenous Use**. How much diluent must be added to the 250 mg or 500 mg vials? _____

8. What stipulation is made for direct IV administration of the 250 mg and 500 mg reconstituted solution? _____

9. Locate the caution pertaining to rapid IV administration. _____

NDC 0025-6589-82

**AMPICILLIN**

*FOR INJECTION, USP*

Use ampicillin for injection to treat and/or prevent infections that are known to be caused by bacteria.

**DIRECTIONS:**
Use only freshly prepared solutions. Use intramuscular and intravenous injections within one hour of preparation.

*For Intramuscular Use*
Dissolve contents of a vial with the amount of sterile water for injection or bacteriostatic water for injection as outlined in the following table.

| Vial Amount | Amount of Diluent to be Added (mL) | Approximate Available Volume (mL) | Approximate Concentration (in mg/mL) |
|---|---|---|---|
| 250 mg | 0.9 | 1 | 250 |
| 500 mg | 1.7 | 2 | 250 |
| 1 g | 3.4 | 4 | 250 |
| 2 g | 6.8 | 8 | 250 |

Ampicillin for injection1g and 2 g vials are intended for intravenous use; however, intramuscular administration is permissible when 250 mg or 500 mg vials are unavailable. In these instances, dissolve in 3.4 or 6.8 mL sterile water for injection or bacteriostatic water for injection respectively. The resulting solution will provide a concentration of 250 mg per mL

*For Direct Intravenous Use*
Add 5 mL sterile water for injection or bacteriostatic water for injection to the 250 and 500 mg vials. Administer slowly over 3 to 5 minutes. Ampicillin for injection, 1 g or 2 g, may also be given by direct intravenous administration. Dissolve in 7.4 or 14.8 mL sterile water for injection or bacteriostatic water for injection, respectively.

Administer slowly over at least 10 to 15 minutes.

CAUTION: More rapid administration may result in convulsive seizures.

**SL SIMULATED LABEL** For Educational Purposes Only

Lot. Exp. Date   354588-23

Delmar/Cengage Learning

**Figure 10-8**

**Answers   1.** Sterile water for injection or bacteriostatic water for injection   **2.** 0.9 mL   **3.** 1.7 mL
**4.** 3.4 mL   **5.** 6.8 mL   **6.** 250 mg per 1 mL   **7.** 5 mL   **8.** Inject slowly over 3 to 5 minutes   **9.** Rapid administration may result in seizures

In this section, you were concentrating specifically on locating vial label and package insert directions for reconstitution of a single strength solution. And you quickly discovered that there is no standard way that this information is presented. But the information is all there somewhere; you must persist until you locate it.

The next section will introduce you to labels and package inserts that contain directions for preparation of multiple strength solutions.

## RECONSTITUTION OF MULTIPLE STRENGTH SOLUTIONS

Some powdered drugs offer a choice of dosage strengths. When this is the case, you must choose the strength most appropriate for the dosage ordered. For example, refer to the penicillin label in Figure 10-9. The dosage strengths that can be obtained are listed on the right.

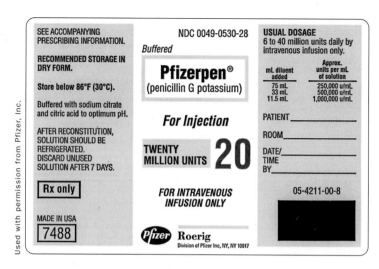

**Figure 10-9**

Notice that three dosage strengths are listed: 250,000 units, 500,000 units, and 1,000,000 units/mL. If the dosage ordered is 500,000 units, the most appropriate strength to mix would be 500,000 units/mL. Read across from this strength, and determine how much diluent must be added to obtain it. The answer is 33 mL. If the dosage ordered is 1,000,000 units, what would be the most appropriate strength to prepare, and how much diluent would this require? The answers are 1,000,000 units/mL and 11.5 mL.

 A multiple strength solution requires that you add one additional piece of information to the label after reconstitution: the dosage strength just mixed.

## Problems 10.8

**Refer to the Pfizerpen® label in Figure 10-9 to answer these additional questions.**

1. If you add 75 mL of diluent to prepare a solution of penicillin, what dosage strength will you print on the label?   _____

2. Does this prepared solution require refrigeration?   _____

3. If you reconstitute it on June 1 at 2 pm, what expiration time and date will you print on the label?   _____

4. What is the total dosage strength of this vial?   _____

5. What else do you print on the label besides the dosage strength just reconstituted?   _____

6. Where will you locate information on the diluent to be used?   _____

**Answers**   **1.** 250,000 units per mL   **2.** Yes   **3.** Exp. June 8 2 pm   **4.** 20 million units
**5.** Your initials   **6.** Package insert

The next problems consist of two simulated vial labels with solution strengths of 500 mg and 1 g and a package insert that gives the directions for their reconstitution.

## Problems 10.9

Refer to the Antibiotic for Intravenous Use labels and insert in Figures 10-10, 10-11, and 10-12. Use both the insert and label information to answer the following questions.

1. How much diluent must be used to reconstitute a 500 mg vial?    _____

2. How much diluent will be needed for a 1 g vial?    _____

3. What kind of diluent is specified?    _____

4. What is the reconstituted dosage per mL of both of these solutions?    _____

5. How long can the solution be used if stored in a refrigerator?    _____

6. If the drug is reconstituted on May 4 at 1350, what expiration date and time will you print on the label?    _____

7. What else must you print on the label?    _____

**Figure 10-10**

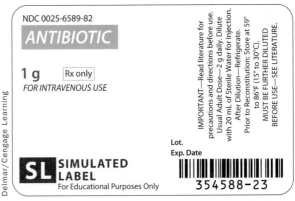

**Figure 10-11**

PREPARATION AND STABILITY
At the time of use, reconstitute by adding either 10 mL of Sterile Water for Injection to the 500-mg vial or 20 mL of Sterile Water for Injection to the 1-g vial of dry, sterile powder. Vials reconstituted in this manner will give a solution of 50 mg/mL. FURTHER DILUTION IS REQUIRED.
After reconstition, the vials may be stored in a refrigerator for 14 days without significant loss of potency. Reconstituted solutions containing 500 mg must be diluted with at least 100 mL of diluent. Reconstituted solutions containing 1g must be diluted with at least 200 mL of diluent, The desired dose, diluted in this manner, should be administered by intermittent intravenous infusion over a period of at least 60 minutes.

**Figure 10-12**

**Answers  1.** 10 mL  **2.** 20 mL  **3.** Sterile water for injection  **4.** 50 mg per mL  **5.** 14 days
**6.** Exp. May 18 1350  **7.** Your initials

## Summary

This concludes the chapter on the reconstitution of powdered drugs. The important points to remember from this chapter are:

- If the medication label does not contain reconstitution directions, these may be located on the medication package insert.

The type and amount of diluent to be used for reconstitution must be exactly as specified in the reconstitution instructions.

If directions are given for both IM and IV reconstitution, be careful to read the correct set for the solution you are preparing.

The person who reconstitutes a drug must initial the vial and print the expiration time and date on the label, unless all the drug is used immediately.

If a solution is prepared using multiple strength medication directions, the strength reconstituted must also be printed on the label.

## Summary Self-Test

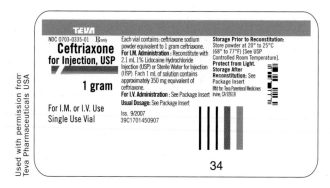

**Figure 10-13**

Refer to the ceftriaxone label in Figure 10-13 to answer the following questions about reconstitution.

1. What is the total dosage of this vial?    _____

2. What volume of diluent must be used for reconstitution?    _____

3. What will be the dosage strength of 1 mL of reconstituted solution?    _____

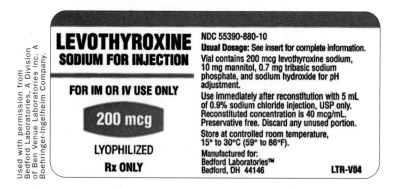

**Figure 10-14**

Refer to the levothyroxine sodium label in Figure 10-14 to answer the following questions.

4. What is the dosage strength of this vial in mcg? In mg?    _____ _____

5. What volume of diluent must you add to prepare the solution for use?    _____

6. What kind of diluent must be used?    _____

7. How long will this reconstituted solution retain its potency?  _____

8. What is the per mL strength of the reconstituted solution?  _____

9. Where will you find average dosage instructions?  _____

**Figure 10-15**

**Refer to the cytarabine label in Figure 10-15 to answer the following questions.**

10. How much diluent is used to reconstitute this solution?  _____

11. What type of diluent?  _____

12. What is the total vial dosage?  _____

13. At what temperature should this medication be stored?  _____

14. What dosage will each 1 mL contain?  _____

15. What is the expiration time of the reconstituted solution?  _____

16. If the solution is reconstituted on Feb 14 at 0840, what expiration date must be printed on the label?  _____

**Figure 10-16**

**Refer to the VFend® I.V. label in Figure 10-16 to answer the following questions.**

17. How much diluent is required to reconstitute this Vfend I.V. solution?  _____

18. What diluent is specified for use?  _____

19. What is the strength of each 1 mL of the reconstituted solution?  _____

20. What is the total dosage of this vial?  _____

**Figure 10-17**

**Refer to the Vantin® Oral Suspension label in Figure 10-17 to answer the following questions.**

21. How much diluent will be required to reconstitute this medication?    _____

22. What type of diluent is listed for reconstitution?    _____

23. How is this diluent to be added?    _____

24. What is the reconstituted dosage strength?    _____

25. How long will the reconstituted Vantin solution retain its potency?    _____

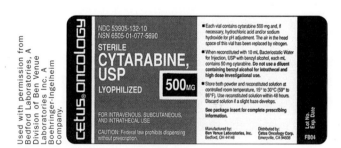

**Figure 10-18**

**Refer to the cytarabine label in Figure 10-18 to answer the following questions.**

26. What is the total strength of this medication?    _____

27. What diluent must be used for reconstitution?    _____

28. How much?    _____

29. What is the dosage per reconstituted mL?    _____

30. How long does the reconstituted cytarabine solution retain its
    potency at room temperature?    _____

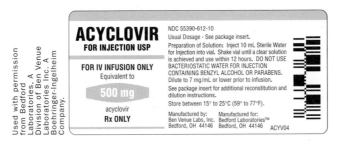

**Figure 10-19**

## Refer to the acyclovir label in Figure 10-19 to answer the following questions for reconstitution.

31. What type of diluent is recommended for reconstitution?   _____

32. How much diluent must be added?   _____

33. What is the total dosage strength of this vial?   _____

34. How soon must this solution be used?   _____

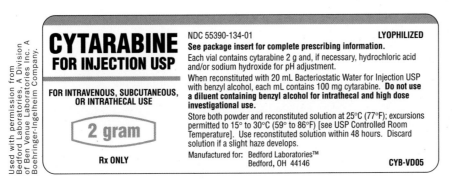

**Figure 10-20**

## Refer to the cytarabine label in Figure 10-20 and answer the following questions.

35. What is the total dosage strength of this vial?   _____

36. What volume of diluent must be added?   _____

37. What kind of diluent must be used?   _____

38. What is the reconstituted dosage strength per mL?   _____

39. How long will this medication retain its potency?   _____

**Figure 10-21**

**Refer to the penicillin G potassium label in Figure 10-21 to answer the following questions.**

40. What is the total dosage strength of this vial?  _____

41. How much diluent must be added to prepare a 100,000 units/mL strength?  _____

42. How much diluent must be added to prepare a 500,000 units/mL strength?  _____

43. How much diluent must be added to prepare a 50,000 units/mL strength?  _____

44. This label has no information on the type of diluent to use. Where will you find this?  _____

45. How must this solution be stored?  _____

46. If reconstituted at 1:10 am on December 18, what must you print on the label?  _____

47. What else must you print on the label?  _____

48. Why print?  _____

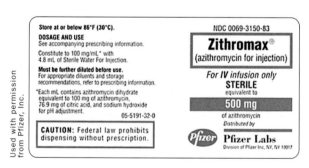

**Figure 10-22**

**Refer to the Zithromax® label in Figure 10-22 to answer the following questions.**

49. What is the generic name for Zithromax?  _____

50. What is the dosage strength of this vial?  _____

51. What diluent is specified for reconstitution?  _____

52. How much diluent is required?  _____

53. What is the reconstituted dosage strength?  _____

**Answer**

1. 1 g
2. 2.1 mL
3. 350 mg/mL
4. 200 mcg; 0.2 mg
5. 5 mL
6. 0.9% sodium chloride
7. must be used immediately
8. 40 mcg/mL
9. package insert
10. 10 mL
11. Bacteriostatic Water for Injection with Benzyl Alcohol
12. 1 gram
13. 25°C (77°F)
14. 100 mg per mL
15. 48 hours
16. Exp. Feb. 16 0840
17. 19 mL
18. Water for Injection
19. 10 mg/mL
20. 200 mg
21. 29 mL
22. Distilled Water
23. Shake the bottle to loosen granules, add half (15 mL) of the distilled water, and shake vigorously to dissolve granules; add balance of water and shake vigorously
24. 100 mg/ 5 mL
25. 14 days
26. 500 mg
27. Bacteriostatic Water with Benzyl Alcohol
28. 10 mL
29. 50 mg per mL
30. 48 hours
31. Sterile Water for Injection
32. 10 mL
33. 500 mg
34. Within 12 hours
35. 2 g
36. 20 mL
37. Bacteriostatic Water for Injection USP with Benzyl Alcohol
38. 100 mg/mL
39. 48 hours
40. One million units
41. 10 mL
42. 1.8 mL
43. 20 mL
44. Package insert
45. Refrigerate
46. Exp. 1:10 am Dec. 25
47. Your initials
48. Space considerations; handwriting is difficult to read
49. azithromycin
50. 500 mg
51. Sterile Water for Injection
52. 4.8 mL
53. 100 mg per mL

## Objectives

**The learner will:**

1. identify insulins in current use.

2. discuss the difference between rapid-, short-, intermediate-, and long-acting insulins.

3. read insulin labels to identify type.

4. read calibrations on 100 units/mL insulin syringes.

5. measure single insulin dosages.

6. measure combined insulin dosages.

# MEASURING INSULIN DOSAGES

Diabetes is one of the fastest-growing health problems in both the United States and Canada, and since the advent of DNA technology in the 1980s, the number of insulin products has almost quadrupled in an effort to keep pace with treatment needs.

This chapter will introduce you to the current insulin preparations available; provide real insulin vial labels to familiarize you with the different insulins; describe the physical appearance of insulins; explain insulin action times in relation to dietary intake; instruct you in the use of specialized insulin syringes; and provide a step-by-step procedure for the combination of Regular and N (NPH) insulin in a single syringe, a skill you may use on an ongoing basis throughout your career.

## TYPES OF INSULIN

Prior to the 1980s, all insulin was produced from animal sources. Today, **all are products of DNA**. The two earliest DNA insulins, **R (Regular)** and **N (NPH)\*** are made from **recombinant DNA** (cut and spliced DNA fragments). Both of these insulins incorporate the "**lin**" of the word insu**lin** in their trade names: Humu**lin**® **R** and Humu**lin**® **N** manufactured by the Eli Lilly Co., and Novo**lin**® **R** and Novo**lin**® **N** from Novo Nordisk. **Regular** insulin is a **clear** solution, and it is **fast acting**, while **N** is **cloudy**, classified as **intermediate acting**, and has a **slower start but longer action**. Regular and N insulin can safely be and often are **combined in a single syringe** to reduce the number of injections an individual must have. They may be combined at first to determine an individual's R and NPH insulin requirements, then ordered in **actual combined insulin preparations**, such as the Humulin and Novolin **70/30** and **50/50** mixes, to provide both a fast and more prolonged action.

Another type of DNA preparation is the **analogs**, which are **chemically altered DNA**. Depending on their structure, the analogs offer an extremely rapid action, or a longer and more balanced control of blood glucose levels. Once again, some of the trade names of these products reflect their

---

*Note: The N intermediate action insulin takes its "N" designation from NPH, the first intermediate action insulin developed in the mid 1930s. The NPH initials represent *neutral protamine Hagedorn,* the chemical structure and name of the developer of NPH, Hans Hagedorn.

origin: the **"log"** of ana**log** is incorporated in two of the frequently used trade-named insulins: Huma**log**® and Novo**log**®. Among the analogs whose trade names do not identify their analog structure are Apidra® (glulisine), Lantis® (glargine), and Levemir® (detemir).

 The -lin ending of regular and N insulin trade names can be used as an additional safeguard in distinguishing them from several of the analogs, which incorporate -log at the end of their trade names.

Unfortunately, most insulin **vials, solutions, and labels look very much alike**, and it is here where the first precaution in insulin preparation must be stressed.

## INSULIN LABEL IDENTIFICATION

Like other medications, insulin preparations have both trade and generic names. Eli Lilly and Novo Nordisk are the major insulin manufacturers; however, there are now other manufacturers producing and marketing insulin. In the insulin label identification problems that follow, you will be asked to identify insulin manufacturers, as well as insulin types and dosages. Some of the labels included are from **insulin pen** preparations: **prefilled, self-injection syringes** that contain **multiple doses** of insulin. To see an excellent demonstration of insulin pen use, go to http://www.levemir-us.com.

### Problems 11.1

Refer to the insulin labels provided to answer the specific questions pertaining to each.

1. What does the R on the label in Figure 11-1 identify?    _____
2. What is the dosage strength of this insulin?    _____
3. What part of the trade name aids in identifying this preparation?    _____

© Novo Nordisk Inc.
Reprinted with permission.
® Novolin is a registered trademark of Novo Nordisk Inc.

Exp. Date/Control:

U-100    NDC 0169-1833-11
10 mL    100 units/mL
*Novolin*® **R**
Regular, Human Insulin Injection (recombinant DNA origin) USP

*Novo Nordisk*®
• Important: see insert
• Keep in a cold place
• Avoid freezing
Novo Nordisk Inc.
Princeton, NJ 08540
1-800-727-6500
Manufactured by
Novo Nordisk A/S
DK-2880 Bagsvaerd
Denmark

**Figure 11-1**

4. Who is the manufacturer of the insulin in Figure 11-2? _____

5. What kind of insulin is this? _____

6. What dosage strength does this insulin have? _____

**Figure 11-2**

7. What does the 70/30 on the label in Figure 11-3 represent? _____

8. What company manufactured this insulin? _____

9. What is the dosage strength of this insulin? _____

**Figure 11-3**

10. What does the 50/50 on the label in Figure 11-4 represent? _____

**Figure 11-4**

11. What is the total volume of the insulin vial in Figure 11-5?      _____

12. What is the dosage strength of this insulin?      _____

13. What is the generic name of this preparation?      _____

14. What does the "log" in this trade name identify?      _____

**Figure 11-5**

15. What is the generic name of the insulin preparation in Figure 11-6?      _____

16. What is the dosage strength?      _____

17. What volume of insulin does this pen contain?      _____

**Figure 11-6**

18. How is the 70% insulin in Figure 11-7 described?      _____

19. What does the 30% represent?      _____

20. What actions does a combined insulin provide?      _____

**Figure 11-7**

21 What is the generic name of the insulin in Figure 11-8? _____

22. What exactly does the 50/50 identify? _____

**Figure 11-8**

23. What is the generic name of the insulin in Figure 11-9? _____

**Figure 11-9**

24. What is the generic name of the insulin in Figure 11-10? _____

25. What is the trade name of this insulin? _____

26. What is the dosage strength of this preparation? _____

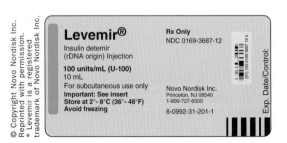

**Figure 11-10**

27. What is the trade name of the insulin in Figure 11-11?   _____

28. What is the generic name?   _____

29. Who manufactures this insulin?   _____

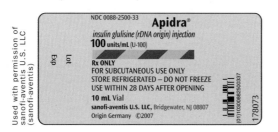

**Figure 11-11**

30. What does the R on the label in Figure 11-12 identify?   _____

31. Is this a short- or long-action insulin?   _____

32. What is the total volume of this vial?   _____

33. What is the dosage strength of this insulin?   _____

**Figure 11-12**

34. What is the generic name of the insulin in the combination preparation in Figure 11-13?   _____

**Figure 11-13**

35. What does the lin in the trade name in Figure 11-14 identify? _____

36. What insulin does the 30% identify? _____

**Figure 11-14**

37. What is the trade name of the insulin label in Figure 11-15? _____

38. What is its generic name? _____

39. What is its dosage strength? _____

40. Who manufactures this insulin? _____

**Figure 11-15**

Diligence in the identification of insulin preparations is critical, as many vials, solutions, and their labels are strikingly similar.

## INSULIN ACTION TIMES

As equally important as insulin type and dosage is **the timing of insulin adminis-tration,** based on **onset of action, peak and duration, and relationship to dietary intake**.

Insulin is classified by action as **rapid, short, intermediate, or long acting**. Refer to the Joslin Diabetes Center chart in Figure 11-16. This provides a summary of all the insulins in current use by action, generic and trade names, onset and peak of action, and duration.

**Pharmacokinetics of Current Insulin Preparations**

| Insulin Type | Product | Onset | Peak | Duration |
|---|---|---|---|---|
| **Rapid-Acting** | | | | |
| Insulin aspart analog | NovoLog | | | |
| Insulin glulisine analog | Apidra | 10 – 30 minutes | 0.5 – 3 hours | 3 – 5 hours |
| Insulin lispro analog | Humalog | | | |
| | | | | |
| **Short-Acting** | | | | |
| Regular insulin | Humulin R | 30 minutes | 1 – 5 hours | 8 hours |
| | Novolin R | | | |
| **Intermediate-Acting** | | | | |
| NPH insulin | Humulin N | 1 – 4 hours | 4 – 12 hours | 14 – 26 hours |
| | Novolin N | | | |
| **Long-Acting ("Basal" – like)** | | | | |
| Insulin detemir | Levemir | 1 – 2 hours | Minimal peak | Up to 24 hours |
| Insulin glargine | Lantus | | | |
| **Premixed Insulin Combinations** | | | | |
| 50% Human Insulin Isophane Suspension (NPH); 50% Regular | | Humulin 50/50 | | |
| 70% Human Insulin Isophane Suspension (NPH); 30% Regular | | Humulin 70/30 | | |
| 70% Human Insulin Isophane Suspension (NPH); 30% Regular | | Novolin 70/30 | | |
| 50% lispro protamine suspension (NPL); 50% lispro | | Humalog Mix 50/50 | | |
| 75% lispro protamine suspension (NPL); 25% lispro | | Humalog Mix 75/25 | | |
| 70% insulin aspart protamine suspension (intermediate) ; 30% aspart | | NovoLog Mix 70/30 | | |

**Figure 11-16**

The **rapid-acting** insulins aspart, glulisine, and lispro, whose onset of action varies from 10 to 30 minutes, **must be followed immediately by a meal**. Failure to imme-diately ingest food would result in a rapidly lowered blood glucose level and **insulin reaction from hypoglycemia**. Also note that these rapid-acting insulins have a peak and duration of from 0.5 to 5 hours. Their action is relatively short.

Next, compare the **short-acting, regular** insulins, Humulin® R and Novolin® R, which have an onset of 30 minutes, a peak of 1–5 hours, and a duration of 8 hours. These also require that the individual **eat shortly after administration**.

 Rapid- and short-acting insulin must be followed immediately by a meal.

The **intermediate-acting** Humulin® N and Novolin® N isophane suspension insulins are moving into the longer action range, with an onset of 1–4 hours, a peak of 4–12 hours, and duration of 14–26 hours. And, finally, the **long-acting** detemir (Levemir®) and glargine (Lantus®) insulins have an onset of 1–2 hours but a sustained minimal peak of up to 24 hours. Their administration is not related to dietary intake. Insulin detemir may be administered once or twice a day, while glargine is administered at night.

> Long-acting insulins are not administered in relation to immediate food ingestion.

The number of diabetic products will continue to increase because of the rapidly rising incidence of Type 2 diabetes. An inhalation insulin, Exubera®, is now available, and two additional new drugs are now in increasing use: Byetta® and Symlin®. Both of the latter act to change the body's response to food, either by promoting insulin secretion, delaying gastric emptying, and/or altering glucose metabolism.

## INSULIN SYRINGES

Think back for a moment to the insulin labels you have just read, and you will recall that all have a dosage strength of **100 units per mL**. You may have also noticed that these vials are additionally labeled **U-100**, which similarly identifies the 100 units per mL strength.

Insulin is administered using special **insulin syringes calibrated in units**. In diameter, these are quite like the smaller TB syringes, but the calibrations are totally different. Insulin syringes are used **only for insulin administration**, and they are available in the **100 unit, 50 unit, and 30 unit sizes** in Figure 11-17. The smaller 30 and 50 unit syringe calibrations are larger, and they provide an added degree of safety in measurement of small dosages.

Because of their small diameter, insulin syringe calibrations and numbering wrap around the small syringe barrel. Refer to the insulin syringes in Figure 11-17 again, and notice the calibrations there. For accurate measurement, you will learn **to rotate insulin syringes side to side to locate the calibration you need and to draw up the insulin dosage ordered**. To make your instruction in measuring insulin dosages easier,

**Figure 11-17a, b and c** | Insulin syringes  **a** 30 unit; **b** 50 unit; **c** 100 unit.

the syringe manufacturers have provided the actual art (the calibrations) they use on their insulin syringes. You will be using these "flattened out" calibrations next for your initial instruction in preparing insulin dosages.

The calibrations for the 50 unit dosage syringes are used in the first problems that follow. Notice that the **first long calibration**, as on all other syringes, identifies **zero** and that **each subsequent calibration measures 1 unit. Each 5 unit calibration is numbered: 5, 10, 15, 20, and so forth.**

## Problems 11.2

Refer to the syringe calibrations for the 50 unit calibrated syringes provided to identify the dosages indicated by the shaded areas and arrows.

1. _____

2. _____

3. _____

**Answers   1.** 11 units   **2.** 15 units   **3.** 22 units

## Problems 11.3

Use the 50 unit calibrations provided to shade in the following dosages. Have your instructor check your accuracy.

1. 33 units

2. 38 units

3. 18 units

**Answers**   Have your instructor check your accuracy.

There are two 100 unit insulin syringes in common use. Refer to the first of these syringe calibrations in Problems 11.4. First, notice the 100 unit capacity and that, in contrast to the smaller dose syringes, only **each 10 unit increment is numbered: 10, 20, 30, and so forth**. Next, notice the number of calibrations in each 10 unit increment, which is 5, indicating that **this syringe is calibrated in 2 unit increments. Odd-numbered units cannot be measured accurately using this syringe.**

## Problems 11.4

Identify the dosages indicated by the shading and arrows on the 100 unit syringes provided.

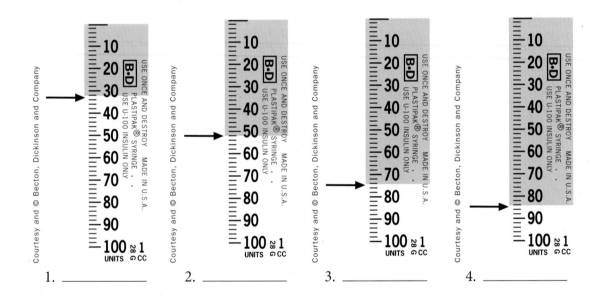

1. _____     2. _____     3. _____     4. _____

**Answers   1.** 32 units   **2.** 52 units   **3.** 74 units   **4.** 84 units

## Problems 11.5

Shade in the syringe calibrations provided to measure the dosages indicated. Have your instructor check your accuracy.

1. 66 units    2. 84 units    3. 28 units    4. 44 units

**Answers**   Have your instructor check your accuracy.

The second type of 100 unit syringe calibration is illustrated in Figure 11-18. Notice that this syringe has a **double scale: the odd numbers are on the left, and the even are on the right**. Each 5 unit increment is numbered, but on **opposite sides** of the syringe. This syringe does have a calibration for each 1 unit increment, but in order to count every calibration to measure a dosage, the syringe would have to be rotated back and forth. This could cause confusion. There is a safer way to read the calibrations. **To measure uneven numbered dosages**—for example, 7, 13, 27, and so forth—**use the uneven (left) scale only; for even-numbered dosages**—such as 6, 10, 56, and so forth—**use the even (right) scale only. Count each calibration (on one side only) as 2 units, because that is what it is measuring.**

**Figure 11-18**

### EXAMPLE 1

To prepare an 89 unit dosage, start at 85 units on the uneven left scale, count the first calibration above this as 87 units and the next as 89 units (**each calibration on the same side measures 2 units**).

### EXAMPLE 2

To measure a 26 unit dosage, use the even-numbered right side calibrations. Start at 20 units, move up one calibration to 22 units, another to 24 units, and one more to 26 units (**each calibration is 2 units**).

## Problems 11.6

Identify the dosages measured on the 100 unit syringe calibrations provided.

1. _____    2. _____    3. _____

**Answers**   **1.** 66 units   **2.** 41 units   **3.** 79 units

## Problems 11.7

Shade in the syringe calibrations provided to identify the following dosages.

1. 55 units                2. 94 units                3. 69 units

**Answers**   Have your instructor check your accuracy.

## COMBINING INSULIN DOSAGES

Insulin-dependent individuals may have one or even several subcutaneous injections of insulin per day. In order to reduce the number of injections as much as possible, it is common to combine two insulins in a single syringe: a short-acting Regular with an intermediate-acting NPH insulin.

 When two insulins are combined in the same syringe, the clear Regular (shortest acting) insulin is drawn up first.

Both insulins will be withdrawn from sealed 10 mL vials. This requires that an amount of air equal to the insulin to be withdrawn be injected into each vial as a preliminary step, to **keep the pressure inside the vials equalized after the insulin is withdrawn**. An additional step concerns preparation of the insulin itself. Regular clear insulin does not need to be mixed, but **N (NPH) is cloudy and precipitates out**. It must be **gently rotated to mix immediately before withdrawal**.

The smallest volume insulin syringe available is used to measure the dosages you need, as their larger calibrations provide additional ease and safety in reading. Examples of the actual step-by-step combination procedure follow.

**EXAMPLE 1**

The order is for a dosage of 10 units of Regular and 48 units of NPH.

**STEP 1**    Locate the correct R and NPH insulin and use an alcohol wipe to cleanse both vial tops.

**STEP 2**    The combined dosage, 10 units of Regular and 48 of NPH, is 58 units. This requires the use of a 100 unit syringe.

**STEP 3**    Draw up 48 units of replacement air for the NPH in the syringe, and insert the needle tip into the NPH vial. Keep the needle tip above the insulin level so as to not inject air into the insulin and possibly distort the dosage. Inject the air and remove the needle.

**STEP 4**    Draw up 10 units of replacement air for the Regular insulin vial. Insert the needle into the vial, again above the insulin level, and inject the air. Draw up the 10 units of Regular insulin.

**STEP 5**    Pick up and gently rotate the NPH vial until the insulin is mixed. Insert the needle back into the vial and draw up the 48 units of NPH.

**STEP 6**    Administer the insulin dosage at once so that the NPH has no chance to precipitate out. Chart the administration.

EXAMPLE 2

A dosage of 16 units Regular and 22 units of NPH has been ordered.

STEP 1    **Locate the correct Regular and NPH insulin and use an alcohol wipe to cleanse both vial tops.**

STEP 2    **The combined dosage, 16 units of Regular and 22 of NPH, totals 38 units. For this administration, you can use a 50 unit volume syringe.**

STEP 3    **Draw up 22 units of replacement air for the NPH in the syringe. Insert the needle tip into the NPH vial. Keep the needle tip above the insulin level so as to not inject air into the insulin and possibly distort the dosage. Inject the air and remove the needle.**

STEP 4    **Draw up 16 units of replacement air for the Regular insulin vial. Insert the needle into the vial, again above the insulin level, and inject the air. Draw up the 16 units of Regular insulin.**

STEP 5    **Pick up and gently rotate the NPH vial until the insulin is mixed. Insert the needle and draw up the 22 units of NPH.**

STEP 6    **Administer the insulin at once so that the NPH has no chance to precipitate out. Chart the administration.**

## INSULIN INJECTION SITES AND TECHNIQUES

Insulin is injected subcutaneously. As with other parenteral medications, the **injection sites must be rotated**, keeping **at least an inch away from each previously used site**. The abdomen has the most rapid absorption, followed by the upper arm. The outer thigh, a full hand's breadth above the knee and below the hip, may be used, but absorption is somewhat slower at this site. Your responsibility is, and will continue to be, to give the correct insulin and dosage at the correct time, taking special care to assure that a meal immediately follows rapid and short-acting insulin injection.

### Problems 11.8

For each of the following combined Regular and NPH insulin dosages, indicate the total volume of the combined dosage and the smallest capacity syringe you can use to prepare it; 30, 50, and 100 unit capacity syringes are available.

|  | Total Volume | Syringe Size |
|---|---|---|
| 1. 28 units Regular, 64 units NPH | _____ | _____ |
| 2. 16 units NPH, 6 units Regular | _____ | _____ |
| 3. 33 units Regular, 41 units NPH | _____ | _____ |
| 4. 21 units Regular, 52 units NPH | _____ | _____ |
| 5. 13 units Regular, 27 units NPH | _____ | _____ |

**Answers**   **1.** 92 units; 100 unit   **2.** 22 units; 30 unit   **3.** 74 units; 100 unit   **4.** 73 units; 100 unit   **5.** 40 units; 50 unit

## Summary

**This concludes the chapter on insulin dosages. The important points to remember from this chapter are:**

- Insulin labels must be read with extreme care because they look very similar.

- Insulin is measured using specially calibrated insulin syringes.

- Insulin syringes are available in 100, 50, and 30 unit capacities.

- The smaller 30 or 50 unit capacity syringes provide a greater degree of safety because of their larger calibrations.

- Each calibration on 30 and 50 unit volume syringes measures 1 unit.

- Calibrations on 100 unit capacity insulin syringes may measure 1 or 2 unit increments, depending on their design.

- The "lin" in the trade names of Regular and N (NPH) insulin identifies their recombinant DNA origin.

- The "log" in several of the analog insulins identifies their chemically altered DNA structure.

- Regular (R) and N (NPH) insulin can be mixed in a single syringe.

- Regular insulin is drawn up first in combination R and N dosages.

- N insulins are cloudy because they contain insoluble particles.

- Because N insulins precipitate out, they must be gently and thoroughly mixed before withdrawal and injected immediately after preparation.

- Insulin is administered subcutaneously.

- The abdomen and upper arm provide the most rapid subcutaneous absorption sites.

- Insulin injection sites are routinely rotated.

## Summary Self-Test

**Use the syringe calibrations provided to measure the following dosages. For combined insulin dosages, use arrows to indicate the exact calibration to be used for each insulin ordered. Have your instructor check your answers.**

1. 37 units Regular

2. 17 units Regular
   12 units NPH

3. 48 units NPH

4. 14 units Regular
58 units NPH

5. 12 units NPH

6. 18 units Regular
8 units NPH

7. 23 units Regular
14 units NPH

8. 8 units Regular
20 units NPH

9. 24 units Regular

10. 57 units NPH

11. 22 units Regular

12. 14 units Regular
44 units NPH

13. 24 units Regular
    27 units NPH

14. 33 units Regular
    10 units NPH

15. 56 units Regular

**Identify the dosages measured on the following syringes.**

16. _____

17. _____

18. _____

19. _____

20. _____

21. _____

22. _____

23. _____

24. _____

25. _____

26. _____

27. _____

28. _____

29. _____

30. _____

**Answers**

| | | | |
|---|---|---|---|
| **1–15.** See instructor | **19.** 73 units | **24.** 76 units | **29.** 43 units |
| **16.** 67 units | **20.** 32 units | **25.** 92 units | **30.** 82 units |
| **17.** 43 units | **21.** 60 units | **26.** 14 units | |
| **18.** 54 units | **22.** 52 units | **27.** 58 units | |
| | **23.** 8 units | **28.** 85 units | |

SECTION 4

# Dosage Calculations

CHAPTER 12
Dimensional Analysis /
Units Conversion / 160

# DIMENSIONAL ANALYSIS/UNITS CONVERSION

## Objectives

The learner will:

1. use dimensional analysis to calculate dosages.

## Prerequisites

Chapters 1–10

You may already be familiar with dimensional analysis (DA) under its official name: **units conversion**, which is used in chemistry, physics, and other scientific calculations. DA was first introduced for clinical dosage calculations in the 1950s using the name dimensional analysis, but it has acquired several other names along the way: the label factor and factor label methods being two.

DA is actually ratio and proportion made simple. Its great virtue is that **it reduces multiple-step calculations to a single equation**. However, to understand the simplicity of DA, it is necessary to look at clinical ratios from a different perspective.

## CLINICAL RATIOS

Clinical ratios provide the components for **all** the calculations you have already learned and will be learning in the remainder of this text. Some examples of ratios you are already familiar with from previous chapters include the following:

> **oral dosages:** 1 tab = 250 mg; 5 mL = 125 mg
> **IM and subcutaneous dosages:** 2 g = 1.5 mL;
>     1 mL = 10 units; 10 mL = 20 mEq
> **metric conversions:** 1000 mcg = 1 mg; 1 g = 1000 mg

In addition, you will be using the following ratios, although it isn't necessary for you to memorize them at this time.

> **IV flow rates:** 80 gtt per min; 100 mL per hr
> **IV set calibrations:** 10 gtt per mL; 15 gtt per mL; 60 gtt per mL
> **time conversions:** 60 min = 1 hr; 1 hr = 60 min

In DA, ratios are written as common fractions.

$$\frac{1 \text{ tab}}{250 \text{ mg}} \qquad \frac{5 \text{ mL}}{125 \text{ mg}} \qquad \frac{2 \text{ g}}{1.5 \text{ mL}}$$

$$\frac{1 \text{ mL}}{10 \text{ units}} \qquad \frac{10 \text{ mL}}{20 \text{ mEq}} \qquad \frac{1000 \text{ mcg}}{1 \text{ mg}}$$

## THE BASIC DA EQUATION

The first step in setting up a DA equation is to **write the unit of measure being calculated**. One commonly calculated measure is mL, so let's begin by using an mL calculation to illustrate the steps involved. Notice that color is used in the first DA examples to help you learn the sequence of ratio entry.

**EXAMPLE 1**     The available dosage strength is **750 mg in 2.5 mL**. How many mL will be needed to prepare a **600 mg** dosage?

Write the mL unit of measure being calculated, followed by an equal sign.

$$\text{mL} =$$

There are two important reasons for identifying the unit of measure being calculated first: it eliminates any confusion over exactly **which** measure is being calculated, and it dictates how the first or "starting" clinical ratio is entered in the equation.

In a DA equation, the unit of measure being calculated is written first, followed by an equal sign.

Next, go back to the problem to **identify the complete clinical ratio that contains mL**. This is provided by the **dosage strength available**, which is **750 mg in 2.5 mL**. Enter this as a common fraction so that **the 2.5 mL** *numerator* matches the mL unit of measure being calculated; **750 mg** becomes the *denominator*.

$$\text{mL} = \frac{2.5 \text{ mL}}{750 \text{ mg}}$$

In a DA equation, the unit of measure being calculated is matched in the numerator of the first clinical ratio entered.

All additional ratios are entered so that **each** *denominator* **is matched in its successive** *numerator*. The **denominator in the first ratio is mg**, so the **next numerator must be mg**. Go back to the problem to discover that this is provided by the **600 mg** dosage to be given. Enter this now as the next numerator to complete this single-step equation.

$$\text{mL} = \frac{2.5 \text{ mL}}{750 \text{ mg}} \times \frac{600 \text{ mg}}{}$$

The unit of measure in each denominator of a DA equation is matched in the successive numerator entered.

All the pertinent clinical ratios have now been entered in this one-step DA equation. The next step is to **cancel the alternate denominator/numerator measurement units (but not their quantities) to be sure they match**. This ensures that the clinical ratios were entered correctly. **After cancellation, only the unit of measure being calculated may remain in the equation.** The denominator/numerator mg/mg units cancel, leaving only the mL unit being calculated remaining in the equation.

$$\text{mL} = \frac{2.5 \text{ mL}}{750 \text{ mg}} \times \frac{600 \text{ mg}}{}$$

Only the unit of measure being calculated may remain in the equation after the denominator/numerator units of measure are cancelled.

Only the mL being calculated remains in the equation. The math can now be done.

$$mL = \frac{2.5 \text{ mL}}{750 \text{ mg}} \times \frac{600 \text{ mg}}{}$$

$$mL = \frac{2.5 \text{ mL}}{\underset{5}{750} \text{ mg}} \times \frac{\overset{4}{600} \text{ mg}}{} \qquad \text{Divide by 150}$$

$$mL = \frac{\overset{2}{10}}{\underset{1}{5}} = 2 \text{ mL}$$

**To obtain a dosage of 600 mg from an available dosage strength of 750 mg in 2.5 mL, you would give 2 mL.**

DA works exactly the same way for every calculation **regardless of the number of ratios entered**. As you can see, there are no complicated rules to memorize. In these simple steps, you have now learned how to use DA for **all** clinical calculations.

**EXAMPLE 2** A dosage of **50,000 units** is ordered to be added to an IV solution. The strength available is **10,000 units in 1.5 mL**. Calculate how many **mL** will contain this dosage.

Write the mL being calculated to the left of the equation followed by an equal sign.

$$mL =$$

Locate the complete ratio containing mL, the 10,000 units in 1.5 mL dosage strength available. Enter this now, with **1.5 mL as the numerator to match the mL being calculated**; 10,000 units becomes the denominator.

$$mL = \frac{1.5 \text{ mL}}{10,000 \text{ units}}$$

The units denominator must be matched in the next numerator. This is provided by the 50,000 units ordered. Enter this now to complete this one-step equation.

$$mL = \frac{1.5 \text{ mL}}{10,000 \text{ units}} \times \frac{50,000 \text{ units}}{}$$

Cancel the alternate denominator/numerator units/units entries to double-check for correct ratio entry. Only the mL being calculated remains in the equation. Do the math.

$$mL = \frac{1.5 \text{ mL}}{10,000 \text{ units}} \times \frac{50,000 \text{ units}}{}$$

$$mL = \frac{1.5 \text{ mL}}{\underset{1}{10,000} \text{ units}} \times \frac{\overset{5}{50,000} \text{ units}}{} \qquad \begin{array}{l}\text{Divide 50,000 by 10,000 to} \\ \text{obtain 5; multiply 1.5 by 5 to} \\ \text{obtain 7.5 mL}\end{array}$$

$$mL = 1.5 \times 5 = 7.5 \text{ mL}$$

**It will require a 7.5 mL volume of the 10,000 units in 1.5 mL solution to prepare the 50,000 units ordered for this IV additive.**

**EXAMPLE 3**   Tablet calculations are not common but would be done the same way using DA.

Scored (breakable) **tablets** with a strength of **0.5 mg** are available to prepare a dosage of **1.25 mg**. How many **tablets** must you give?

Enter the tab being calculated to the left of the equation followed by an equal sign.

$$\text{tab} =$$

The tab unit being calculated is matched by the tab strength available, 0.5 mg in 1 tab. Enter this as the first ratio, with 1 tab as the numerator; 0.5 mg becomes the denominator.

$$\text{tab} = \frac{1 \text{ tab}}{0.5 \text{ mg}}$$

The mg denominator must be matched in the next numerator. This is provided by the 1.25 mg ordered. Enter this to complete the equation.

$$\text{tab} = \frac{1 \text{ tab}}{0.5 \text{ mg}} \times \frac{1.25 \text{ mg}}{}$$

Cancel the alternate denominator/numerator mg units of measure to check that you have entered the ratios correctly. Only the tab being calculated remains in the equation. Do the math.

$$\text{tab} = \frac{1 \text{ tab}}{0.5 \; \cancel{\text{mg}}} \times \frac{1.25 \; \cancel{\text{mg}}}{}$$

$$\text{tab} = \frac{1 \text{ tab}}{\underset{2}{\cancel{50} \; \cancel{\text{mg}}}} \times \frac{\overset{5}{\cancel{125} \; \cancel{\text{mg}}}}{}$$   Eliminate the decimal points; reduce the numbers

$$\text{tab} = \frac{5}{2} = 2\tfrac{1}{2} \text{ tab}$$

**To obtain the 1.25 mg dosage ordered, 2½ tab must be given.**

Let's stop for a moment now and take a look at what happens if the ratios are incorrectly entered in a DA equation. We'll **assume that the units of measure have not been entered with their quantities** and that the **entries have been mixed up.** The correct equation will be shown alongside for comparison.

**EXAMPLE 4**   A drug label reads **100 mg per 2 mL**. The medication order is for **130 mg**. How many **mL** must you prepare?

| Correct | Incorrect |
|---------|-----------|

$$\text{mL} = \frac{2 \text{ mL}}{100 \text{ mg}} \times \frac{130 \text{ mg}}{} = \textbf{2.6 mL} \qquad \text{mL} = \frac{100}{2} \times \frac{130}{} = \textbf{6500 mL}$$

In the incorrect equation, the starting ratio is upside down, and since the units of measure were not entered with their quantities, there is no way to catch this.

The safety step of cancellation to check ratio entry cannot be done. But notice something else: The answer, 6500 mL, is impossible. If the entries in a DA equation are mixed up, the numbers are often so outrageous that you will know instantly that you have made a mistake. **But mistakes are not always this obvious, so stick to the step-by-step calculation rules**. There is a reason for every one of them. Let's look at a few more examples.

**EXAMPLE 5**   How many **mL** will you draw up to prepare a **1.2 g** dosage if the solution available is labeled **2 g in 3 mL**?

Write the mL unit being calculated to the left of the equation followed by an equal sign. Enter the starting ratio, 2 g in 3 mL, with 3 mL as the numerator to match the mL being calculated; 2 g becomes the denominator.

$$mL = \frac{3\ mL}{2\ g}$$

Match the g denominator in the next numerator with the 1.2 g ordered to complete the equation.

$$mL = \frac{3\ mL}{2\ g} \times \frac{1.2\ g}{}$$

Cancel the alternate denominator/numerator g units of measure to double-check that the entries are correct. Only the mL being calculated remains.

$$mL = \frac{3\ mL}{2\ \cancel{g}} \times \frac{1.2\ \cancel{g}}{}$$

Do the math, expressing fractional answers to the nearest tenth.

$$mL = \frac{3\ mL}{2\ \cancel{g}} \times \frac{1.2\ \cancel{g}}{} = \textbf{1.8 mL}$$

**The 1.2 g dosage ordered is contained in 1.8 mL of the 2 g in 3 mL solution available.**

**EXAMPLE 6**   Medication with a strength of **0.75 mg per mL** is available to prepare a dosage of **2 mg**. Calculate the mL this will require.

Write the mL being calculated to the left of the equation followed by an equal sign.

$$mL =$$

The mL being calculated is provided for the first ratio by the 0.75 mg per mL dosage strength available. Enter 1 mL as the numerator and 0.75 mg as the denominator.

$$mL = \frac{1\ mL}{0.75\ mg}$$

The mg denominator must now be matched. This is provided by the 2 mg dosage ordered. Enter this now to complete this one-step equation.

$$mL = \frac{1\ mL}{0.75\ mg} \times \frac{2\ mg}{}$$

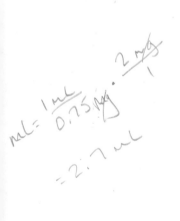

Cancel the alternate denominator/numerator mg units of measure to check for correct ratio entry, then do the math.

$$mL = \frac{1 \text{ mL}}{0.75 \text{ mg}} \times \frac{2 \text{ mg}}{} = 2.67 = \textbf{2.7 mL}$$

**It will require 2.7 mL of the 0.75 mg in 1 mL dosage available to administer the 2 mg ordered.**

## Problems 12.1

Calculate these dosages using DA. Express mL answers to the nearest tenth.

1. A dosage of 0.3 g has been ordered. The strength available is 0.4 g in 1.5 mL.  _1.1mL_

2. A dosage strength of 0.8 mg in 2 mL is to be used to prepare a 0.5 mg dosage.  _1.3 mL_

3. Prepare a 1.8 mg dosage from a solution labeled 2 mg in 3 mL.  _2.7 mL_

4. The order is for 1500 mg. You have available a 1200 mg per mL solution.  _1.3 mL_

5. A dosage strength of 0.2 mg in 1.5 mL is available. Give 0.15 mg.  _____

6. The strength available is 1000 mg in 3.6 mL. Prepare a 600 mg dosage.  _____

7. A 10,000 units dosage has been ordered. The strength available is 8000 units in 1 mL.  _____

8. An IV additive has a dosage strength of 20 mEq per 20 mL. A dosage of 15 mEq has been ordered.  _____

9. A 200,000 units dosage must be prepared from a 150,000 units in 2 mL strength.  _____

10. An IV additive order is for 400 mg. The solution available has a strength of 500 mg in 20 mL.  _____

**Answers   1.** 1.1 mL   **2.** 1.3 mL   **3.** 2.7 mL   **4.** 1.3 mL   **5.** 1.1 mL   **6.** 2.2 mL   **7.** 1.3 mL   **8.** 15 mL **9.** 2.7 mL   **10.** 16 mL

You now know the basics of using DA in calculations. **But how do you know if the answer you obtain is correct?** The answer to this question is provided by the key points already covered.

- **If** the unit being calculated is correctly identified to the left of the equation.

- **If** the starting ratio is entered so that its numerator matches the unit of measure being calculated.

- **If** the unit of measure in each denominator is matched in each successively entered numerator.

- **If** the only unit of measure remaining after cancellation is the same as the unit of measure being calculated.
- **If** the quantities have been correctly entered.
- **If** the math has been double-checked and is correct.

**THEN THE ANSWER WILL BE CORRECT.**

A tall order? Not really. You are doing a clinical dosage calculation. All you must do is carefully follow each step, and the answer will be correct.

In addition, **don't divorce your previous learning and reasoning from the calculation process.** You already know that **most IM dosages are contained in a 0.5–3 mL volume,** that **IV additives may be contained in larger volumes,** and that **large numbers of tab/cap are unusual** in dosages. **If you get an unreasonable answer to a calculation, you must question it.** In time, you will know the average dosages of all the drugs you give and another safety component will be added to your repertoire, but for now, concentrate on the simple mechanics of calculation you have just been taught. Don't shortcut these steps, and you'll do just fine.

## EQUATIONS REQUIRING METRIC CONVERSIONS

The major advantage of DA is that it allows multiple ratios to be entered in a single equation. This is especially useful when a drug is ordered in one unit of measure—for example, mg—but is labeled in another—for example, g or mcg.

There are two ways to handle a conversion. Sometimes, it will be easier to do the conversion before setting up the equation. In other instances, you may elect to incorporate the conversion into an equation. For practice purposes, let's look at how **conversion ratios**—for example, **1 g = 1000 mg** or **1 mg = 1000 mcg**—are entered in a DA equation.

> **EXAMPLE 1**   The IM dosage ordered is **275 mg**. The drug available is labeled **0.5 g per 2 mL**. How many **mL** must you give?

Enter the mL to be calculated to the left of the equation. Locate the ratio containing mL, the 0.5 g per 2 mL dosage strength, and enter it, with 2 mL as the numerator; 0.5 g becomes the denominator.

$$mL = \frac{2 \, mL}{0.5 \, g}$$

When you refer back to the problem, you will not find a g measure to match the starting ratio g denominator. The dosage to be given is in mg. So, a **conversion ratio between g and mg** is needed: 1 g = 1000 mg. Enter this now, with **1 g as the numerator to match the g of the previous denominator;** 1000 mg becomes the new denominator.

$$mL = \frac{2 \, mL}{0.5 \, g} \times \frac{1 \, g}{1000 \, mg}$$

The final entry, the 275 mg dosage to be given, will automatically fall into its correct position as it is entered as the final numerator to match the mg of the previous denominator. The equation is now complete.

$$ \text{mL} = \frac{2\ \text{mL}}{0.5\ \text{g}} \times \frac{1\ \text{g}}{1000\ \text{mg}} \times \frac{275\ \text{mg}}{} $$

Cancel the alternate denominator/numerator g/g and mg/mg units of measure to double-check the ratio entry. Only the mL being calculated remains. Do the math.

$$ \text{mL} = \frac{2\ \text{mL}}{0.5\ \cancel{\text{g}}} \times \frac{1\ \cancel{\text{g}}}{1000\ \cancel{\text{mg}}} \times \frac{275\ \cancel{\text{mg}}}{} = 1.1\ \text{mL} $$

**To give a dosage of 275 mg, you must prepare 1.1 mL of the 0.5 g in 2 mL strength solution.**

**EXAMPLE 2**    The drug label reads **800 mcg in 1.5 mL**. The IM order is for **0.6 mg**.

Enter the mL to be calculated followed by an equal sign to the left of the equation. Locate the ratio containing mL, 800 mcg in 1.5 mL. Enter 1.5 mL as the numerator to match the mL being calculated; 800 mcg becomes the denominator.

$$ \text{mL} = \frac{1.5\ \text{mL}}{800\ \text{mcg}} $$

There is no mcg measure in the problem, which is your clue to the necessity for a conversion ratio. Enter the 1000 mcg = 1 mg conversion ratio, with 1000 mcg as the numerator to match the mcg of the previous denominator; 1 mg becomes the denominator.

$$ \text{mL} = \frac{1.5\ \text{mL}}{800\ \text{mcg}} \times \frac{1000\ \text{mcg}}{1\ \text{mg}} $$

The mg denominator is now matched by the 0.6 mg dosage to be given, and completes the equation.

$$ \text{mL} = \frac{1.5\ \text{mL}}{800\ \text{mcg}} \times \frac{1000\ \text{mcg}}{1\ \text{mg}} \times \frac{0.6\ \text{mg}}{} $$

Cancel the alternate denominator/numerator mcg/mcg and mg/mg units of measure to check for correct ratio entry. Only the mL being calculated should remain in the equation. Do the math.

$$ \text{mL} = \frac{1.5\ \text{mL}}{800\ \cancel{\text{mcg}}} \times \frac{1000\ \cancel{\text{mcg}}}{1\ \cancel{\text{mg}}} \times \frac{0.6\ \cancel{\text{mg}}}{} = 1.12 = \textbf{1.1 mL} $$

**To give a dosage of 0.6 mg from the available 1.5 mL per 800 mcg strength, you must prepare 1.1 mL.**

**EXAMPLE 3**   Prepare a **0.5 mg** dosage from an available strength of **200 mcg per mL**.

Enter the mL being calculated to the left of the equation followed by an equal sign. Enter the 1 mL in 200 mcg dosage as the starting ratio, with 1 mL as the numerator to match the mL being calculated; 200 mcg becomes the denominator.

$$mL = \frac{1 \text{ mL}}{200 \text{ mcg}}$$

A mcg to mg conversion ratio is needed. Enter 1000 mcg as the numerator to match the mcg in the previous denominator; 1 mg becomes the new denominator.

$$mL = \frac{1 \text{ mL}}{200 \text{ mcg}} \times \frac{1000 \text{ mcg}}{1 \text{ mg}}$$

The mg denominator is now matched by the 0.5 mg dosage ordered to complete the equation.

$$mL = \frac{1 \text{ mL}}{200 \text{ mcg}} \times \frac{1000 \text{ mcg}}{1 \text{ mg}} \times \frac{0.5 \text{ mg}}{}$$

Cancel the alternate mcg/mcg and mg/mg units of measure to double-check for correct ratio entry. Only the mL unit being calculated remains in the equation. Do the math.

$$mL = \frac{1 \text{ mL}}{200 \text{ mcg}} \times \frac{1000 \text{ mcg}}{1 \text{ mg}} \times \frac{0.5 \text{ mg}}{} = 2.5 \text{ mL}$$

**A 0.5 mg dosage requires a 2.5 mL volume of the 200 mcg per mL strength solution available.**

**EXAMPLE 4**   The medication has a strength of **0.5 g in 1.5 mL**. Prepare **750 mg**.

Enter the mL to be calculated to the left of the equation followed by an equal sign. Enter the starting ratio, the 1.5 mL in 0.5 g dosage available, with 1.5 mL as the numerator, to match the mL being calculated; 0.5 g becomes the denominator.

$$mL = \frac{1.5 \text{ mL}}{0.5 \text{ g}}$$

There is no g dosage in the problem, which signals the need for a conversion ratio. Enter the 1 g = 1000 mg conversion ratio, with 1 g as the numerator, to match the g denominator of the starting ratio; 1000 mg becomes the new denominator.

$$mL = \frac{1.5 \text{ mL}}{0.5 \text{ g}} \times \frac{1 \text{ g}}{1000 \text{ mg}}$$

Enter the dosage ordered, 750 mg, as the final numerator to match the mg in the previous denominator. The equation is complete.

$$mL = \frac{1.5 \text{ mL}}{0.5 \text{ g}} \times \frac{1 \text{ g}}{1000 \text{ mg}} \times \frac{750 \text{ mg}}{}$$

Cancel the alternate g/g and mg/mg units of measure to check the accuracy of ratio entry, then complete the math.

$$mL = \frac{1.5 \text{ mL}}{0.5 \text{ g}} \times \frac{1 \text{ g}}{1000 \text{ mg}} \times \frac{750 \text{ mg}}{} = 2.25 = 2.3 \text{ mL}$$

**A 750 mg dosage requires 2.3 mL of the 0.5 g in 1.5 mL medication.**

## Problems 12.2

**Calculate these dosages using DA. Express mL answers to the nearest tenth.**

1. Prepare 0.1 g of an IM medication from a strength of 200 mg per mL.   <u>0.5 mL</u>

2. A drug label reads 0.1 g in 2 mL. Prepare a 130 mg dosage.   _____

3. An oral solution has a strength of 500 mg in 5 mL. Prepare a 0.6 g dosage.   _____

4. Prepare a 0.75 g dosage from a 250 mg per mL strength solution.   <u>3 mL</u>

5. Prepare 500 mg for IM injection from an available strength of 1 g per 3 mL.   _____

6. A dosage of 85 mg is ordered, and the drug available is labeled 0.1 g in 1.5 mL.   _____

7. The strength available is 500 mcg in 1.5 mL. Prepare a 0.75 mg dosage.   _____

8. A dosage of 1500 mg has been ordered. The solution available is 0.5 g per mL.   _____

9. The dosage strength available is 200 mcg per mL. A 0.5 mg dosage has been ordered.   _____

10. The dosage ordered is 0.2 g. Tablets available are labeled 80 mg.   _____

*Handwritten notes in right margin:*

$$\frac{1\,mL}{200\,mg} \cdot \frac{1000\,mg}{1\,g} \cdot 0.1\,g$$

$$\frac{1\,mL}{250\,mg} \cdot \frac{1000\,mg}{1\,g} \cdot 0.75$$

**Answers   1.** 0.5 mL   **2.** 2.6 mL   **3.** 6 mL   **4.** 3 mL   **5.** 1.5 mL   **6.** 1.3 mL   **7.** 2.3 mL   **8.** 3 mL
**9.** 2.5 mL   **10.** 2½ tab

## Summary

This completes your introduction to clinical calculations using dimensional analysis. The important points to remember from this chapter are:

- The unit of measure being calculated is written first to the left of the equation, followed by an equal sign.

- All ratios entered must include the quantity **and** the unit of measure.

- The numerator in the starting ratio must be in the same measurement unit as the unit of measure being calculated.

- The unit of measure in each denominator must be matched in the numerator of each successive ratio entered.

- Metric system conversions can be made by incorporating a conversion ratio directly into the DA equation.

- The unit of measure in each alternate denominator and numerator must cancel, leaving only the unit of measure being calculated remaining in the equation.

- The numerator of the starting ratio is never cancelled.

## Summary Self-Test

**Calculate these dosages using DA. Express mL answers to the nearest tenth (or hundredth where indicated) using the medication labels provided. Measure the dosages you calculate on the syringes provided. Have your answers checked by your instructor to be sure you have calculated and measured the dosages correctly.**

**Dosage Ordered**                                                              **mL Needed**

1. terbutaline sulfate 800 mcg                                        _____

2. furosemide 15 mg                                                        _____

3. Vistaril® 70mg                                                            _____

## Dosage Ordered                                      ## mL Needed

4. fentanyl citrate 0.15 mg                            _____

5. naloxone 350 mcg                                    _____

6. clindamycin 225 mg                                  _____

7. Robinul® 75 mcg (calculate to the nearest hundredth)   _____

**Dosage Ordered**                                                      **mL Needed**

8. midazolam HCl 4 mg                                            _____

9. Inapsine® 3mg                                                 _____

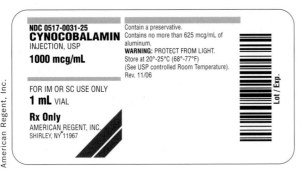

10. cyanocobalamin 800 mcg                                       _____

## Dosage Ordered                                                   ## mL Needed

11. potassium acetate 16 mEq for IV additive                       _____

12. calcium gluconate 0.93 mEq for an IV additive                  _____

13. morphine sulfate 1.5 mg                                        _____

14. heparin sodium 450 units (calculate to the nearest hundredth)  _____

**Dosage Ordered**

**mL Needed**

15. droperidol 4 mg

_____

16. Dilantin® 0.1 g

_____

17. medroxyprogesterone 0.9 g

_____

18. gentamicin 70 mg

_____

## Dosage Ordered

**mL Needed**

19. Vistaril® 120 mg

_____

20. sodium chloride 60 mEq for an IV additive

_____

21. atropine sulfate 150 mcg

_____

**Dosage Ordered**                                                **mL Needed**

22. meperidine 75 mg                                        _____

23. fentanyl citrate 80 mcg                                  _____

24. celestone 10 mg                                          _____

## Dosage Ordered                                                           ## mL Needed

**25.** morphine sulfate 20 mg

_____

**26.** gentamicin 0.1 g

_____

**27.** Dilantin® 0.15 g

_____

**28.** doxorubicin HCl 16 mg for an IV additive

_____

**Dosage Ordered**                                                      **mL Needed**

29. meperidine HCl 30 mg                                          _____

30. methotrexate 40 mg                                            _____

31. midazolam HCl 3 mg                                            _____

## Dosage Ordered                                          ## mL Needed

32. ondansetron 3 mg                                        _____

33. dexamethasone 5 mg                                      _____

34. hydroxyzine HCl 40 mg                                   _____

**Dosage Ordered**

**mL Needed**

35. Ketorolac tromethamine 20mg

_____

36. nalbuphine HCl 30 mg

_____

37. morphine 15 mg

_____

## Dosage Ordered

**mL Needed**

38. cyanocobalamin 750 mcg

_____

39. aminophylline 0.4 g for an IV additive

_____

40. Dilantin® 125 mg

_____

| **Dosage Ordered** | **mL Needed** |
|---|---|

### 41. Ketorolac 25 mg

_____

### 42. Vistaril 50 mg

_____

### 43. gentamicin 0.1 g

_____

### 44. Robinul® 180 mcg

_____

## Dosage Ordered

**mL Needed**

### 45. hydroxyzine HCl 70 mg

_____

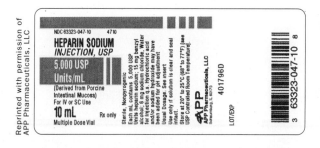

### 46. Bicillin® C-R 400,000 units

_____

### 47. heparin sodium 1500 units (calculate to the nearest hundredth)

_____

### 48. potassium chloride 20 mEq for an IV additive

_____

**Dosage Ordered**                                                    **mL Needed**

49. Inapsine® 4.5 mg                                    _____

50. epinephrine 1.4 mg                                  _____

51. Nubain 15 mg                                        _____

52. furosemide 15 mg                                    _____

## Dosage Ordered

## mL Needed

**53.** dexamethasone 6000 mcg

_____

**54.** phenytoin Na 0.1 g

_____

**55.** lidocaine HCl 15 mg

_____

**Answers**

| | | | |
|---|---|---|---|
| **1.** 0.8 mL | **14.** 0.45 mL | **28.** 8 mL | **42.** 2 mL |
| **2.** 1.5 mL | **15.** 1.6 mL | **29.** 1.2 mL | **43.** 2 mL |
| **3.** 1.4 mL | **16.** 2 mL | **30.** 1.6 mL | **44.** 0.9 mL |
| **4.** 3 mL | **17.** 2.3 mL | **31.** 0.6 mL | **45.** 1.4 mL |
| **5.** 0.9 mL | **18.** 1.8 mL | **32.** 1.5 mL | **46.** 0.7 mL |
| **6.** 1.5 mL | **19.** 2.4 mL | **33.** 1.3 mL | **47.** 0.3 mL |
| **7.** 0.38 mL | **20.** 15 mL | **34.** 1.6 mL | **48.** 10 mL |
| **8.** 0.8 mL | **21.** 1.5 mL | **35.** 1.3 mL | **49.** 1.8 mL |
| **9.** 1.2 mL | **22.** 0.8 mL | **36.** 1.5 mL | **50.** 1.4 mL |
| **10.** 0.8 mL | **23.** 1.6 mL | **37.** 1.5 mL | **51.** 0.8 mL |
| **11.** 8 mL | **24.** 1.7 mL | **38.** 0.8 mL | **52.** 1.5 mL |
| **12.** 2 mL | **25.** 1.3 mL | **39.** 16 mL | **53.** 1.5 mL |
| **13.** 1.5 mL | **26.** 2.5 mL | **40.** 2.5 mL | **54.** 2 mL |
| | **27.** 3 mL | **41.** 1.7 mL | **55.** 0.8 mL |

SECTION

# 5

## Dosage Calculation from Body Weight and Body Surface Area

CHAPTER **13**
Adult and Pediatric
Dosages Based on Body
Weight / 188

CHAPTER **14**
Adult and Pediatric Dosages
Based on Body Surface
Area / 203

# ADULT AND PEDIATRIC DOSAGES BASED ON BODY WEIGHT

## Objectives

The learner will:

1. convert body weight from lb to kg.

2. convert body weight from kg to lb.

3. calculate dosages using mcg/mg per kg, or per lb.

4. determine if dosages ordered are within the normal range.

Body weight is a major factor in calculating drug dosages for both adults and children. It is the **most** important determiner of dosages for infants and neonates, whose ability to metabolize drugs is not fully developed. The dosage that will produce optimum therapeutic results for any particular individual, either child or adult, depends not only on dosage but on individual variables, including drug sensitivities and tolerance, age, weight, sex, and metabolic, pathologic, or psychologic conditions.

The prescriber will order the drug and dosage. However, it is a nursing responsibility to check each dosage to be sure the order is correct. Each drug label or drug package insert provides specific dosage details, but more complete information is readily available in drug formularies, the *PDR*, and other medical references. The hospital pharmacist is the ultimate resource for information.

Individualized dosages may be calculated in terms of mcg or mg per kg or lb per day. The total daily dosage may be administered in divided (more than one) dosages; for example, every 6 hours or every 8 hours.

Because body weight is critical in calculating infant and neonatal dosages, measurement is usually done using a weight scale calibrated in kg. Adult weights may be recorded in either kg or lb, and occasionally, conversions between these two measures are necessary.

### CONVERTING LB TO KG

If body weight is recorded in lb, but the drug literature lists dosage per kg, a conversion from lb to kg will be necessary. There are 2.2 lb in 1 kg. This means that **kg body weights are smaller than lb weights**, so **the conversion from lb to kg is made by dividing body weight by 2.2**. For ease of calculation, fractional lb may be converted to the nearest quarter and written as decimal fractions instead of oz: ¼ lb (4 oz) as 0.25, ½ lb (8 oz) as 0.5, and ¾ lb (12 oz) as 0.75. If this kind of accuracy is critical, the prescribing orders should so indicate.

**EXAMPLE 1**   A child weighs 41 lb 12 oz. Convert to kg.

41 lb 12 oz = 41.75 ÷ 2.2 = 18.97 = **19 kg**

The kg weight should be a smaller number than 41.75 because you are dividing, and 19 kg is.

**EXAMPLE 2**   Convert the weight of a 144½ lb adult to kg.

144½ lb = 144.5 ÷ 2.2 = 65.68 = **65.7 kg**

**EXAMPLE 3**   Convert the weight of a 27¼ lb child to kg.

27¼ lb = 27.25 ÷ 2.2 = 12.38 = **12.4 kg**

## Problems 13.1

Convert these body weights. Round to the nearest tenth kg.

1. 58¾ lb   = __26.7__ kg          6. 134½ lb  = _____ kg
2. 63½ lb   = __28.9__ kg          7. 112¾ lb  = _____ kg
3. 163¼ lb  = __74.2__ kg          8. 73¼ lb   = _____ kg
4. 39¾ lb   = __18.1__ kg          9. 121½ lb  = _____ kg
5. 100¼ lb  = _____ kg         10. 92¾ lb   = _____ kg

---

**Answers   1.** 26.7 kg   **2.** 28.9 kg   **3.** 74.2 kg   **4.** 18.1 kg   **5.** 45.6 kg   **6.** 61.1 kg   **7.** 51.3 kg
**8.** 33.3 kg   **9.** 55.2 kg   **10.** 42.2 kg

---

## CONVERTING KG TO LB

There are 2.2 lb in 1 kg. To convert from kg to lb, **multiply by 2.2**. Because you are multiplying, **the answer in lb will be larger than the kg** being converted. Express weight to the nearest tenth lb.

**EXAMPLE 1**   A child weighs 23.3 kg. Convert to lb.

23.3 kg = 23.3 × 2.2 = 51.26 = **51.3 lb**

The answer must be larger because you are multiplying, and it is.

**EXAMPLE 2**   Convert an adult weight of 73.4 kg to lb.

73.4 kg = 73.4 × 2.2 = 161.48 = **161.5 lb**

**EXAMPLE 3**   Convert the weight of a 14.2 kg child to lb.

14.2 kg = 14.2 × 2.2 = 31.24 = **31.2 lb**

## Problems 13.2

**Convert kg to lb. Round to the nearest tenth lb.**

1. 21.3 kg = __46.9__ lb
2. 99.2 kg = __218.2__ lb
3. 28.7 kg = __63.1__ lb
4. 71.4 kg = __157.1__ lb
5. 30.8 kg = __67.8__ lb

6. 43.7 kg = _____ lb
7. 63.8 kg = _____ lb
8. 57.1 kg = _____ lb
9. 84.2 kg = _____ lb
10. 34.9 kg = _____ lb

**Answers**  **1.** 46.9 lb  **2.** 218.2 lb  **3.** 63.1 lb  **4.** 157.1 lb  **5.** 67.8 lb  **6.** 96.1 lb  **7.** 140.4 lb
**8.** 125.6 lb  **9.** 185.2 lb  **10.** 76.8 lb

## CALCULATING DOSAGES FROM DRUG LABEL INFORMATION

Information you will need to calculate dosages from body weight will be on the actual drug label or on the drug package insert.

Calculating the dosage is a two-step procedure. First, the **total daily dosage** is calculated. Then it is **divided by the number of doses per day** to obtain the actual dose administered at one time.

Let's start by looking at some oral antibiotic labels that contain the mg/kg/day dosage guidelines.

**EXAMPLE 1**    Refer to the information written sideways on the right of the sample antibiotic label in Figure 13-1 for children's dosages. Notice that the dosage is **20 mg/kg/day (or 40 mg/kg/day in otitis media)**. This dosage is to be given in **divided doses every 8 hours**—or a total of 3 doses (24 hr ÷ 8 hr = 3 doses).

**Figure 13-1**

Once you have located the dosage information, you can move ahead and calculate the dosage. Let's assume you are checking the dosage ordered for an **18.2 kg** child. Start by calculating the **recommended daily dosage range**.

Lower daily dosage  =  **20 mg/kg**

20 mg × 18.2 kg (weight of child)  =  **364 mg/day**

Upper daily dosage  =  **40 mg/kg**

40 mg × 18.2 kg  =  **728 mg/day**

**The recommended range for this 18.2 kg child is 364–728 mg/day.**
The drug is to be given in three divided doses.

Lower dosage   364 mg ÷ 3  =  **121 mg per dose**

Upper dosage   728 mg ÷ 3  =  **243 mg per dose**

**The per dose dosage range is 121 mg to 243 mg per dose every 8 hours.**

Now that you have the dosage range for this child, you are able to assess the accuracy of physician orders. Let's look at some orders and see how you can use the dosage range you just calculated.

1. **If the order is to give 125 mg every 8 hours, is this within the recommended dosage range?**
   Yes, 125 mg is within the average range of 121–243 mg per dose.

2. **If the order is to give 375 mg every 8 hours, is this within the recommended dosage range?**
   No, this is an overdosage. The maximum recommended dosage is 243 mg per dose. The 375 mg dose should not be given; the prescriber must be called and the order questioned.

3. **If the order is for 75 mg every 8 hours, is this an accurate dosage?**
   The recommended lower limit for an 18.2 kg child is 121 mg. Although 75 mg might be **safe**, it will probably be **ineffective**. Notify the prescriber that the dosage appears to be too low.

4. **If the order is for 250 mg every 8 hours, is this accurate?**
   Because 243 mg per dose is the recommended upper limit, 250 mg is essentially within normal range. The drug strength is 125 mg per 5 mL, and a 250 mg dosage is 10 mL. The prescriber has probably ordered this dosage based on the available dosage strength and for ease of preparation.

5. **If the dosage ordered is 125 mg every 4 hours, is this an accurate dosage?**
   In this order, the **frequency of administration** does not match the recommended dosage of every 8 hours The total daily dosage of 750 mg (125 mg × 6 doses = 750 mg) is slightly, but not significantly, higher than the 728 mg maximum. There may be a reason the prescriber ordered the dosage every 4 hours, but call to verify it.

> To determine the safety of an ordered dosage, use body weight to calculate the dosage range ordered, and compare this with the recommended dosage range in mg/kg/day (or mg/lb/day). Assessment must also include the frequency of dosage ordered.

The difference between 4 mg and 6 mg is much more critical than the difference between 243 mg and 250 mg because the drug potency is obviously greater.

Additional factors that must be considered are age, weight, and medical condition. Although these factors cannot be dealt with at length, keep in mind that **the younger, the older, or more compromised by illness an individual is, the more critical a discrepancy is likely to be.**

Discrepancies in dosages are much more significant if the number of mg or mcg ordered is small.

## Problems 13.3

Refer to the Biaxin® Granules label in Figure 13-2 to answer the questions for a 20 lb child.

1. What is the child's body weight in kg to the nearest tenth?   _9.1 kg_
2. What is the recommended dosage in mg per day for this child?   _136.5 mg_
3. How many mg will this be per dose?   _68.3 mg_
4. The order is to give 62.5 mg twice a day.  Is this dosage reasonable?   _____
5. How many mL would you need to administer this dosage?   _____
6. How much water must you add as diluent to prepare this oral suspension?   _____

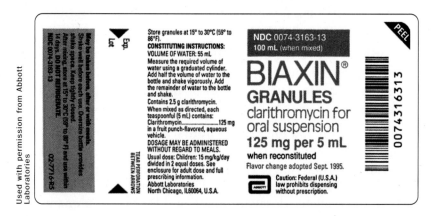

**Figure 13-2**

**Answers**   **1.** 9.1 kg   **2.** 136.5 mg/day   **3.** 68.3 mg/dose   **4.** Yes   **5.** 2.5 mL   **6.** 55 mL

## CALCULATING DOSAGES FROM DRUG LITERATURE

The labels you have just been reading were from oral syrups and suspensions, but the same calculation steps are necessary for dosages to be administered by the IV or IM route. Parenteral labels are much smaller in size and usually do not include dosage recommendations. To obtain these, you will have to refer to the **drug package inserts,** the *PDR,* or **similar references**. These references will contain extensive details about each drug's chemistry, actions, adverse reactions, recommended administration, and so on, so it will be necessary for you to search for and select the information you need under the heading **Dosage and Administration.** In the following exercises, the searching has been done for you, and only those excerpts necessary for your calculations are shown.

## Problems 13.4

**Refer to the cefazolin package insert in Figure 13-3 to locate the information for pediatric dosages.**

1. What is the dosage range in mg/kg/day for mild-to-moderate infections?                                                    _____

2. What is the dosage range for mild-to-moderate infections in mg/lb/day?                                                    _____

3. The total dosage will be divided into how many doses per day?     _____

4. In severe infections, what is the maximum daily dosage recommended in mg/kg?                                              _____

   In mg/lb?                                                        _____

**Figure 13-3**

Answers   **1.** 25 mg–50 mg   **2.** 10 mg–20 mg   **3.** 3–4 doses per day   **4.** 100 mg/kg; 45 mg/lb

## Problems 13.5

**Use the information you just obtained from Figure 13-3 to do the calculations for a child who weighs 35 lb and has a moderately severe infection.**

1. What is the lower daily dosage range?                             _____

2. What is the upper daily dosage range?

3. If the medication is given in 4 divided dosages, what will the per dosage range be? _____

4. If a dosage of 125 mg is ordered every 6 hours, will you need to question it? _____

---

**Answers   1.** 350 mg/day   **2.** 700 mg/day   **3.** 87.5 mg to 175 mg per dose   **4.** No; within normal range

---

## Problems 13.6

**Refer to the dosage information in Figure 13-4 to answer the following questions about adult IV dosages.**

1. What is the recommended daily dosage range for serious infections? _____

2. In how many divided doses should this daily dosage be given? _____

3. What is the maximum daily dosage? _____

4. Calculate the daily dosage range in g for a 176 lb adult. _____

5. If this dosage is to be given every 6 hours, what will this individual's dosage range be? _____

6. If a dosage of 2 g is ordered, what initial assessment would you make about it? _____

7. If a dosage of 10 g is ordered every 6 hours, what assessment would you make? _____

---

Used with permission from Novartis AG

**DOSAGE AND ADMINISTRATION**

MEZLIN® (sterile mezlocillin sodium) may be administered intravenously or intramuscularly. For serious infections, the intravenous route of administration should be used. Intramuscular doses should not exceed 2g per injection.

The recommended adult dosage for serious infections is 200-300 mg/kg per day given in 4 to 6 divided doses. The usual dose is 3g given every 4 hours (18g/day) or 4g given every 6 hours (16g/day). For life-threatening infections, up to 350 mg/kg per day may be administered, but the total daily dosage should ordinarily not exceed 24g.
[See table below.]
For patients with life-threatening infections, 4g may be administered every 4 hours (24g/day).

**Figure 13-4**

---

**Answers   1.** 200–300 mg/kg   **2.** 4 to 6 doses; every 6 or 4 hours   **3.** 24 g   **4.** 16–24 g   **5.** 4–6 g
**6.** The dosage is too low   **7.** The dosage is too high

## Problems 13.7

Refer to the dosage recommendations for the antineoplastic agent in Figure 13-5 to answer the following questions for treatment of testicular tumors in a patient weighing 240 lb.

1. What is the recommended daily dosage range in mcg/kg? _____

2. How often is this dosage to be given and for how long? _____ _____

3. What is the daily dosage range in mcg for this patient? In mg? (Calculate kg weight to the nearest tenth.) _____ _____

4. If a dosage of 3 mg IV is ordered every morning, does this need to be questioned? _____

Used with permission of Bayer Corporation

**MITHRACIN®** ℞
(plicamycin)
**FOR INTRAVENOUS USE**

**DOSAGE**
The daily dose of Mithracin is based on the patient's body weight. If a patient has abnormal fluid retention such as edema, hydrothorax or ascites, the patient's ideal weight rather than actual body weight should be used to calculate the dose.
**Treatment of Testicular Tumors:** In the treatment of patients with testicular tumors the recommended daily dose of Mithracin (plicamycin) is 25 to 30 mcg (0.025–0.030 mg) per kilogram of body weight. Therapy should be continued for a period of 8 to 10 days unless significant side effects or toxicity occur during therapy. A course of therapy consisting of more than 10 daily doses is not recommended. Individual daily doses should not exceed 30 mcg (0.030 mg) per kilogram of body weight.

**Figure 13-5**

**Answers** **1.** 25–30 mcg/kg **2.** Once a day; 8–10 days **3.** 2728–3273 mcg/day; 2.7–3.3 mg/day
**4.** No; within normal range

## Problems 13.8

Refer to the Rocephin™ literature in Figure 13-6 to answer the following questions on pediatric dosages.

1. What is the dosage in mg/kg/day for acute bacterial otitis media? _____

2. What is the dosage range for skin structure infections? _____

3. What is the initial dosage for meningitis? _____

4. What will the initial dosage be for a child with meningitis weighing 12.6 kg? In mg? In g? _____

5. What is the twice-daily dosage in mg for this child to follow the initial dose? _____

6. What will the initial meningitis dosage be for a child weighting 19½ lb? _____

7. How many days must rocephin therapy be continued for meningitis after the initial dose? _____

### ROCEPHIN DOSAGE FOR CHILDREN

*PEDIATRIC PATIENTS*: For the treatment of skin and skin structure infections, the recommended total daily dose is 50 to 75 mg/kg given once a day (or in equally divided doses twice a day). The total daily dose should not exceed 2 grams.

For the treatment of acute bacterial otitis media, a single intramuscular dose of 50 mg/kg (not to exceed 1 gram) is recommended (see **INDICATIONS AND USAGE**).

For the treatment of serious miscellaneous infections other than meningitis, the recommended total daily dose is 50 to 75 mg/kg, given in divided doses every 12 hours. The total daily dose should not exceed 2 grams.

In the treatment of meningitis, it is recommended that the initial therapeutic dose be 100 mg/kg (not to exceed 4 grams). Thereafter, a total daily dose of 100 mg/kg/day (not to exceed 4 grams daily) is recommended. The daily dose may be administered once a day (or in equally divided doses every 12 hours). The usual duration of therapy is 7 to 14 days.

**Figure 13-6**

Rocephin information is available online at **http://www.rxlist.com/rocephin-drug.htm**.

**Answers   1.** 50 mg/kg   **2.** 50–75 mg/kg once a day or equally divided dosages twice a day
**3.** 100 mg/kg not to exceed 4 g   **4.** 1260 mg; 1.26 g   **5.** 630 mg   **6.** 887 mg   **7.** 7–14 days

## Summary

**This concludes the chapter on calculation and assessment of dosages based on body weight. The important points to remember from this chapter are:**

- Dosages are frequently ordered on the basis of weight, especially for children.

- Dosages may be recommended based on mcg or mg per kg or lb per day, usually administered in divided doses.

- Body weight may need to be converted from kg to lb or lb to kg to correlate with dosage recommendations.

- To convert lb to kg, divide by 2.2; to convert kg to lb, multiply by 2.2.

- Calculating dosage is a two-step procedure: first, calculate the total daily dosage for the weight; then, divide this by the number of doses to be administered.

- To check the accuracy of a prescriber's order, calculate the correct dosage and compare it with the dosage ordered.

- Dosage discrepancies are much more critical if the dosage range is low—for example, 2–5 mg—as opposed to high—for example, 250–500 mg.

- Factors that make discrepancies particularly serious are age, low body weight, and severity of medical condition.

- If the drug label does not contain all the necessary information for safe administration, additional information should be obtained from drug package inserts, the PDR, drug formularies, or the hospital pharmacist.

## Summary Self-Test

**Read the dosage labels and literature provided to answer the questions.**

*19.6 kg*

1. A 43 lb child has an order for oral cefaclor. What is the daily dosage for this child?   *390.1 mg*

2. What is the per dose dosage?   *130 mg*

3. Is an order for 250 mg of cefaclor every 8 hours correct for this child?   *no, too high*

4. A 140 lb adult has an order for IV methylprednisolone. Calculate this patient's per dose dosage.   *63.6 kg*   *1.9 g*

5. How often is this dosage to be given?   *every 4-6 hours*

6. Children's dosages are smaller. What is the lowest mg/kg dosage recommended?   *<0.5 mg every 24 hours*

7. Calculate the lowest daily dosage for a child weighing 43 lb.   *9.8 mg*

8. When given intravenously what period of time is specified for the Solu-Medrol administration?   *>30 minutes*

**SOLU-MEDROL®**
brand of methylprednisolone sodium succinate sterile powder
(methylprednisolone sodium succinate for injection, USP)
For Intravenous or Intramuscular Administration

**DOSAGE AND ADMINISTRATION**
When high dose therapy is desired, the recommended dose of SOLU-MEDROL Sterile Powder (methylprednisolone sodium succinate) is 30 mg/kg administered intravenously over at least 30 minutes. This dose may be repeated every 4 to 6 hours for 48 hours.

Dosage may be reduced for infants and children but should be governed more by the severity of the condition and response of the patient than by age or size. It should not be less than 0.5 mg per kg every 24 hours.

Used with permission of Pfizer Inc.

9. Refer to the penicillin V potassium oral solution label and identify the dosage strength in mg.    _____

10. What is the dosage strength in units?    _____

11. This medication is shipped in powdered form. How much diluent is needed for reconstitution?    _____

12. What kind of diluent?    _____

13. What dosage in mg/kg is specified for infants?    _____

14. If an infant weighs 6.2 kg, what will the dosage range be?    _____

15. What will the dosage range be for a 16 lb infant?    _____

16. A 7.9 kg infant has an order for 125 mg every 8 hours. Calculate the per dose dosage based on this infant's body weight. Is the penicillin dosage ordered correct?    _____  _____

NDC 0025-6589-82

**PENICILLIN V POTASSIUM**

**125 mg (200,000 units)**
*For Oral Solution U.S.P.*    Rx only

**per 5 mL  when mixed as directed;
200 mL after mixing**

**Do Not Use If Caked**

SL **SIMULATED LABEL**
For Educational Purposes Only

Contains penicillin V potassium equivalent to 5 grams penicillin V in a dry mixture.

Each 5 mL teaspoon of prepared solution yields penicillin V potassium equivalent to 125 mg (200,000 units) penicillin V.

DIRECTIONS FOR PREPARATION

Use 117 mL of water to prepare 200 mL oral solution. Loosen powder then add water and shake vigorously.
Usual dosage: Adults and children — 1 to 2 teaspoons, given three or four times per day. Infants —15 to 56 mg/kg body weight daily, given in three to six divided doses. See insert for detailed information.
Store at room temperature in dry form.

Lot.
Exp. Date

354588-23

Delmar/Cengage Learning

17. Cefaclor oral suspension has been ordered for a child weighing 100 lb. Calculate the daily dose.    _____

18. What will the per dose dosage be?    _____

19. Would a 5 mL dosage every 8 hours be reasonable for this child?    _____

20. How is this oral cefaclor suspension to be reconstituted?    _____

21. What precautions did you learn about pouring and administering suspensions such as cefaclor?    _____

**R RANBAXY**
NDC 63304-**956**-01

**CEFACLOR**
For Oral Suspension USP

**250 mg/5 mL**

**75 mL** (when mixed)
SHAKE WELL BEFORE USE

**Rx only**

Used with permission of Ranbaxy Pharmaceuticals Inc.

22. Refer to the acyclovir sodium injection insert to locate the adult and adolescent dosage in mg/kg.                                      _____

23. What will the dosage be per dose for an adult with mucosal herpes simplex weighing 61.4 kg?                                      _____

24. What would the dosage be for an adolescent with herpes simplex encephalitis weighing 180 lb?                                      _____

25. What mg/kg dosage is recommended for an infant with herpes simplex encephalitis?                                      _____

26. Read the literature to locate the time period recommended for intravenous infusion.                                      _____

27. There are bold print precautions regarding parenteral administration on this insert. What are they?                                      _____

---

# ACYCLOVIR SODIUM

### INJECTION

**DOSAGE AND ADMINISTRATION:**
**CAUTION - AVOID RAPID OR BOLUS INTRAVENOUS INJECTION. (see WARNINGS and PRECAUTIONS).**

**AVOID INTRAMUSCULAR OR SUBCUTANEOUS INJECTION (see WARNINGS).**
**Initiate therapy as early as possible following onset of signs and symptoms of herpes infections.**
Do not exceed a dose equivalent to 20 mg/kg every 8 hours for any patient.

**DOSAGE IN HERPES SIMPLEX INFECTION:**
*MUCOSAL AND CUTANEOUS HERPES SIMPLEX (HSV-1 and HSV-2) INFECTIONS IN IMMUNOCOMPROMISED PATIENTS:*

**Adults and Adolescents 12 years of age and older:** 5 mg/kg infused at a constant rate over 1 hour, every 8 hours for 7 days.

**Children under 12 years of age:** 10 mg/kg infused at a constant rate over 1 hour, every 8 hours for 7 days.

**DOSAGE IN SEVERE INITIAL CLINICAL EPISODES OF HERPES GENITALIS:**
**Adults and Adolescents 12 years of age and older:** 5 mg/kg infused at a constant rate over 1 hour, every 8 hours for 5 days.

**DOSAGE IN HERPES SIMPLEX ENCEPHALITIS:**
**Adults and Adolescents 12 years of age and older:** 10 mg/kg infused at a constant rate over 1 hour, every 8 hours for 10 days.

**Children 3 months to 12 years of age:** 20 mg/kg infused at a constant rate over 1 hour, every 8 hours for 10 days.

**Administration**
Further dilute the calculated dose in an appropriate intravenous solution at a volume selected for administration during each 1 hour infusion. Infusion concentrations of approximately 7 mg/mL or lower are recommended. Clinical studies reveal that the average 70 kg adult received between 60 and 150 mL of fluid per dose. Higher concentrations (e.g.,10 mg/mL) may produce phlebitis or inflammation at the injection site upon inadvertent extravasation. Standard, commercially available electrolyte and glucose solutions are suitable for intravenous administration; biologic or colloidal fluids (e.g., blood products, protein solutions, etc.) are not recommended.
   Once diluted, each dose should be used within 24 hours.
   Visually inspect for particulate matter and discoloration prior to administration, whenever solution and container permit.

NDC 0025-6589-82

354588-23

Delmar/Cengage Learning

Lot.
Exp. Date

**SL** SIMULATED LABEL
For Educational Purposes Only

---

28. A 198 lb adult is to be treated with IV ticarcillin disodium for bacterial septicemia. What is the daily dosage range in mg for this patient?                                      _____

29. If the drug is administered every 4 hours, what will the per dose be in g?                                      _____

30. Do you need to question a per dose dosage of 4 g of ticarcillin every 4 hours for this patient?                                      _____

---

## TICARCILLIN DISODIUM
### FOR INTRAMUSCULAR OR INTRAVENOUS ADMINISTRATION

**DOSAGE AND ADMINISTRATION**
In serious urinary tract and systemic infections, intravenous therapy in the higher doses should be used. Intramuscular injections should not exceed 2 grams per injection.

**Adults:**

| | |
|---|---|
| Bacterial septicemia | 200 to 300 mg/kg/day by I.V. infusion in divided doses every four or six hours. |
| Respiratory tract infection | Usual dose is 3 grams every four hours (18 grams/day) or 4 grams every six hours |
| Skin and soft-tissue infection | (16 grams/day) depending on weight and the severity of the infection. |
| Intra-abdominal infection | |
| Infections of the female pelvis and genital tract | |

| | |
|---|---|
| Urinary tract infections | |
| Complicated: | Give 150 to 200 mg/kg/day by I.V. infusion every four to six hours in divided doses. Recommended dosage for average (70 kg) adult: 3 grams four times daily. |
| Uncomplicated: | Give 1 gram I.M. or direct I.V. every six hours. |

**354588-23**

NDC 0025-6589-82

Lot.
Exp. Date

Delmar/Cengage Learning

**SL SIMULATED LABEL**
For Educational Purposes Only

---

31. Refer to the VFEND® package insert information to locate the IV maintenance dosage in mg/kg every 12 hours (written with the abbreviation q12h, now slated for deletion) for invasive aspergillosis. _____

32. What would the daily IV dosage be for an individual weighing 92.7 kg? _____

33. What would the daily oral dosage be for this same 92.7 kg individual? _____

34. What will a single IV maintenance dosage be for the same 92.7 kg individual? _____

35. Locate the VFEND information on the maximum rate of administration for intravenous administration. _____

36. There is a bold type and capitalized warning for IV administration of VFEND on this insert. What is it? _____

---

## VFEND® I.V.
(voriconazole) for Injection
## VFEND® Tablets
(voriconazole)
## VFEND® (voriconazole) for Oral Suspension

**DESCRIPTION**
VFEND® (voriconazole), a triazole antifungal agent, is available as a lyophilized powder for solution for intravenous infusion, film-coated tablets for oral administration, and as a powder for oral suspension.

**DOSAGE AND ADMINISTRATION**
**Administration**
VFEND Tablets or Oral Suspension should be taken at least one hour before, or one hour following, a meal.

VFEND I.V. for Injection requires reconstitution to 10 mg/mL and subsequent dilution to 5 mg/mL or less prior to administration as an infusion, at a maximum rate of 3 mg/kg per hour over 1–2 hours (see Intravenous Administration).
**NOT FOR IV BOLUS INJECTION**

### Recommended Dosing Regimen

| Infection | Loading dose | Maintenance Dose | |
|---|---|---|---|
| | IV | IV | Oral[a] |
| Invasive Aspergillosis | 6 mg/kg q12h for the first 24 hours | 4 mg/kg q12h | 200 mg q12h |
| Candidemia in nonneutropenic patients and other deep tissue Candida infections | 6 mg/kg q12h for the first 24 hours | 3–4 mg/kg q12h[b] | 200 mg q12h |
| Esophageal Candidiasis | c | c | 200 mg q12h |
| Scedosporiosis and Fusariosis | 6 mg/kg q12h for the first 24 hours | 4 mg/kg q12h | 200 mg q12h |

Used with permission of Pfizer Inc.

FZC-P01

# FLUCONAZOLE INJECTION

### For Intravenous Infusion Only
### Rx ONLY
### DESCRIPTION

Fluconazole, the first of a new subclass of synthetic triazole antifungal agents, is available as a sterile solution for intravenous use in glass vials.

**Dosage and Administration in Children:**
The following dose equivalency scheme should generally provide equivalent exposure in pediatric and adult patients:

| Pediatric Patients | Adults |
|---|---|
| 3 mg/kg | 100 mg |
| 6 mg/kg | 200 mg |
| 12*mg/kg | 400 mg |

*Some older children may have clearances similar to that of adults. Absolute doses exceeding 600 mg/day are not recommended. Experience with fluconazole in neonates is limited to pharmacokinetic studies in premature newborns. (See **CLINICAL PHARMACOLOGY**.) Based on the prolonged half-life seen in premature newborns (gestational age 26 to 29 weeks), these children, in the first two weeks of life, should receive the same dosage (mg/kg) as in older children, but administered every 72 hours. After the first two weeks, these children should be dosed once daily. No information regarding fluconazole pharmacokinetics in full-term newborns is available.

*Oropharyngeal candidiasis:* The recommended dosage of fluconazole for oropharyngeal candidiasis in children is 6 mg/kg on the first day, followed by 3 mg/kg once daily. Treatment should be administered for at least 2 weeks to decrease the likelihood of relapse.

*Esophageal candidiasis:* For the treatment of esophageal candidiasis, the recommended dosage of fluconazole in children is 6 mg/kg on the first day, followed by 3 mg/kg once daily. Doses up to 12 mg/kg/day may be used based on medical judgment of the patient's response to therapy. Patients with esophageal candidiasis should be treated for a minimum of three weeks and for at least 2 weeks following the resolution of symptoms.

*Systemic Candida infections:* For the treatment of candidemia and disseminated *Candida* infections, daily doses of 6 to 12 mg/kg/day have been used in an open, noncomparative study of a small number of children.

*Cryptococcal meningitis:* For the treatment of acute cryptococcal meningitis, the recommended dosage is 12 mg/kg on the first day, followed by 6 mg/kg once daily. A dosage of 12 mg/kg once daily may be used, based on medical judgment of the patient's response to therapy. The recommended duration of treatment for initial therapy of cryptococcal meningitis is 10 to 12 weeks after the cerebrospinal fluid becomes culture negative. For suppression of relapse of cryptococcal meningitis in children with AIDS, the recommended dose of fluconazole is 6 mg/kg once daily.

37. Refer to the fluconazole injection insert to locate the first day dosage for a child with esophageal candidiasis.   _____

38. What is the dosage recommendation for subsequent days?   _____

39. How long must treatment for this condition be continued?   _____

40. What will the first dose be for a child weighing 18.2 kg?   _____

41. What will the subsequent dosage be for this same 18.2 kg child?   _____

42. How often will this dosage be administered?   _____

43. What is the maximum mg/kg dosage recommended if the child has a particularly severe infection?   _____

44. What would the first dose of fluconazole be for a child weighing 72 lb?   _____

**Answers**

1. 390 mg
2. 130 mg/dose
3. No, too high
4. 1908 mg/dose
5. Every 4 to 6 hours for 48 hours
6. 0.5 mg/kg every 24 hours
7. 9.8 mg/day
8. At least 30 minutes
9. 125 mg/5 mL
10. 200,000 units/ 5 mL
11. 117 mL
12. Water
13. 15–56 mg/kg
14. 93–347 mg
15. 110–409 mg/daily
16. 40–147 mg/dose; the 125 ordered is correct
17. 910 mg/day
18. 303 mg/dose
19. Yes
20. Add 53 mL water in 2 portions. Shake well after each addition until mixed.
21. Shake well to mix completely before pouring; administer immediately to prevent settling out.
22. 5 mg/kg
23. 307 mg
24. 818 mg
25. 20 mg/kg
26. 1 hour
27. No rapid or bolus injection; no intramuscular or subcutaneous injection
28. 18,000–27,000 mg daily
29. 3–4.5 g/dose
30. No
31. 4 mg/kg
32. 742 mg daily
33. 400 mg daily
34. 371 mg/dose
35. 3 mg/kg per hour over 1–2 hours
36. Not for IV bolus injection
37. 6 mg/kg
38. 3 mg/kg
39. Minimum of three weeks and at least two weeks following resolution of symptoms
40. 109 mg
41. 55 mg
42. Once daily
43. 12 mg/kg/day
44. 196 mg

# ADULT AND PEDIATRIC DOSAGES BASED ON BODY SURFACE AREA

Body surface area (BSA or SA) is a major factor in calculating dosages for a number of drugs, because many of the body's physiologic processes are more closely related to body surface than they are to weight. Body surface is used extensively to calculate dosages of antineoplastic agents for cancer chemotherapy, and for patients with severe burns. However, an increasing number of other drugs is also calculated using BSA. The nursing responsibility for checking dosages based on BSA varies widely in clinical facilities; therefore, this chapter covers all three essentials: calculation of BSA, calculation of dosages based on BSA, and assessment of physician orders based on BSA.

Body surface is calculated in **square meters (m²)** using the patient's **weight and height** and a calculator that has **square root ($\sqrt{\phantom{x}}$)** capabilities. Two formulas are used by physicians and pharmacists: one using kg and cm measurements, and another using lb (pound) and in (inch) measurements. We'll look at these separately.

## CALCULATING BSA FROM kg AND cm

The safest way to calculate BSA is by using a time-tested formula with kilogram and centimeter measurements.

$$BSA = \sqrt{\frac{wt(kg) \times ht(cm)}{3600}}$$

## Objectives

**The learner will:**

1. calculate BSA using formulas for weight and height.

2. use BSA to calculate dosages.

3. assess the accuracy of dosages prescribed on the basis of BSA.

**EXAMPLE 1** Calculate the BSA of a man who weighs **104 kg** and whose height is **191 cm**. Express BSA to the nearest hundredth.

$$\sqrt{\frac{104(\text{kg}) \times 191(\text{cm})}{3600}}$$

$$= \sqrt{5.517}$$

$$= 2.348 = \textbf{2.35 m}^2$$

**Calculators vary in the way a square root must be obtained**. Here is how the BSA was calculated in this example and throughout the chapter:

$$104. \times 191. \div 3600. = 5.517, \text{ then immediately enter } \sqrt{\phantom{x}}$$

Practice with your own calculator to determine how to calculate a square root. Be careful to **insert periods after all whole numbers** or you may obtain a wrong answer from preset decimal placement.

　　**The m² BSA is rounded to hundredths**. Answers may vary slightly depending on how your calculator is set. Consider answers within 2–3 hundredths correct. Fractional weights and heights are also used in calculations. Refer to Examples 2 and 3.

**EXAMPLE 2** Calculate the BSA of an adolescent who weighs **59.1 kg** and is **157.5 cm** in height. Express BSA to the nearest hundredth.

$$\sqrt{\frac{59.1(\text{kg}) \times 157.5(\text{cm})}{3600}}$$

$$= \sqrt{2.585}$$

$$= 1.607 = \textbf{1.61 m}^2$$

**EXAMPLE 3** A child is **96.2 cm** tall and weighs **15.17 kg**. What is his BSA in m² to the nearest hundredth?

$$\sqrt{\frac{15.17(\text{kg}) \times 96.2(\text{cm})}{3600}}$$

$$= \sqrt{0.4053}$$

$$= 0.636 = \textbf{0.63 m}^2$$

## Problems 14.1

**Calculate the BSA in m². Express answers to the nearest hundredth.**

1. An adult weighing 59 kg whose height is 160 cm.　_____

2. A child weighing 35.9 kg whose height is 63.5 cm.　_____

3. A child weighing 7.7 kg whose height is 40 cm.　_____

4.  An adult weighing 92 kg whose height is 178 cm.   _____

5.  A child weighing 46 kg whose height is 102 cm.   _____

**Answers**   **1.** 1.62 m²   **2.** 0.8 m²   **3.** 0.29 m²   **4.** 2.13 m²   **5.** 1.14 m²

## CALCULATING BSA FROM lb AND in

The formula for calculating BSA from lb and in measurements is equally easy to use. **The only difference is the denominator, which is 3131.**

$$BSA = \sqrt{\frac{wt(lb) \times ht(in)}{3131}}$$

EXAMPLE 1   Calculate BSA to the nearest hundredth for a child who is **24 in** tall and weighs **34 lb**.

$$\sqrt{\frac{34(lb) \times 24(in)}{3131}}$$

$$= \sqrt{0.260}$$

$$= 0.510 = \mathbf{0.51\ m^2}$$

EXAMPLE 2   Calculate BSA to the nearest hundredth for an adult who is **61.3 in** tall and weighs **142.7 lb**.

$$\sqrt{\frac{142.7(lb) \times 61.3(in)}{3131}}$$

$$= \sqrt{2.793}$$

$$= 1.671 = \mathbf{1.67\ m^2}$$

EXAMPLE 3   A child weighs **105 lb** and is **51 in** tall. Calculate BSA to the nearest hundredth.

$$\sqrt{\frac{105(lb) \times 51(in)}{3131}}$$

$$= \sqrt{1.710}$$

$$= 1.307 = \mathbf{1.31\ m^2}$$

## Problems 14.2

**Determine the BSA. Express answers to the nearest hundredth.**

1.  A child weighing 92 lb who measures 35 in.   _____

2.  An adult who weighs 175 lb and who is 67 in tall.   _____

3.  An adult who is 70 in tall and weighs 194 lb.   _____

4. A child who weighs 72.4 lb and is 40.5 in tall. _____

5. A child who measures 26 in and weighs 36 lb. _____

**Answers** **1.** 1.01 m² **2.** 1.94 m² **3.** 2.08 m² **4.** 0.97 m² **5.** 0.55 m²

## DOSAGE CALCULATION BASED ON BSA

Once you know the BSA in m², dosage calculation is straight multiplication.

**EXAMPLE 1**  Dosage recommended is **5 mg per m²**. The child has a BSA of **1.1 m²**.

$$1.1 (m^2) \times 5 mg = \textbf{5.5 mg}$$

**EXAMPLE 2**  The recommended child's dosage is 25–50 mg/m². The child has a BSA of **0.76 m²**.

**Lower dosage**   $0.76 (m^2) \times 25 mg = 19 mg$

**Upper dosage**   $0.76 (m^2) \times 50 mg = 38 mg$

**The dosage range is 19–38 mg.**

### Problems 14.3

Determine the dosage for the following drugs. Express answers to the nearest whole number.

1. The recommended child's dosage is 5–10 mg/m².
   The BSA is 0.43 m². _____

2. A child with a BSA of 0.81 m² is to receive a drug with a recommended dosage of 40 mg/m². _____

3. Calculate the recommended dosage of 20 mg/m² for a child with a BSA of 0.51 m². _____

4. An adult is to receive a drug with a recommended dosage of 20–40 units/m². The BSA is 1.93 m². _____

5. The adult recommended dosage is 3–5 mg/m².
   Calculate dosage for 2.08 m². _____

**Answers** **1.** 2–4 mg **2.** 32 mg **3.** 10 mg **4.** 39–77 units **5.** 6–10 mg

## ASSESSING ORDERS BASED ON BSA

In situations where you will have to check a dosage against m² recommendations, you will be referring to drug package inserts, medication protocols, or the *Physicians' Desk Reference* (*PDR*) to determine what the dosage should be.

**EXAMPLE 1**   Refer to the vinblastine information insert in Figure 14-1 and calculate the **first dose** for an adult whose BSA is **1.66 m²**. Calculations are to the nearest whole number.

Recommended first dose  $=$  3.7 mg/m²

$1.66(\text{m}^2) \times 3.7 \text{ mg} = 6.14 = \textbf{6 mg}$

**EXAMPLE 2**   A child with a BSA of 0.96 m² is to receive her **fourth dose** of vinblastine.

Recommended fourth dose  $=$  6.25 mg/m²

$0.96(\text{m}^2) \times 6.25 \text{ mg} = \textbf{6 mg}$

# cetus oncology

## STERILE VINBLASTINE SULFATE, USP

### DOSAGE AND ADMINISTRATION

Caution:  It is extremely important that the needle be properly positioned in the vein before this product is injected.

If leakage into surrounding tissue should occur during intravenous administration of vinblastine sulfate, it may cause considerable irritation.  The injection should be discontinued immediately, and any remaining portion of the dose should then be introduced into another vein.  Local injection of hyaluronidase and the application of moderate heat to the area of leakage help disperse the drug and are thought to minimize discomfort and the possibility of cellulitis.

There are variations in the depth of the leukopenic response which follows therapy with vinblastine sulfate.  For this reason, it is recommended that the drug be given no more frequently than *once every 7 days*.  It is wise to initiate therapy for adults by administering a single intravenous dose  of 3.7 mg/M² of body surface area (bsa); the initial dose for children should be 2.5 mg/M².  Thereafter, white-blood-cell counts should be made to determine the patient's sensitivity to vinblastine sulfate.  A reduction of 50% in the dose of vinblastine is recommended for patients having a direct serum bilirubin value above 3 mg/100 mL.  Since metabolism and excretion are primarily hepatic, no modification is recommended for patients with impaired renal function.

A simplified and conservative incremental approach to dosage *at weekly intervals* may be outlined as follows:

|  | Adults |  | Children |  |
|---|---|---|---|---|
| First dose | 3.7 | mg/M² bsa | 2.5 | mg/M² bsa |
| Second dose | 5.5 | mg/M² bsa | 3.75 | mg/M² bsa |
| Third dose | 7.4 | mg/M² bsa | 5 | mg/M² bsa |
| Fourth dose | 9.25 | mg/M² bsa | 6.25 | mg/M² bsa |
| Fifth dose | 11.1 | mg/M² bsa | 7.5 | mg/M² bsa |

The above-mentioned increases may be used until a maximum dose (not exceeding 18.5 mg/M² bsa for adults and 12.5 mg/M² bsa for children) is reached.  The dose should not be increased after that dose which reduces the white-cell count to approximately 3000 cells/mm³.  In some adults, 3.7 mg/M² bsa may produce this leukopenia; other adults may require more than 11.1mg/M² bsa; and, very rarely, as much as 18.5 mg/M² bsa may be necessary.  For most adult patients, however, the weekly dosage will prove to be 5.5 to 7.4 mg/M² bsa.

**Figure 14-1**

## Problems 14.4

Calculate the following dosages of vinblastine to the nearest whole number from the information available in Figure 14-1.

1. Calculate the dosage for an adult's third dose. The patient's BSA is 1.91 m². _____
2. Calculate the child's first dosage for a patient with a BSA of 1.2 m². _____
3. Calculate the adult's fifth dosage. The BSA is 1.53 m². _____
4. Calculate the child's second dosage for a BSA of 1.01 m². _____
5. Calculate the adult's second dose for a BSA of 2.12 m². _____

**Answers 1.** 14 mg **2.** 3 mg **3.** 17 mg **4.** 4 mg **5.** 12 mg

## Problems 14.5

Refer to Figure 14-2 for BiCNU® to locate the following information. Express all dosages to the nearest whole number.

1. What is the dosage per m² if the drug is to be given in a single dose? _____
2. If the patient has a BSA of 1.91 m², what will the daily dosage range be? _____
3. If the order for this patient is a single dosage of 325 mg, is there any need to question it? _____
4. If the dosage ordered is 450 mg, is there any need to question it? _____

# BiCNU ®
## (carmustine for injection)

**DOSAGE AND ADMINISTRATION**
The recommended dose of BiCNU as a single agent in previously untreated patients is 150 to 200 mg/m² intravenously every 6 weeks. This may be given as a single dose or divided into daily injections such as 75 to 100 mg/m² on 2 successive days. When BiCNU is used in combination with other myelosuppressive drugs or in patients in whom bone marrow reserve is depleted, the doses should be adjusted accordingly.

**Figure 14-2**

**Answers 1.** 150–200 mg/m² **2.** 287–382 mg **3.** No **4.** Yes, too high

## Problems 14.6

**Refer to the package insert for the antineoplastic medication bleomycin in Figure 14-3 to answer the following questions.**

1. Locate the dosage information on Hodgkin's disease and identify the dosage per m². _____

2. This insert also identifies the dosage per kg. What is this dosage? _____

3. Calculate the unit dosage based on m² for an adult with a BSA of 1.73 m². _____

4. How often is dosage recommended? _____

**BLEOMYCIN FOR INJECTION USP**

BLE-P03

**Rx ONLY**

To reduce the development of drug-resistant bacteria and maintain the effectiveness of bleomycin and other antibacterial drugs, bleomycin should be used only to treat or prevent infections that are proven or strongly suspected to be caused by bacteria.

**WARNING**

It is recommended that bleomycin be administered under the supervision of a qualified physician experienced in the use of cancer chemotherapeutic agents. Appropriate management of therapy and complications is possible only when adequate diagnostic and treatment facilities are readily available.

Pulmonary fibrosis is the most severe toxicity associated with bleomycin. The most frequent presentation is pneumonitis occasionally progressing to pulmonary fibrosis. Its occurrence is higher in elderly patients and in those receiving greater than 400 units total dose, but pulmonary toxicity has been observed in young patients and those treated with low doses.

A severe idiosyncratic reaction consisting of hypotension, mental confusion, fever, chills, and wheezing has been reported in approximately 1% of lymphoma patients treated with bleomycin.

**DOSAGE AND ADMINISTRATION**

**Because of the possibility of an anaphylactoid reaction, lymphoma patients should be treated with 2 units or less for the first two doses. If no acute reaction occurs, then the regular dosage schedule may be followed.**

The following dose schedule is recommended:

**Squamous cell carcinoma, non-Hodgkin's lymphoma, testicular carcinoma**—0.25 to 0.50 units/kg (10 to 20 units/m²) given intravenously, intramuscularly, or subcutaneously weekly or twice weekly.

**Hodgkin's Disease**—0.25 to 0.50 units/kg (10 to 20 units/m²) given intravenously, intramuscularly, or subcutaneously weekly or twice weekly. After a 50% response, a maintenance dose of 1 unit daily or 5 units weekly intravenously or intramuscularly should be given.

Pulmonary toxicity of bleomycin appears to be dose related with a striking increase when the total dose is over 400 units. Total doses over 400 units should be given with great caution.

**Note: When bleomycin for injection is used in combination with other antineoplastic agents, pulmonary toxicities may occur at lower doses.**

Improvement of Hodgkin's Disease and testicular tumors is prompt and noted within 2 weeks. If no improvement is seen by this time, improvement is unlikely Squamous cell cancers respond more slowly, sometimes requiring as long as 3 weeks before any improvement is noted.

**Malignant Pleural Effusion**–60 units administered as a single dose bolus intrapleural injection (see **Administration: Intrapleural**).

**Figure 14-3**

**Answers   1.** 10–20 units/m²   **2.** 0.25 to 0.5 units/kg   **3.** 17–35 units   **4.** Weekly or twice weekly

## Problems 14.7

**Refer to the mitomycin package insert information in Figure 14-4 to answer the following questions.**

1. This preparation is a combination of two different drugs. It is shipped in powdered form. How much diluent must be added to prepare a mitomycin 40 mg and mannitol 80 mg dosage strength? _____

2. What kind of diluent is specified? _____

3. What dosage is required in m²? _____

4. What mitomycin dosage will be required for an individual with a BSA of 1.73? _____

5. How will this be administered? _____

Used with permission from Bedford Laboratories, A Division of Ben Venue Laboratories Inc. A Boehringer-Ingelheim Company.

**BEDFORD**
L A B O R A T O R I E S™

# MITOMYCIN FOR INJECTION, USP
## Rx ONLY.

**DOSAGE AND ADMINISTRATION**

Mitomycin should be given intravenously only, using care to avoid extravasation of the compound. If extravasation occurs, cellulitis, ulceration, and slough may result.

Each vial contains either mitomycin 5 mg and mannitol 10 mg, or mitomycin 20 mg and mannitol 40 mg, or mitomycin 40 mg and mannitol 80 mg. To administer, add Sterile Water for Injection, 10 mL 40 mL, or 80 mL, respectively. Shake to dissolve. If product does not dissolve immediately, allow to stand at room temperature until solution is obtained.

After full hematological recovery (see guide to dosage adjustment) from any previous chemotherapy, the following dosage schedule may be used at 6- to 8-week intervals:

   20 mg/m² intravenously as a single dose via a functioning intravenous catheter.

Because of cumulative myelosuppression, patients should be fully reevaluated after each course of mitomycin, and the dose reduced if the patient has experienced any toxicities. Doses greater than 20 mg/m² have not been shown to be more effective and are more toxic than lower doses.

**Figure 14-4**

**Answers** **1.** 80 mL  **2.** Sterile Water for Injection  **3.** mitomycin 20 mg/m²  **4.** 35 mg
**5.** Intravenously as a single dose via a functioning intravenous catheter

## Summary

**This concludes the chapter on dosage calculation based on BSA. The important points to remember from this chapter are:**

 The BSA in m² is calculated from a patient's weight and height.

 BSA is more important than weight alone in calculating some drug dosages because many physiologic processes are more closely related to surface area than they are to weight.

 BSA is calculated in square meters (m²) using a formula.

 Two formulas for calculation of BSA are available:

Using kg and cm: $\sqrt{\dfrac{wt(kg) \times ht(cm)}{3600}}$     Using lb and in: $\sqrt{\dfrac{wt(lb) \times ht(in)}{3131}}$

 After the BSA has been obtained, it can be used to calculate specific drug dosages and assess accuracy of physician orders.

## Summary Self-Test

**Use the formula method to calculate the following BSAs. Express m² to the nearest hundredth.**

1. The weight is 58 lb and the height is 36 in.                                    _____

2. An adult weighing 74 kg and measuring 160 cm.                                   _____

3. A child who is 14.2 kg and measures 64 cm.                                      _____

4. An adult weighing 69 kg whose height is 170 cm.                                 _____

5. An adolescent who is 55 in and 103 lb.                                          _____

6. A child who is 112 cm and weighs 25.3 kg.                                       _____

7. An adult who weighs 55 kg and measures 157.5 cm.                                _____

8. An adult who weighs 65.4 kg and is 132 cm in height.                            _____

9. A child whose height is 58 in and whose weight is 26.5 lb.                      _____

10. A child whose height is 60 cm and weight is 13.6 kg.                           _____

**Read the drug insert information provided in Figure 14-5 to answer the following questions. Calculate dosages to the nearest whole number.**

11. Read the information on children's dosage to calculate the daily dosage for a 6-year-old child whose BSA is 0.78 m².                                              _____

12. If a dosage of 4 mg is ordered for this 6-year-old child, would you question it?                                              _____

13. What would the daily dosage be for a 4-year-old child whose BSA is 0.29 m²?                                              _____

14. What would the daily dosage be for a 5-year-old child with a BSA of 0.51 m²?                                              _____

# Antibiotic

**DOSAGE AND ADMINISTRATION**

DOSAGE SHOULD BE INDIVIDUALIZED ACCORDING TO THE NEEDS AND THE RESPONSE OF THE PATIENT.
Each tablet contains 4 mg of antibiotic.

*Pediatric Patients*

*Age 2 to 6 years*
The total daily dosage for pediatric patients may be calculated on the basis of body weight or body area using approximately 0.25 mg/kg/day or 8 mg per square meter of body surface (8 mg/m²).
The usual dose is 2 mg (½ tablet) two or three times a day, adjusted as necessary to the size and response of the patient. The dose is not to exceed 12 mg a day.

*Age 7 to 14 years*
The usual dose is 4 mg (1 tablet) two or three times a day, adjusted as necessary to the size and response of the patient. The dose is not to exceed 16 mg a day.

*Adults*
The total daily dose for adults should not exceed 0.5 mg/kg/day.
The therapeutic range is 4 to 20 mg a day, with the majority of patients requiring 12 to 16 mg a day. An occasional patient may require as much as 32 mg a day for adequate relief. It is suggested that dosage be initiated with 4 mg (1 tablet) three times a day and adjusted according to the size and response of the patient.

Delmar/Cengage Learning.

**Figure 14-5**

### Refer to Figure 14-6 to answer the following questions.

15. A patient is to be treated with the drug carboplatin for ovarian carcinoma. Her BSA is 1.61 m$^2$. What will her dosage be?    _____

16. Another patient with ovarian cancer, who weighs 130 lb and measures 62 in, is to receive carboplatin. What is her BSA?    _____

17. What dosage of carboplatin will she require?    _____

18. Carboplatin is given in conjunction with cyclophosphamide. What is the recommended m$^2$ dosage for this drug?    _____

19. Calculate the BSA of a third patient who is receiving therapy for ovarian cancer. She weighs 53.2 kg and measures 150.3 cm.    _____

20. What will the companion dosage of cyclophosphamide be for this patient?    _____

Manufactured by:
Ben Venue Laboratories, Inc.
Bedford, OH 44146

Manufactured for:
Bedford Laboratories™
Bedford, OH 44146

**Patient Information**
## CARBOplatin for Injection

Read this entire leaflet carefully.
**Keep it for future reference.**

This information will help you learn more about CARBOplatin for Injection. It cannot, however, cover all the possible warnings or side effects relating to CARBOplatin, and it does not list all of the benefits and risks of CARBOplatin. Your doctor should always be your first choice for detailed information about your medical condition and your treatment. Be sure to ask your doctor about any questions you may have.

**DOSAGE AND ADMINISTRATION**

**NOTE: Aluminum reacts with carboplatin causing precipitate formation and loss of potency, therefore, needles or intravenous sets containing aluminum parts that may come in contact with the drug must not be used for the preparation or administration of carboplatin.**

**Single Agent Therapy**

Carboplatin for injection, as a single agent, has been shown to be effective in patients with recurrent ovarian carcinoma at a dosage of 360 mg/m$^2$ IV on day 1 every 4 weeks (alternatively see **Formula Dosing**). In general, however, single intermittent courses of carboplatin should not be repeated until the neutrophil count is at least 2000 and the platelet count is at least 100,000.

**Combination Therapy with Cyclophosphamide**

In the chemotherapy of advanced ovarian cancer, an effective combination for previously untreated patients consists of:
Carboplatin injection—300 mg/m$^2$ IV on day 1 every four weeks for six cycles (alternatively see **Formula Dosing**).
Cyclophosphamide—600 mg/m$^2$ IV on day 1 every four weeks for six cycles. For directions regarding the use and administration of cyclophosphamide please refer to its package insert. (See **CLINICAL STUDIES**.)

**Figure 14-6**

| Answers | | | |
|---|---|---|---|
| **1.** 0.82 m$^2$ | **6.** 0.89 m$^2$ | **12.** Yes; too low | **18.** 600 mg |
| **2.** 1.81 m$^2$ | **7.** 1.55 m$^2$ | **13.** 2 mg per day | **19.** 1.49 m$^2$ |
| **3.** 0.50 m$^2$ | **8.** 1.55 m$^2$ | **14.** 4 mg | **20.** 894 mg |
| **4.** 1.81 m$^2$ | **9.** 0.70 m$^2$ | **15.** 580 mg | |
| **5.** 1.35 m$^2$ | **10.** 0.48 m$^2$ | **16.** 1.6 m$^2$ | |
| | **11.** 6 mg per day | **17.** 576 mg | |

# SECTION 6

# Intravenous Calculations

**CHAPTER 15**
Introduction to IV Therapy  /  214

**CHAPTER 16**
IV Flow Rate Calculation  /  229

**CHAPTER 17**
Calculating IV Infusion and
Completion Times  /  247

**CHAPTER 18**
IV Medication and Titration
Calculations  /  262

**CHAPTER 19**
Heparin Infusion
Calculations  /  276

# INTRODUCTION TO IV THERAPY

## Objectives

The learner will:

1. differentiate between primary, secondary, peripheral, and central IV lines.

2. explain the function of IV drip chambers, roller and slide clamps, and on-line and indwelling injection ports.

3. differentiate between heparin flush and heparin admixture dosage strengths.

4. differentiate between volumetric pumps, syringe pumps, and PCAs.

5. identify the abbreviations used for IV fluid orders.

The calculations associated with IV therapy will be easier to understand if you have some general understanding of IV therapy. Intravenous fluid and medication administration is one of the most challenging of all nursing responsibilities. There are currently estimated to be over 200 different manufactured IV fluids, and at least as many additives are used with IV fluids, including medications, electrolytes, and nutrients. In addition, there are hundreds of different types of IV administration sets and components, and dozens of different models of electronic infusion devices (EIDs) to infuse and monitor IV fluids. This would appear to make the entire subject of IV therapy overwhelming, but it is not. This chapter presents the essentials in understandable segments and will provide you with an excellent base of instruction upon which to build. Let's begin by looking at a basic sterile IV setup, which is referred to as a primary line.

## PRIMARY LINE

Refer to Figure 15-1, which shows a typical primary IV line connecting an IV fluid bag or bottle to the needle or cannula in a vein. The IV **tubing is connected to the IV solution bag** (using sterile technique), and the bag is hung on an IV stand.

**Close all roller clamps on the IV tubing before connecting it to the solution bag. This step prevents air bubbles from entering the tubing.**

The **drip chamber**, Figure 15-1A, is then squeezed to **half-fill** it with fluid. This level is very important because **IV flow rates are set and monitored by counting the drops falling in this chamber**. If the chamber is too full, the drops cannot be counted. On the other hand, if the outlet at the bottom of the chamber is not completely covered, air can enter the tubing during infusions and, subsequently, the vein and circulatory system. So, the half-full fluid level is extremely important.

**The correct fluid level for IV drip chambers is half-full to allow drops to be counted and prevent air from entering the tubing.**

**Figure 15-1** | IV tubing and solution bag. Courtesy of Abbott Laboratories.

Next, notice Figure 15-1B, the **roller clamp**. This is adjusted while the drops falling in the drip chamber are counted to **set the flow rate**. It provides an extremely accurate control of rate. A second type of clamp, Figure 15-1C, called a **slide clamp**, is present on all IV tubings. The **slide clamp** can be used to **temporarily stop an IV without disturbing the rate set** on the roller clamp.

Next, notice Figure 15-1D, the **injection port**. Rubber ports are located in several locations on the tubing, typically near the cannula end, drip chamber, and middle of the line, and also on most IV solution bags. **Ports allow injection of medication directly into the line or bag** or the **attachment to the primary line of secondary IV lines** containing compatible IV fluids or medications.

**Intravenous fluids run by gravity flow.** This necessitates that the IV solution bag be hung **above the patient's heart level** to exert sufficient pressure to infuse. Three feet above heart level is considered an average height.

> The higher an IV bag is hung, the greater the pressure and the faster the IV will infuse.

This pressure differential also means that if the flow rate is adjusted while the patient is lying in bed, it will slow down if he or she sits or stands, and, in fact, it changes slightly with each turn from side to side. For this reason, **monitoring IV flow rate is ongoing,** officially **done every hour,** but routinely checked **after each major position change.**

There are two additional terms relating to primary lines that you must know. If an arm or hand (or, less commonly, leg) vein is used for an infusion, it is referred to as a **peripheral line.** This is to distinguish it from a **central line,** which uses a special catheter whose tip is located centrally **in a deep chest vein.** Central lines may access the chest vein directly through the chest wall, via a neck vein, or through a peripheral vein in the arm or leg.

## SECONDARY LINE

Secondary lines attach to the primary line at an injection port. They are used primarily **to infuse medications,** frequently on an intermittent basis; for example, every 6–8 hours. They may also be used to infuse other compatible IV fluids. Secondary lines are commonly referred to as **IV piggybacks.** They are abbreviated **IVPB.** Refer to Figure 15-2, which illustrates a primary and secondary line setup.

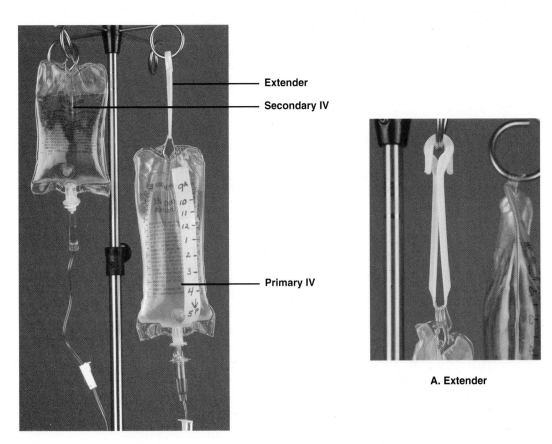

**Figure 15-2** | Primary and secondary IV setup. Courtesy of Abbott Laboratories.

The IVPB is connected to a port located below the drip chamber on the primary line. Notice that **the IVPB bag is hanging higher than the primary**. This gives it greater pressure and causes it to **infuse first**. Each IVPB set includes a plastic or metal **extender**, in Figure 15-2A, which is used to lower the primary solution bag to obtain this pressure differential. The flow rate for the IVPB is set by a separate roller clamp located on the secondary line. When the IVPB bag has emptied, the primary line will automatically resume its flow. Secondary medication bags are usually much smaller than primary bags. Fifty, 100, 150, 200, and 250 mL bags are frequently used.

Another type of secondary medication setup is provided by Abbott Laboratories **ADD-Vantage System**® (Figure 15-3). In this system, a specially designed IV fluid bag that contains a **medication vial port** is used. The medication vial containing the ordered drug and dosage is inserted into the port, and the drug (frequently in powdered form) is mixed using IV fluid as the diluent, as illustrated in Figure 15-4. The vial contents are then displaced back into the solution bag and thoroughly mixed in the total solution before infusion. The vial remains in the solution bag port throughout the infusion, making it possible to cross-check the vial label for drug and dosage at any time.

**Figure 15-3** | ADD-Vantage System® Courtesy of Abbott Laboratories.

If a drug is not available in either a prepackaged or ADD-Vantage format, it is often prepared and labeled by the hospital pharmacy. And, finally, an IV medication may be prepared, added to the appropriate IV fluid, thoroughly mixed, labeled and initialed, and administered by the nurse who initiates the infusion.

A

B

C

D

**Figure 15-4** | ADD-Vantage® System **A**, The ADD-Vantage® medication vial is opened first. **B**, The medication vial port on the IV bag is opened. **C**, The vial top is inserted into the IV bag port and twisted to lock tightly in place. **D**, The vial stopper is removed "inside" the IV bag, and the medication and solution are thoroughly mixed before infusion. Courtesy of Abbott Laboratories.

## VOLUME-CONTROLLED BURETTES

For greater accuracy in the measurement of **small-volume** IV medications and fluids, a **calibrated burette chamber** such as the one shown in Figure 15-5 may be used. The total capacity of burettes varies from 100 to 150 mL, calibrated in 1 mL increments. Many burettes are calibrated to deliver very small drops (microdrops), which also contributes to their accuracy. Burettes are most often referred to by their trade names; for example, Buretrols®, Solusets®, or Volutrols®. Burette chambers are most often connected to a secondary solution bag and used as a secondary line, but they can also be primary lines. When medication is ordered, it is injected into the burette through its injection port. The exact amount of IV fluid is then added as a diluent. After thorough mixing, the flow rate is set using a separate clamp on the burette line. Burettes are used extensively in pediatric and intensive care units, where medication dosages and fluid volumes are critical.

## INDWELLING INFUSION PORTS/ INTERMITTENT LOCKS

When a continuous IV is not necessary, but intermittent IV medication administration is, an **infusion port adapter** (Figure 15-6) can be attached to an indwelling cannula in a vein. Infusion ports are frequently referred to as **heplocks** or **saline locks (or ports)**. This terminology evolved because the ports must be irrigated with 1–2 mL of sterile saline every 6–8 hours, or with a heparin lock flush solution (100 units/mL) to prevent clotting and blockage. To infuse medication, the port top is cleansed and the medication line is attached. When the infusion is complete, the line is disconnected until the next dosage is due. Ports are also used for **direct injection of medication using a syringe**, which is called an **IV push** or **bolus**.

Heparin anticoagulant therapy will be discussed in detail in a later chapter, where you will learn that heparin is most commonly diluted in large volume intravenous solutions for administration. **The heparin vial dosage strengths available for IV dilution range from 1000 to 50,000 units/mL.** Stop now, and think about the **enormous difference in dosage strengths between heparin flush solutions and intravenous admixture dosages: 10 to 100 units/mL for a flush; 1000 to 50,000 units/mL for IV admixes.**

These large differences in dosage strength demonstrate why **extreme caution is necessary in heparin flush dosage preparation.**

Delmar/Cengage Learning.

**Figure 15-5** | A calibrated burette chamber.

Delmar/Cengage Learning.

**Figure 15-6** | An infusion port adapter.

## HEPARIN FLUSH DOSAGE ALERT

Heparin flush solutions used to maintain patent (open) indwelling infusion ports come in **two dosage strengths: 10 units/mL and 100 units/mL.** Refer to the Heparin Lock Flush vial label in Figure 15-7 and identify its 10 units/mL strength.

In early 2008 errors in heparin flush dosages became national news when actor Dennis Quaid publicized the near-death of his newborn twins by not one, but two successive errors in flush dosages, which caused the newborns to almost hemorrhage to death.

Thanks to Mr. Quaid, this error was taken all the way to a Congressional hearing to publicize the danger. Similar heparin vial size and label colors were cited as contributing to the errors. But the fact remains that **these errors in dosage were caused by failure to correctly identify label dosage strengths,** not vial size or label color.

**Figure 15-7**

 The average heparin flush dosage strength is 10 units and never exceeds 100 units.

## Problems 15.1

**Answer the questions about IV administration sets as briefly as possible.**

1. What is the correct fluid level for an IV drip chamber? _____

2. Which clamp is used to regulate IV flow rate? _____

3. When might a slide clamp be used? _____

4. What is a peripheral line? _____

5. What is a central line? _____

6. What is the common abbreviation for an intravenous piggyback? _____

7. Is the IVPB a primary or secondary line? _____

8. What must the height of a primary solution bag be when a secondary bag is infusing? _____

9. When is a saline lock used? _____

10. What are the two strengths of heparin
    flush solutions available? _____

**Answers** **1.** Middle of chamber   **2.** Roller clamp   **3.** Stop the IV temporarily without disturbing
the rate set on the roller clamp   **4.** Arm or leg vein   **5.** IV catheter inserted into a deep chest vein
**6.** IVPB   **7.** Secondary   **8.** Lower than secondary bag   **9.** For intermittent infusions when a
continuous IV is not necessary   **10.** 10 units/mL and 100 units/mL

## VOLUMETRIC PUMPS

Refer now to Figure 15-8 of the Alaris® SE Dual pump. Notice that the IV tubing
with the AccuSlide® flow regulator has been inserted into the channels on the right
and left. The center pumping mechanism maintains the desired flow rates.

All volumetric pumps look similar, and may physically resemble the Alaris SE
pump, but the **functions of different models vary widely**. Some models continue to
pump fluids even if an IV infiltrates, whereas others have a built-in pressure sensor
that will sound an alarm if a resultant increased infusion resistance pressure occurs.
Some models sound an alarm when the solution has completely infused; other
models do not.

Because of the wide variation in pump models and their functions, caution is
mandatory when they are used. It is estimated that a significant number of IV medication errors results from errors in pump programming.

 Hospital or clinical in-service education is required for the use of all
infusion devices.

**Figure 15-8** | Alaris® SE Dual Pump, with Guardrails. Courtesy of
Cardinal Health, Inc., 2008. All rights reserved.

**Figure 15-9** | Outlook™ 200 Safety Infusion System. Courtesy of B. Braun Medical, Inc.

Infusion devices are also widely used for IV medication administration, and their precautions in use apply less to the difficulty of the skill than in becoming familiar with the particular infusion model being used. A single hospital or clinic could realistically have a dozen different models in use, and it is an ongoing nursing responsibility to learn how to use each particular model.

 **Double-checking of programming is mandatory in the use of infusion devices.**

Because errors in infusion device programming are a factor in IV medication errors, it is mandatory that all programming be double-checked. A new generation of sophisticated infusion safety systems has built-in libraries of usual drug dosages, offers customizable drug libraries for facility-specific needs, and is capable of alerting users to programming errors outside hospital-defined parameters. The B. Braun Outlook™ 200 illustrated in Figure 15-9 is one example. Another dose-specific pump is the Alaris System with Guardrails® Suite MX of safety software shown in Figure 15-10, a lightweight, modular platform that integrates infusion, patient monitoring, and clinical best-practice guidelines. As you can clearly see from the photograph, this is an infusion device that requires in-service instruction and certification to use.

**Figure 15-10** | Alaris® PC System. Courtesy of Cardinal Health, 2008. All rights reserved.

**Figure 15-11** | Perfusor® Basic. Courtesy of B. Braun Medical, Inc.

## SYRINGE PUMPS

Syringe pumps, as their name implies, are devices that **use a syringe to administer medications or fluids** (Figure 15-11). Syringe pumps are particularly valuable when **drugs that cannot be mixed with other solutions or medications must be administered at a controlled rate over a short period of time**; for example, 5, 10, or 20 minutes. The drug is measured in the syringe, which is inserted into the device, and the medication is infused at the rate set.

## PATIENT-CONTROLLED ANALGESIA (PCA) DEVICES

PCA devices allow a patient to **self-administer medication to control pain**. A prefilled syringe or medication bag containing pain medication is inserted into the device (Figure 15-12), and the **dosage and frequency of administration ordered are set**. The patient presses the control button as medication is needed, and the medication is administered and recorded by the PCA.

The device also keeps a record of the number of times a patient **attempts** to use it and thus provides a record of the effectiveness of the dosage prescribed. If a patient's pain is not being relieved, new orders must be obtained and the PCA reset to administer the new dosage.

 All electronic devices must be monitored frequently to be sure they are functioning properly.

Is the IV infusing at the rate that was set? Is the patient who activates a PCA getting relief of pain? If not, is it possible the PCA itself is malfunctioning? Electronic devices have been in use for many years and are relatively trouble-free, but if the desired goal is not being obtained, in the absence of other obvious reasons, **the possibility of malfunction must always be considered**.

**Figure 15-12** | Syndeo PCA (patient-controlled analgesia syringe pump). Courtesy of Baxter Medication Delivery.

## Problems 15.2

**Answer the questions about infusion devices as briefly as possible.**

1. What is the function of a volumetric pump? _____

2. List two major precautions in the use of volumetric pumps. _____

3. When might a syringe pump be used? _____

4. What is a PCA? _____

**Answers** **1.** To administer IVs at a controlled rate **2.** Accurate programming; rate and site monitoring
**3.** To infuse small volumes of drugs that are not compatible with other drugs and/or fluids
**4.** Patient-controlled analgesia device

# INTRODUCTION TO IV FLUIDS

Intravenous fluids are prepared in plastic solution bags or glass bottles in volumes ranging from 50 mL (bags only) to 1000 mL. The 500 and 1000 mL sizes are the most commonly used. The bags and bottles are labeled with the **complete name** of the fluid they contain, and the fine print under the solution name identifies the exact amount of each component of the fluid. **Orders and charting**, however, are done **using abbreviations**.

In IV fluid abbreviations, D identifies dextrose; W identifies water; S identifies saline; NS identifies normal saline; and numbers identify percentage (%) strengths.

Solutions may be abbreviated in different ways; for example, D5W, 5%D/W, D5%W, or other combinations. But the **initials and percentage have the identical meaning regardless of the way they are abbreviated**. Normal saline solutions are frequently written with the 0.9, or % sign included; for example, D5 0.9NS, or D5 0.9%S. Solutions with different percentages of saline are also available: 0.45%, often written as 1/2 (0.45% is half of 0.9%), and 0.225%, sometimes written as 1/4 (¼ of 0.9) are examples. Some typical orders might be abbreviated D5 1/2S or D5 1/4NS.

Another commonly used solution is **Ringer's lactate**, a balanced electrolyte solution, which is also called Lactated Ringer's Solution. As you would now expect, this solution is abbreviated **RL, LR**, or **RLS**. Electrolytes may also be added to the basic fluids (DW and DS) just discussed. One electrolyte so commonly added that it must be mentioned is **potassium chloride**, which is abbreviated **KCl**. It is measured in milliequivalents (**mEq**).

## Problems 15.3

List the components and percentage strengths of the IV solutions.

1. D10NS _____

2. D5NS _____

3. D2.5 1/2S _____

4. D5 1/4S _____

5. D20W _____

6. D5NS 20 mEq KCl _____

7. D5RL _____

**Answers**  **1.** 10% dextrose in 0.9% saline  **2.** 5% dextrose in normal (0.9%) saline  **3.** 2.5% dextrose in 0.45% saline  **4.** 5% dextrose in 0.225% saline  **5.** 20% dextrose in water  **6.** 5% dextrose in 0.9% saline with 20 mEq potassium chloride  **7.** 5% dextrose in Ringer's lactate solution

## PERCENTAGES IN IV FLUIDS

You will recall that **percent means grams of drug per 100 mL of fluid**. This means that a 5% dextrose solution will have 5 g of dextrose in each 100 mL. A 500 mL bag of a 5% solution will contain 5 g × 5, or 25 g of dextrose, whereas 500 mL of a 10% solution contains 10 g × 5, or 50 g of dextrose. The fine print on IV labels always lists the name and amount of all ingredients.

The Ringer's lactate solution in Figure 15-13 illustrates this very well. Take a minute to read the components of this solution.

The point being made here is that **percentages make IV fluids significantly different from each other**. As with drugs, reading labels and making sure the IVs are administered as ordered is critically important.

**Figure 15-13** | IV Solution label: D$_s$LR.

## PARENTERAL NUTRITION

One of the options available for providing nutrition when a patient is unable to eat is to **administer a nutrient solution via a central vein**. This is referred to as parenteral nutrition. The solutions infused are generally of a high caloric content and contain varying percentages of glucose, amino acids, and/or fat emulsions. A number of abbreviations/descriptions are used for parenteral nutrients. Some of the more common are **total parenteral nutrition (TPN), partial parenteral nutrition (PPN), and hyperalimentation (nutrition in excess of maintenance needs)**. There is a noticeable difference in fluids that contain lipids (fat, intralipids) in that they are **opaque-white** in appearance, not unlike nonfat milk. These fluids are normally **infused slowly,** but **not usually over a period of more than 24 hours because they can spoil and support bacterial growth**. All precautions applicable to IVs in general apply equally to parenteral nutrients, with more care necessary for the IV site to prevent infection. Flow rate and infusion time calculations covered in subsequent chapters are also applicable for parenteral nutrition solutions.

## CALCULATING gtt/min FLOW RATES FROM mL/hr ORDERED

The flow rate in **gtt/min** is calculated from the **calibration of the IV set being used**, either 10, 15, 20, or 60 gtt/mL, and the **mL/hr ordered**. You will immediately notice a difference from the previous DA calculations you have learned because **this calculation includes two values: gtt and min**. However, the DA calculation steps are identical.

**EXAMPLE 1**    Calculate a **gtt/min** flow rate to infuse **125 mL/hr** using a set calibrated at **10 gtt/mL**.

- Enter the **gtt/min** to be calculated as a **common fraction** followed by an equal sign.

$$\frac{gtt}{min} =$$

- **Begin ratio entries as if you were calculating only the gtt numerator.** Locate the ratio containing gtt—the 10 gtt/mL set calibration. Enter 10 gtt as the numerator to match the gtt numerator being calculated; 1 mL becomes the denominator.

$$\frac{gtt}{min} = \frac{10 \ gtt}{1 \ mL}$$

- Match the mL denominator with the 125 mL of the 125 mL/hr ordered; 1 hr becomes the denominator.

$$\frac{gtt}{min} = \frac{10 \ gtt}{1 \ mL} \times \frac{125 \ mL}{1 \ hr}$$

- **Enter a 1 hr equals 60 min conversion ratio,** with 1 hr as the numerator and 60 min as the denominator. Notice that **the min being calculated falls automatically into place** as the final denominator to complete the equation.

$$\frac{gtt}{min} = \frac{10 \ gtt}{1 \ mL} \times \frac{125 \ mL}{1 \ hr} \times \frac{1 \ hr}{60 \ min}$$

- Cancel the mL, mL and hr, and hr denominator/numerators to check for correct ratio entry. Do the math.

$$\frac{gtt}{min} = \frac{10 \ gtt}{1 \ mL} \times \frac{125 \ mL}{1 \ hr} \times \frac{1 \ hr}{60 \ min} = 20.8 = \textbf{21 gtt/min}$$

**To infuse 125 mL/hr using a 10 gtt/mL infusion set, the flow rate is 21 gtt/min.**

 Flow rates are rounded to the nearest whole gtt.

**EXAMPLE 2**    A **20 gtt/mL** set is used to infuse **90 mL/hr**. Calculate the **gtt/min** flow rate.

- Enter the gtt/min to be calculated followed by an equal sign.

$$\frac{gtt}{min} =$$

- Enter the 20 gtt/mL infusion set ratio with 20 gtt to match the gtt numerator being calculated; 1 mL becomes the denominator.

$$\frac{gtt}{min} = \frac{20\ gtt}{1\ mL}$$

- Match the mL denominator with the 90 mL of the mL/hr ordered; 1 hr is the new denominator.

$$\frac{gtt}{min} = \frac{20\ gtt}{1\ mL} \times \frac{90\ mL}{1\ hr}$$

- Enter a 1 hr equals 60 min conversion ratio, with 1 hr as the numerator and 60 min as the denominator, to complete the equation.

$$\frac{gtt}{min} = \frac{20\ gtt}{1\ mL} \times \frac{90\ mL}{1\ hr} \times \frac{1\ hr}{60\ min}$$

- Cancel the mL, mL and hr, and hr denominator/numerators to check for correct ratio entry. Do the math.

$$\frac{gtt}{min} = \frac{20\ gtt}{1\ \cancel{mL}} \times \frac{90\ \cancel{mL}}{1\ \cancel{hr}} \times \frac{1\ \cancel{hr}}{60\ min} = \textbf{30 gtt/min}$$

**To infuse 90 mL/hr using a set calibrated at 20 gtt/mL, the rate is 30 gtt/min.**

---

**EXAMPLE 3**    Calculate the **gtt/min** rate to infuse **2500 mL** in **24 hr** using a **15 gtt/mL** infusion set.

- Enter the gtt/min to be calculated followed by an equal sign.

$$\frac{gtt}{min} =$$

- Enter the 15 gtt/mL infusion set ratio with 15 gtt to match the gtt numerator being calculated; 1 mL becomes the denominator.

$$\frac{gtt}{min} = \frac{15\ gtt}{1\ mL}$$

- Enter the 2500 mL/24 hr ordered with 2500 mL as the numerator to match the previous mL denominator. Enter 24 hr as the new denominator.

$$\frac{gtt}{min} = \frac{15\ gtt}{1\ mL} \times \frac{2500\ mL}{24\ hr}$$

- Enter a 1 hr equals 60 min conversion ratio, with 1 hr as the numerator and 60 min as the denominator, to complete the equation.

$$\frac{gtt}{min} = \frac{15\ gtt}{1\ mL} \times \frac{2500\ mL}{24\ hr} \times \frac{1\ hr}{60\ min}$$

- Cancel the mL, mL and hr, and hr denominator/numerators to check for correct ratio entry. Do the math.

$$\frac{gtt}{min} = \frac{15\ gtt}{1\ \cancel{mL}} \times \frac{2500\ \cancel{mL}}{24\ \cancel{hr}} \times \frac{1\ \cancel{hr}}{60\ min} = 26.04 = \textbf{26 gtt/min}$$

**To infuse 2500 mL in 24 hr using a 15 gtt/mL calibrated infusion set, the rate is 26 gtt/min.**

**EXAMPLE 4**   Calculate the **gtt/min** rate to infuse **2000 mL** in **10 hr** using a **10 gtt/mL** IV infusion set.

- Enter the gtt/min to be calculated followed by an equal sign.

$$\frac{gtt}{min} =$$

- Enter the 10 gtt/mL infusion set ratio with 10 gtt as the numerator to match the gtt numerator being calculated; 1 mL becomes the denominator.

$$\frac{gtt}{min} = \frac{10\ gtt}{1\ mL}$$

- Enter the 2000 mL in 10 hr ordered with 2000 mL as the numerator to match the previous mL denominator; 10 hr is the next denominator to be matched.

$$\frac{gtt}{min} = \frac{10\ gtt}{1\ mL} \times \frac{2000\ mL}{10\ hr}$$

- Enter a 1 hr equals 60 min conversion ratio, with 1 hr as the numerator and 60 min as the denominator, to complete the equation.

$$\frac{gtt}{min} = \frac{10\ gtt}{1\ mL} \times \frac{2000\ mL}{10\ hr} \times \frac{1\ hr}{60\ min}$$

- Cancel the mL, mL and hr, and hr denominator/numerators to check for correct ratio entry. Do the math.

$$\frac{gtt}{min} = \frac{10\ gtt}{1\ \cancel{mL}} \times \frac{2000\ \cancel{mL}}{10\ \cancel{hr}} \times \frac{1\ \cancel{hr}}{60\ min} = 33.3 = \textbf{33 gtt/min}$$

**To infuse 2000 mL in 10 hr using a 10 gtt/mL calibrated infusion set, the rate is 33 gtt/min.**

## Problems 16.2

**Calculate gtt/min flow rates. Round to the nearest whole gtt.**

1. An IV of 2000 mL is to infuse in 12 hr using a 10 gtt/mL set. — 27.8 gtt/min

2. 3500 mL are ordered to infuse in 24 hr using a set calibrated at 20 gtt/mL. — 49 gtt/min

3. Infuse 500 mL in 3 hr using a 15 gtt/mL set. — _____

4. A volume of 1500 mL is to infuse in 5 hr using a 15 gtt/mL set. — _____

5. 1750 mL are ordered to infuse in 9 hr using a 20 gtt/mL set. — 65 gtt/min

6. An IV of 2500 mL is to infuse in 18 hr on a set calibrated at 10 gtt/mL. — _____

7. A 3000 mL volume is to infuse in 24 hr on a set calibrated at 20 gtt/mL. — 42 gtt/min

8. A volume of 2750 mL is to infuse in 22 hr on a 15 gtt/mL set. — 31 gtt/min

9. An IV of 750 mL is ordered to infuse in 8 hr on a 10 gtt/mL set. — 16 gtt/min

10. A volume of 1250 mL is to infuse in 12 hr using a 15 gtt/mL set. — 26 gtt

**Answers   1.** 28 gtt/min   **2.** 49 gtt/min   **3.** 42 gtt/min   **4.** 75 gtt/min   **5.** 65 gtt/min   **6.** 23 gtt/min
**7.** 42 gtt/min   **8.** 31 gtt/min   **9.** 16 gtt/min   **10.** 26 gtt/min

## FORMULA AND DIVISION FACTOR METHODS OF FLOW RATE CALCULATION

The **formula** and **division factor** methods are intrinsically related because **the division factor is derived from the formula method**. Let's start by looking at the formula method.

The formula method has a limitation in that it can **only be used if the flow rate is expressed as mL/hr (60 min) or less**; for example, 110 mL/60 min or 125 mL/60 min. It is especially suitable for small-volume infusions to be completed in less than 60 min; for example, 30 mL in 20 min.

$$\text{Flow Rate} = \frac{\text{mL/hr Volume} \times \text{Set Calibration}}{\text{Time (60 min or less)}}$$

**EXAMPLE 1**   An IV of 500 mL is ordered to infuse at **125 mL/hr.** Calculate the **gtt/min** rate for a set calibrated at **10 gtt/mL.**

- **Convert the hr rate to 60 min.**

$$\frac{125(\text{mL}) \times 10(\text{gtt/mL})}{60 \ (\text{min})}$$

- **Calculate the gtt/min rate.**

$$\frac{125 \times 10}{60} = 20.8 = \textbf{21 gtt/min}$$

**EXAMPLE 2** Administer an IV medication of **100 mL** in **40 min** using a set calibrated at **15 gtt/mL**.

$$\frac{100 \text{ mL} \times 15 \text{ gtt/mL}}{40 \text{ min}} = 37.5 = \textbf{38 gtt/min}$$

**EXAMPLE 3** A **75 mL** volume of IV medication is ordered to infuse in **45 min**. The set is calibrated at **20 gtt/mL**.

$$\frac{75 \text{ mL} \times 20 \text{ gtt/mL}}{45 \text{ min}} = 33.3 = \textbf{33 gtt/min}$$

## Problems 16.3

Calculate the flow rate in gtt/min to the nearest whole drop using the formula method.

1. Administer an IV of 110 mL/hr using a set calibrated at 20 gtt/mL.   _37 gtt/min_

2. A 500 mL IV solution is ordered to infuse at 200 mL/hr using a set calibrated at 15 gtt/mL.   _50 gtt/min_

3. A volume of 80 mL is to be infused in 20 min using a 10 gtt/mL set.   _40 gtt/min_

4. An IV of 1000 mL is ordered to infuse at 150 mL/hr using a 10 gtt/mL calibrated set.   _25 gtt/min_

5. An IV rate of 90 mL/hr is ordered using a 15 gtt/mL calibrated set.   _23 gtt/min_

6. An IV of 500 mL is to infuse at 120 mL/hr using a 20 gtt/mL calibrated set.   _40 gtt/min_

7. A total of 90 mL is to infuse at 100 mL/hr using a 20 gtt/mL set.   _____

8. A 15 gtt/mL set is used to infuse 120 mL at 80 mL/hr.   _____

9. A rate of 60 mL/hr is ordered for a volume of 250 mL using a 10 gtt/mL set.   _____

10. A medication volume of 50 mL is to infuse at 20 mL/hr using a 20 gtt/mL set.   _____

**Answers** **1.** 37 gtt/min  **2.** 50 gtt/min  **3.** 40 gtt/min  **4.** 25 gtt/min  **5.** 23 gtt/min
**6.** 40 gtt/min  **7.** 33 gtt/min  **8.** 20 gtt/min  **9.** 10 gtt/min  **10.** 7 gtt/min

When an IV is ordered to infuse in **more than 1 hour**, the formula method can still be used. However, it is necessary to add a preliminary step and determine the **mL/hr** the ordered volume will represent.

**EXAMPLE 1**   Calculate the gtt/min flow rate for an IV of **1000 mL** to infuse in **8 hr** on a set calibrated at **20 gtt/mL**.

- **Convert 1000 mL/8 hr to mL/hr.**

  1000 mL/8 hr = 1000 ÷ 8 = **125 mL/hr (60 min)**

- **Calculate the gtt/min flow rate.**

  $$\frac{125 \text{ (mL)} \times 20 \text{ (gtt/mL)}}{60 \text{ (min)}} = 41.6 = \textbf{42 gtt/min}$$

**EXAMPLE 2**   Calculate the gtt/min flow rate for a volume of **2500 mL** to infuse in **24 hr** on a set calibrated at **10 gtt/mL**.

- **Convert 2500 mL/24 hr to mL/hr.**

  2500 mL/24 hr = 2500 ÷ 24 = **104 mL/hr (60 min)**

- **Calculate the gtt/min flow rate.**

  $$\frac{104 \text{ mL} \times 10 \text{ gtt/mL}}{60 \text{ min}} = 17.3 = \textbf{17 gtt/min}$$

**EXAMPLE 3**   An IV of **1200 mL** is to infuse in **16 hr** on a set calibrated at **15 gtt/mL**.

  1200 mL/16 hr = 1200 ÷ 16 = **75 mL/hr (60 min)**

  $$\frac{75 \text{ mL} \times 15 \text{ gtt/mL}}{60 \text{ min}} = 18.7 = \textbf{19 gtt/min}$$

## Problems 16.4

**Calculate the gtt/min flow rate using the formula method.**

1. A volume of 2000 mL to infuse in 24 hr on a set calibrated at 15 gtt/mL. _21 gtt/min_

2. A volume of 300 mL to infuse in 6 hr on a 60 gtt/mL microdrip set. _50_

3. A volume of 500 mL to infuse in 4 hr on a 15 gtt/mL calibrated set. _31_

4. A 10 hr infusion of 1200 mL using a 20 gtt/mL set. _40_

5. An infusion of 500 mL in 5 hr on a set calibrated at 10 gtt/mL. _17_

6.  A 2000 mL volume to infuse in 18 hr using a
    20 gtt/mL set.                                    _____

7.  A 10 gtt/mL set to infuse 400 mL in 4 hr.        _____

8.  An 8 hr infusion of 1500 mL to use a set calibrated
    at 15 gtt/mL.                                      _____

9.  A volume of 250 mL to infuse in 2 hr using a
    20 gtt/mL set.                                     _____

10. A 5 hr infusion of 750 mL using a 10 gtt/mL set.  _____

**Answers  1.** 21 gtt/min  **2.** 50 gtt/min  **3.** 31 gtt/min  **4.** 40 gtt/min  **5.** 17 gtt/min  **6.** 37 gtt/min
**7.** 17 gtt/min  **8.** 47 gtt/min  **9.** 42 gtt/min  **10.** 25 gtt/min

## DIVISION FACTOR METHOD

The **division factor** is derived from the formula method, and it is invaluable for
use in clinical facilities where **all the macrodrip infusion sets have the same
calibration**—either 10, 15, or 20 gtt/mL. Once again, **this method can only be
used if the rate is expressed in mL/hr (60 min)**. Let's start by looking at how the
division factor is obtained.

EXAMPLE          Administer an IV at **125 mL/hr**. The set calibration is **10 gtt/mL**.
                 Calculate the gtt/min rate. Express the hr rate as 60 min.

$$\frac{125(\text{mL}) \times \overset{1}{\cancel{10}}(\text{gtt/mL})}{\underset{6}{\cancel{60}}(\text{min})} = 20.8 = \textbf{21 gtt/min}$$

Look at the completed equation, and notice that because the time is restricted to
60 min, **the set calibration (10) will be divided into 60 (min) to obtain a constant
number (6). This constant (6) is the division factor for a 10 gtt/mL calibrated set.**

The division factor can be obtained for any IV set by dividing
60 by the calibration of the set.

Problems 16.5

Determine the division factor for these IV sets.
1. 20 gtt/mL    ____3____
2. 15 gtt/mL    ____4____
3. 60 gtt/mL    ____1____
4. 10 gtt/mL    ____6____

**Answers  1.** 3  **2.** 4  **3.** 1  **4.** 6

Once the division factor is known, **the gtt/min rate can be calculated in one step by dividing the mL/hr rate by the division factor**. Look again at the example.

$$\frac{125(\text{mL}) \times \overset{1}{\cancel{10}}(\text{gtt/mL})}{\underset{6}{\cancel{60}}(\text{min})} = 20.8 = \textbf{21 gtt/min}$$

or $125(\text{mL/hr}) \div \textbf{6} = 20.8 = \textbf{21 gtt/min}$

**The 125 mL/hr flow rate divided by the division factor 6 gives the same 21 gtt/min rate.**

The gtt/min flow rate can be calculated for mL/hr IV orders in one step by dividing the mL/hr to be infused by the division factor of the administration set.

**EXAMPLE 1**   Infuse an IV at **100 mL/hr** using a set calibrated at **10 gtt/mL**.

**Determine the division factor:**   $60 \div 10 = \textbf{6}$

**Calculate the flow rate:**   $100 \text{ mL} \div 6 = 16.6 = \textbf{17 gtt/min}$

**EXAMPLE 2**   Infuse an IV at **125 mL/hr** using a set calibrated at **15 gtt/mL**.

$60 \div 15 = 4$                $125 \text{ mL} \div 4 = 31.2 = \textbf{31 gtt/min}$

**EXAMPLE 3**   A set calibrated at **20 gtt/mL** is used to infuse **90 mL per hr**.

$60 \div 20 = 3$                $90 \text{ mL} \div 3 = \textbf{30 gtt/min}$

## Problems 16.6

Calculate the flow rates in gtt/min using the division factor method.

1. A rate of 110 mL/hr via a set calibrated at 20 gtt/mL.   _____
2. A set is calibrated at 15 gtt/mL. Infuse at 130 mL/hr.   _____
3. To infuse 150 mL/hr using a 10 gtt/mL set.   _____
4. A set calibrated at 20 gtt/mL to infuse 45 mL/hr.   _____
5. A 75 mL/hr volume with a set calibrated at 15 gtt/mL.   _____
6. A rate of 130 mL/hr using a 10 gtt/mL set.   _____
7. A 200 mL rate using a 15 gtt/mL set.   _____
8. A rate of 120 mL/hr using a 10 gtt/mL set.   _____
9. A 100 mL/hr rate using a 20 gtt/mL set.   _____
10. A rate of 125 mL/hr using a 15 gtt/mL set.   _____

**Answers**   **1.** 37 gtt/min   **2.** 33 gtt/min   **3.** 25 gtt/min   **4.** 15 gtt/min   **5.** 19 gtt/min
**6.** 22 gtt/min   **7.** 50 gtt/min   **8.** 20 gtt/min   **9.** 33 gtt/min   **10.** 31 gtt/min

All the preceding examples and problems using the division factor were for **macrodrip** sets. Let's now look at what happens when a **microdrip** set calibrated at **60 gtt/mL** is used.

**EXAMPLE**   Infuse at **50 mL/hr** using a **60 gtt/mL** microdrip.

$$60 \div 60 = 1 \qquad\qquad 50 \text{ mL} \div 1 = \textbf{50 gtt/min}$$

Because the set calibration is 60 and the division factor is based on 60 min (1 hr), the division factor is 1. So, **for microdrip sets, the gtt/min flow rate will be identical to the mL/hr ordered**.

 When a 60 gtt/mL microdrip set is used, the flow rate in gtt/min is identical to the volume in mL/hr to be infused.

## Problems 16.7

Calculate gtt/min rates for a microdrip.

1. 120 mL/hr  _____
2. 90 mL/hr  _____
3. 100 mL/hr  _____
4. 75 mL/hr  _____
5. 80 mL/hr  _____

6. 110 mL/hr  _____
7. 60 mL/hr  _____
8. 45 mL/hr  _____
9. 70 mL/hr  _____
10. 130 mL/hr  _____

**Answers**  **1.** 120 gtt/min  **2.** 90 gtt/min  **3.** 100 gtt/min  **4.** 75 gtt/min  **5.** 80 gtt/min
**6.** 110 gtt/min  **7.** 60 gtt/min  **8.** 45 gtt/min  **9.** 70 gtt/min  **10.** 130 gtt/min

The division factor can also be used to calculate the flow rate of **any volume that can be expressed in mL/hr**. Larger volumes can be divided, and smaller volumes can be multiplied and expressed in mL/hr. This does require the conversion step you used earlier.

**EXAMPLE 1**   2400 mL/24 hr = 2400 ÷ 24 = **100 mL/hr**

**EXAMPLE 2**   1800 mL/8 hr = 1800 ÷ 8 = **225 mL/hr**

**EXAMPLE 3**   10 mL/30 min = 10 × 2 (2 × 30 min) = **20 mL/hr**

**EXAMPLE 4**   15 mL/20 min = 15 × 3 (3 × 20 min) = **45 mL/hr**

## REGULATING FLOW RATE

Manual flow rates are regulated by **counting the number of drops falling in the drip chamber**. The standard procedure for counting is to hold a watch next to the drip chamber and actually **count the number of drops falling**. The roller clamp is adjusted during the count until the required rate has been set. A 15 sec count is most commonly used because there is less chance of attention wandering during the count. This means that the ordered gtt/min (60 sec) rate must be divided by 4 to obtain the 15 sec drip count (60 sec ÷ 4 = 15 sec).

**EXAMPLE 1**   An IV is to run at a rate of **60 gtt/min**. What will the 15 sec count be?

60 gtt/min ÷ 4 = **15 gtt**

**Adjust the rate to 15 gtt/15 sec.**

**EXAMPLE 2**   A 70 **gtt/min** IV rate is ordered. What will the 15 sec count be?

70 gtt/min ÷ 4 = 17.5 = **18 gtt**

**Adjust the rate to 18 gtt/15 sec.**

**EXAMPLE 3**   Adjust an IV to a rate of **50 gtt/min** using a 15 sec count.

50 gtt/min ÷ 4 = **13 gtt**

**Adjust the rate to 13 gtt/15 sec.**

### Problems 16.8

**Answer the questions about 15 sec drip rates.**

1. The 15 second count of an IV flow rate is 7 gtt. A 29 gtt/min rate is required. Is this rate correct?   _____

2. You are to regulate a newly started IV to deliver 67 gtt/min. Using a 15 second count, how would you set the flow rate?   _____

3. An IV is to run at 48 gtt/min. What must the 15 second drip rate be?   _____

4. How many gtt will you count in 15 sec if the rate is 55 gtt/min?   _____

5. An IV is to run at 84 gtt/min. What will the 15 sec rate be?   _____

6. What must the 15 sec count be to infuse 80 gtt/min?   _____

7. A 110 gtt/min rate is ordered. What must the 15 sec count be?   _____

8. A 100 gtt/min rate is ordered. What must the 15 sec count be?   _____

9. A rate of 90 gtt/min is ordered. Is a count of 15 gtt in 15 sec correct? _____

10. An IV is infusing at a rate of 30 gtt in 15 sec. A rate of 120 gtt/min was ordered. Is this rate correct? _____

**Answers  1.** Yes  **2.** 17 gtt/15 sec  **3.** 12 gtt/15 sec  **4.** 14 gtt/15 sec  **5.** 21 gtt/15 sec
**6.** 20 gtt/15 sec  **7.** 28 gtt/15 sec  **8.** 25 gtt/15 sec  **9.** No, too slow  **10.** Yes

Individual clinical facilities and/or states/provinces may require a 30 or 60 sec (1 min) count. When a 60 sec count is required, particular care must be taken not to let your attention wander during the count, which can easily happen in this longer time frame. A 60 sec count will require a 1 min count, whereas a 30 sec count will require the gtt/min rate to be divided by 2 (60 sec ÷ 2 = 30 sec).

**EXAMPLE 1**    An IV is to be infused at 56 gtt/min. What is the 30 sec rate?

56 gtt/min ÷ 2 = 28 gtt

**Adjust the rate to 28 gtt/30 sec.**

**EXAMPLE 2**    A rate of 72 gtt/min has been ordered. What will the 30 sec count be?

72 gtt/min ÷ 2 = 36 gtt

**Adjust the rate to 36 gtt/30 sec.**

## Problems 16.9

**Calculate a 30 sec flow rate count.**

1. An IV to be run at a rate of 48 gtt/min.   _____
2. An IV ordered to infuse at 52 gtt/min.   _____
3. An IV to infuse at 120 gtt/min.   _____
4. An infusion rate of 90 gtt/min.   _____
5. An IV to infuse at 100 gtt/min.   _____

**Answers  1.** 24 gtt/30 sec  **2.** 26 gtt/30 sec  **3.** 60 gtt/30 sec  **4.** 45 gtt/30 sec  **5.** 50 gtt/30 sec

## CORRECTING OFF-SCHEDULE RATES

Because positional changes can alter the rate slightly, IVs occasionally infuse ahead of or behind schedule. When this occurs, the usual procedure is to **recalculate the flow rate using the volume and time remaining** and to **adjust the rate accordingly**. However, each situation must be individually evaluated, especially if the discrepancy is large. **If too much fluid has infused, immediately assess the individual's response** to the increased intake and take appropriate action. **If too little fluid has infused**, it will be necessary to **assess the individual's ability to tolerate an increased rate** because many medications and fluids have restrictions on the rate of administration. Both of these factors must be considered before rates can be increased to "catch up." In addition, **most clinical facilities will have specific policies to cover over- or under infusion due to altered flow rates, and you will be responsible for knowing these**.

The following are some examples of how the rate can be recalculated. Because IVs are usually checked hourly, the focus will first be on recalculation using exact hours. Some recalculations have also been included using fractions of hours rounded to the nearest quarter hour: 15 min = 0.25 hr, 30 min = 0.5 hr, and 45 min = 0.75 hr. These equivalents are close enough for uncomplicated infusions because the exact time of completion is not totally predictable. IVs needing exact infusion would be monitored by electronic infusion devices.

**EXAMPLE 1**   An IV of **1000 mL** was ordered to infuse over **10 hr** at a rate of **25 gtt/min**. The set calibration is **15 gtt/mL**. After **5 hr**, a total of 650 mL have infused instead of the **500 mL** ordered. Recalculate the new gtt/min flow rate to complete the infusion on schedule.

**Time remaining**   10 hr − 5 hr = **5 hr**

**Volume remaining**   1000 mL − 650 mL = **350 mL**

350 mL ÷ 5 hr = **70 mL/hr**

Set calibration is **15 gtt/mL**.

70 ÷ 4(division factor) = 17.5 = **18 gtt/min**

**Slow the rate from 25 gtt/min to 18 gtt/min.**

**EXAMPLE 2**   An IV of **800 mL** was to infuse over **8 hr** at **20 gtt/min**. After **4 hr 15 min** only **300 mL** have infused. Recalculate the **gtt/min** rate to complete on schedule. The set calibration is **15 gtt/mL**.

**Time remaining**   8 hr − 4.25 hr = **3.75 hr**

**Volume remaining**   800 mL − 300 mL = **500 mL**

500 mL ÷ 3.75 hr = 133.3 = **133 mL/hr**

Set calibration is **15 gtt/mL**.

133 ÷ 4(division factor) = 33.2 = **33 gtt/min**

**Increase the rate to 33 gtt/min.**

**EXAMPLE 3**   An IV of **500 mL** is infusing at **28 gtt/min**. It was to complete in **3 hr**, but after **1½ hr**, only **175 mL** have infused. Recalculate the **gtt/min** rate to complete the infusion on schedule. Set calibration is **10 gtt/mL**.

**Time remaining**   3 hr − 1.5 hr = **1.5 hr**

**Volume remaining**   500 mL − 175 mL = **325 mL**

325 mL ÷ 1.5 hr = 216.6 = **217 mL/hr**

Set calibration is **10 gtt/mL**.

$217 \div 6(\text{division factor}) = 36.1 = \textbf{36 gtt/min}$

**Increase the rate to 36 gtt/min.**

---

**EXAMPLE 4**

A volume of **250 mL** was to infuse **56 gtt/min** in **1½ hr** using a set calibrated at **20 gtt/mL**. After **30 min, 175 mL** have infused. Recalculate the flow rate.

**Time remaining**   1.5 hr − 30 min = **1 hr**

**Volume remaining**   250 mL − 175 mL = **75 mL**

Set calibration is **20 gtt/mL**.

$75 \div 3(\text{division factor}) = \textbf{25 gtt/min}$

**Decrease the rate to 25 gtt/min.**

## Problems 16.10

**Recalculate flow rates for infusions to complete on schedule.**

1. An IV of 500 mL was ordered to infuse in 3 hr using a 15 gtt/mL set. With 1½ hr remaining, you discover that only 150 mL is left in the bag. At what rate will you need to reset the flow?   _____

2. An IV of 1000 mL was scheduled to run in 12 hr. After 4 hr, only 220 mL have infused. The set calibration is 20 gtt/mL. Recalculate the rate for the remaining solution.   _____

3. An IV of 1000 mL was ordered to infuse in 8 hr. With 3 hr of infusion time left, you discover that 600 mL have infused. The set delivers 20 gtt/mL. Recalculate the drip rate, and indicate how many drops you will count in 15 sec to set the new rate.   _____   _____

4. An IV of 750 mL was ordered to run in 6 hr with a set calibrated at 10 gtt/mL. After 2 hr, you notice that 300 mL have infused. Recalculate the flow rate, and indicate how many drops you will count in 15 sec to reset the rate.

   _____   _____

5. An IV of 800 mL was started at 9 am to infuse in 4 hr. At 10 am 150 mL have infused. The set is calibrated at 15 gtt/mL. Recalculate the flow rate in gtt/min.   _____

6. An IV of 600 mL was to infuse in 5 hr. After 2 hr, 400 mL have infused. Recalculate the gtt/min rate to complete on time. A 20 gtt/mL set is being used.   _____

7. A volume of 250 mL was to infuse in 2 hr. With 1 hr left, 70 mL have infused. Calculate a new gtt/min rate to complete on time using a 15 gtt/mL set.   _____

8. An infiltrated IV is restarted with a volume of 420 mL to complete in 3 hr. Calculate the gtt/min rate for a 20 gtt/mL set. What will the new 30 sec count be?   _____   _____

9. After 1 hr 30 min, 350 mL of a 1000 mL IV has infused. It was ordered to complete in 4 hr using a set calibrated at 15 gtt/mL. Calculate the gtt/min rate to complete on time.   _____

10. A total of 300 mL of an ordered 1000 mL in 10 hr infusion has completed in 4.5 hr. The set calibration is 15 gtt/mL. What gtt/min rate is necessary to complete on time? Calculate the 15 sec count to deliver this rate.   _____   _____

**Answers**   **1.** 25 gtt/min   **2.** 33 gtt/min   **3.** 44 gtt/min; 11 gtt/15 sec   **4.** 19 gtt/min; 4–5 gtt/15 sec   **5.** 54 gtt/min   **6.** 22 gtt/min   **7.** 45 gtt/min   **8.** 47 gtt/min; 23–24 gtt/30 sec   **9.** 65 gtt/min   **10.** 32 gtt/min; 8 gtt/15 sec

## Summary

**This concludes the chapter on IV flow rate calculation and monitoring. The important points to remember from this chapter are:**

- IVs are ordered as mL/hr to be administered.

- Manual flow rates are counted in gtt/min.

- IV tubings are calibrated in gtt/mL.

- Macrodrip IV sets have a calibration of 10, 15, or 20 gtt/mL.

- Microdrip sets have a calibration of 60 gtt/mL.

- The formula for calculating flow rates is

$$\frac{mL/hr \ Volume \times Set \ Calibration}{Time \, (60 \ min \ or \ less)}$$

- The division factor method can be used to calculate flow rates only if the volume to be administered is specified in mL/hr (60 min).

- The division factor is obtained by dividing 60 by the set calibration.

- Flow rate by the division factor method is determined by dividing the mL/hr to be administered by the division factor.

- Because microdrip sets have a calibration of 60 gtt/mL, their division factor is 1, and the flow rate in gtt/min is the same as the mL/hr ordered.

- If an IV runs ahead of or behind schedule, a possible procedure is to use the time and mL remaining to calculate a new flow rate.

- If an IV is determined to have infused ahead of schedule, immediate assessment of the individual's tolerance to the excess fluid is required and appropriate action should be taken.

- If a rate must be increased to compensate for running behind schedule, the type of fluid being infused and the individual's ability to tolerate an increased rate must be assessed.

# Summary Self-Test

**Answer as briefly as possible.**

1. Determine the division factor for the following IV sets.

   a) 60 gtt/mL _____

   b) 15 gtt/mL _____

   c) 20 gtt/mL _____

   d) 10 gtt/mL _____

2. How is the flow rate determined in the division factor method? _____

3. The division factor method can only be used if the volume to be administered is expressed in . . . _____

4. An IV is to infuse at 50 gtt/min. How will you set it using a 15 sec count? _____

5. You are to adjust an IV at a rate of 60 gtt/min. What will the 15 sec count be? _____

**Calculate the flow rate in gtt/min.**

6. An infusion of 2000 mL has been ordered to run 16 hr. The set calibration is 10 gtt/mL. _____

7. The order is for 500 mL in 8 hr. The set is calibrated at 15 gtt/mL. _____

8. Administer 150 mL in 3 hr. A microdrip is used. _____

9. 1500 mL has been ordered to infuse in 12 hr. Set calibration is 20 gtt/mL. _____

10. An IV medication of 30 mL is to be administered in 30 min using a 15 gtt/mL set. _____

11. Administer 100 mL in 1 hr using a 15 gtt/mL set. _____

12. Infuse 500 mL in 6 hr. Set calibration is 10 gtt/mL. _____

13. The order is to infuse a liter in 10 hr. At the end of 8 hr, you notice that there are 500 mL left. What would the new flow rate need to be to finish on schedule if the set calibration is 10 gtt/mL? _____

14. An IV was started at 9 am with orders to infuse 500 mL in 6 hr. At noon, the IV infiltrated with 350 mL left in the bag. At 1 pm, the IV was restarted. The set calibration is 20 gtt/mL. Calculate the new flow rate to deliver the infusion on time. _____

15. A 50 mL IV is to infuse in 15 min. The set calibration is 15 gtt/mL. After 5 min, the IV contains 40 mL. Calculate the flow rate to deliver the volume on time. _____

16. An IV of 1000 mL is ordered to run at 25 mL/hr using a microdrip set. _____

17. An infusion of 800 mL has been ordered to run in 5 hr. Set calibration is 10 gtt/mL. _____

18. Administer 1500 mL in 8 hr using a set calibrated at 20 gtt/mL. _____

19. The order is for 750 mL to run in 6 hr. Set calibration is 15 gtt/mL. _____

20. An IV of 1000 mL was ordered to run in 8 hr. After 4 hr, only 250 mL have infused. The set calibration is 20 gtt/mL. Recalculate the rate for the remaining solution to complete on time.   _____

21. The order is to infuse 50 mL in 1 hr. The set calibration is a microdrip.   _____

22. An IV of 500 mL is to infuse in 6 hr using a set calibrated at 10 gtt/mL.   _____

23. Infuse 120 mL in 1 hr. Set calibration is 10 gtt/mL.   _____

24. Administer 12 mL in 22 min using a microdrip set.   _____

25. A patient is to receive 3000 mL in 20 hr. Set is calibrated at 20 gtt/mL.   _____

26. Infuse 1 liter in 5 hr using a set calibration of 15 gtt/mL.   _____

27. A total of 1180 mL is to infuse in 12 hr using a set calibrated at 20 gtt/mL.   _____

28. A volume of 150 mL is to infuse in 30 min. At the end of 20 min, you discover that 100 mL have infused. The set calibration is 10 gtt/mL. Should the flow rate be adjusted? If so, what is the new rate?

    _____   _____

29. The order is for 1000 mL in 5 hr. The set calibration is 20 gtt/mL.   _____

30. Infuse 15 mL in 14 min using a 20 gtt/mL set.   _____

31. The order is for 1000 mL in 10 hr using a 20 gtt/mL calibration.   _____

32. A microdrip is used to administer 12 mL in 17 min.   _____

33. Infuse 2750 mL in 20 hr using a 10 gtt/mL set.   _____

34. An IV of 1800 mL is to infuse in 15 hr using a 15 gtt/mL set.   _____

35. Infuse 600 mL in 6 hr with a 10 gtt/mL set.   _____

36. Administer 22 mL in 18 min using a mirodrip set.   _____

37. An order of 1800 mL is to infuse in 10 hr. Set calibration is 20 gtt/mL.   _____

38. Infuse 8 mL in 9 min using a microdrip.   _____

39. Infuse 4000 mL in 20 hr. A 20 gtt/mL set is used.   _____

40. An IV of 500 mL that was to infuse in 2 hr is discovered to have only 150 mL left after 30 min. Recalculate the flow rate. Set calibration is 15 gtt/mL.   _____

| **Answers** | **10.** 15 gtt/min | **22.** 14 gtt/min | **33.** 23 gtt/min |
|---|---|---|---|
| **1.** a) 1  b) 4  c) 3  d) 6 | **11.** 25 gtt/min | **23.** 20 gtt/min | **34.** 30 gtt/min |
| **2.** mL/hr ÷ division factor | **12.** 14 gtt/min | **24.** 33 gtt/min | **35.** 17 gtt/min |
| **3.** mL/hr (mL/60 min) | **13.** 42 gtt/min | **25.** 50 gtt/min | **36.** 73 gtt/min |
| | **14.** 58 gtt/min | **26.** 50 gtt/min | **37.** 60 gtt/min |
| **4.** 13 gtt/15 sec | **15.** 60 gtt/min | **27.** 33 gtt/min | **38.** 53 gtt/min |
| **5.** 15 gtt/15 sec | **16.** 25 gtt/min | **28.** No, rate is correct at 50 gtt/min | **39.** 67 gtt/min |
| **6.** 21 gtt/min | **17.** 27 gtt/min | | **40.** 25 gtt/min |
| **7.** 16 gtt/min | **18.** 63 gtt/min | **29.** 67 gtt/min | |
| **8.** 50 gtt/min | **19.** 31 gtt/min | **30.** 21 gtt/min | |
| **9.** 42 gtt/min | **20.** 63 gtt/min | **31.** 33 gtt/min | |
| | **21.** 50 gtt/min | **32.** 42 gtt/min | |

# CALCULATING IV INFUSION AND COMPLETION TIMES

There are a number of reasons for calculating IV infusion and completion times: to know when an IV solution will complete so that additional solutions ordered can be prepared in advance and ready to hang; to discontinue an IV when it has completed; and to label an IV bag with start, progress, and completion times so that the infusion can be monitored and adjusted to keep it on schedule. Knowing the infusion time is also important because laboratory studies are sometimes made before, during, or after specified amounts of IV solutions have infused. The infusion time may be calculated in hours and/or minutes, depending on the type and amount of solution ordered.

## CALCULATING INFUSION TIME FROM mL/hr ORDERED

The infusion time is calculated for each bag/bottle to be hung and infused. The largest capacity IV solution bag or bottle is 1000 mL, but 500 mL, 250 mL, and 50 mL bags are also commonly used. Calculations for odd-numbered volumes remaining when an IV infiltrates are also routinely done. **Infusion time is calculated by dividing the volume being infused by the mL/hr rate ordered.**

Because most IVs take several hours to infuse, the unit of time being calculated most often includes hours (hr) and minutes (min).

 **IV infusion time is calculated by dividing the volume to be infused by the mL/hr flow rate.**

**EXAMPLE 1**   Calculate the infusion time for an IV of **500 mL** to infuse at **50 mL/hr.**

**Infusion Time = volume ÷ mL/hr rate**

= 500 mL ÷ 50 mL/hr = **10 hr**

**The infusion time for an IV of 500 mL infusing at 50 mL/hr is 10 hr.**

## Objectives

The learner will calculate:

1. infusion times.

2. completion times using international/military and standard time.

3. infusion time to label IV bag/bottle with start, progress, and completion times.

**EXAMPLE 2**   The order is to infuse **1000 mL** at **75 mL/hr**. Calculate the infusion time.

1000 mL ÷ 75 mL/hr = **13.33 hr**

In this example, the 13 represents hr, whereas the **.33 represents the fraction of an additional hr.**

 Fractional hr are converted to min by multiplying 60 min by the fraction obtained.

**Calculate min by multiplying 60 min by the fractional .33 hr.**

60 min/hr × .33 hr = 19.8 = **20 min**

**The infusion time is 13 hr 20 min.**

**EXAMPLE 3**   An IV of **1000 mL** is to infuse at **90 mL/hr**. Calculate the infusion time.

1000 mL ÷ 90 mL/hr = **11.11 hr**

**Remember that .11 represents the fraction of an additional hr. Convert this to min by multiplying 60 min by .11**

60 min/hr × .11 hr = 6.6 = **7 min**

**The infusion time is 11 hr 7 min.**

**EXAMPLE 4**   Calculate the infusion time for **750 mL** at a rate of **80 mL/hr**.

750 mL ÷ 80 mL/hr = **9.38 hr**

60 min/hr × .38 hr = 22.8 = **23 min**

**The infusion time is 9 hr 23 min.**

**EXAMPLE 5**   A rate of **75 mL/hr** is ordered for a volume of **500 mL**. Calculate the infusion time.

500 mL ÷ 75 mL/hr = **6.67 hr**

60 min/hr × .67 hr = 40.2 = **40 min**

**The infusion time is 6 hr 40 min.**

## Problems 17.1

**Calculate the infusion times.**

1. An IV of 900 mL to infuse at 80 mL/hr.
2. A volume of 250 mL to infuse at 30 mL/hr.
3. An infusion of 180 mL to run at 25 mL/hr.
4. A volume of 1000 mL ordered at 60 mL/hr.

5. An IV of 150 mL to infuse at 80 mL/hr.     _1 hr 52.5 min._

6. An infusion of 1000 mL at 125 mL/hr.     _____

7. A rate of 120 mL/hr for 500 mL.     _____

8. A volume of 800 mL at 60 mL/hr.     _____

9. An IV of 250 mL at 80 mL/hr.     _____

10. A rate of 135 mL/hr for 750 mL.     _____

**Answers  1.** 11 hr 15 min  **2.** 8 hr 20 min  **3.** 7 hr 12 min  **4.** 16 hr 40 min  **5.** 1 hr 53 min
**6.** 8 hr  **7.** 4 hr 10 min  **8.** 13 hr 20 min  **9.** 3 hr 8 min  **10.** 5 hr 34 min
**Note:** Answers may vary due to rounding or calculator setting, so variations of 1–2 min may be considered correct.

## CALCULATING INFUSION COMPLETION TIMES

The **completion time is the actual hour and/or minute an infusion bag or bottle will complete or empty**. Completion times are calculated in either **international/military time** using the 24-hour clock, or **standard time**, depending on individual clinical facility policy.

 The completion time is calculated by adding the infusion time to the time the IV was started.

An example is the addition of an infusion time of 90 min to a 0515 international/military or 5:15 am standard time when an IV was started.

## INTERNATIONAL/MILITARY TIME CALCULATIONS

**EXAMPLE 1**   An IV started at **0400** is to complete in **2 hr 30 min**. Calculate the completion time.

- **Add the 2 hr 30 min infusion time to the 0400 start time**

$$
\begin{array}{r}
0400 \\
+ \quad 230 \\
\hline
0630
\end{array}
$$

**The completion time is 0630.**

**EXAMPLE 2**   An IV started at **0750** is to complete in **5 hr 10 min**. Calculate the completion time.

- **Add the 5 hr 10 min infusion time to the 0750 start time.**

$$
\begin{array}{r}
0750 \\
+ \quad 510 \\
\hline
1260
\end{array}
$$

**Change the 60 min to 1 hr and add to 1200 = 1300**

**The completion time is 1300.**

> **EXAMPLE 3**   An IV started at **2250** is to complete in **4 hr 20 min**. Calculate the completion time.
>
> - **Add the infusion time to the start time.**
>
> $$\begin{array}{r} 2250 \\ +\ \ 420 \\ \hline 2670 \end{array}$$
>
> **Change the 70 min to 1 hr 10 min = 2710**
>
> **Deduct 24 hr from 2710 = 0310**
>
> **The completion time is 0310.**

## Problems 17.2

Calculate the international/military completion times.

1. An IV started at 0415 to infuse in 1 hr 30 min.  _____
2. An infusion started at 1735 to complete in 2 hr 40 min.  _____
3. An IV to complete in 1 hr 14 min that was started at 0025.  _____
4. An IV started at 2300 to complete in 3 hr 40 min.  _____
5. An infusion time of 6 hr 20 min for an infusion started at 0325.  _____
6. An IV started at 0445 to complete in 3 hr 20 min.  _____
7. A medication infusion started at 0740 to complete in 90 min.  _____
8. An IV medication started at 1247 to complete in 45 min.  _____
9. An IV started at 1430 to complete in 4 hr.  _____
10. An IV started at 1605 to complete in 3 hr 30 min.  _____

**Answers  1.** 0545  **2.** 2015  **3.** 0139  **4.** 0240  **5.** 0945  **6.** 0805  **7.** 0910  **8.** 1332
**9.** 1830  **10.** 1935

## STANDARD TIME CALCULATIONS

> **EXAMPLE 1**   An IV medication will infuse in **20 minutes**. It is now **6:14 pm**. When will it complete?
>
> - **Add the 20 minutes infusion time to the 6:14 pm start time.**
>
> 6:14 pm + **20 min** = **6:34 pm**
>
> **The completion time will be at 6:34 pm.**

> **EXAMPLE 2**   An IV is to infuse in **2 hr 33 min**. It is now **4:43 pm**. When will it complete?
>
> - **Add the 2 hr 33 min infusion time to the 4:43 start time.**
>
> $$\begin{array}{r} 4:43 \text{ pm} \\ +\ 2:33 \\ \hline 6:76 \end{array}$$

Change the 76 min to 1 hr 16 min to make the completion time 7:16 pm.

**The infusion will complete at 7:16 pm.**

**EXAMPLE 3**   An IV infusion time is **13 hr 20 min**. What is its completion time if it was started at **10:45 am**?

- **Add the 13 hr 20 min infusion time to the 10:45 am start time.**

$$
\begin{array}{r}
10{:}45 \text{ am} \\
+\ \underline{13{:}20} \\
23{:}65
\end{array}
$$

Change the 65 min to 1 hr 5 min = 24:05. Subtract 12 hr.

**The completion time will be 12:05 am.**

**EXAMPLE 4**   A IV with an infusion time of **10 hr 7 min** is started at **9:42 am**. When will it complete?

- **Add the 10 hr 7 min infusion time to the 9:42 am start time.**

$$
\begin{array}{r}
9{:}42 \text{ am} \\
+\ \underline{10{:}07} \\
19{:}49
\end{array}
$$

Subtract 12 hr to make the completion time 7:49 pm.

**The completion time will be 7:49 pm.**

**EXAMPLE 5**   An IV with an infusion time of **12 hr 30 min** is started at **2:10 am**. When will it complete?

- **Add the 12 hr 30 min infusion time to the 2:10 am start time.**

$$
\begin{array}{r}
2{:}10 \text{ am} \\
+\ \underline{12{:}30} \\
14{:}40
\end{array}
$$

Subtract 12 hr to make the time 2:40 pm.

**The completion time will be 2:40 pm.**

## Problems 17.3

**Calculate IV completion using standard time.**

1. An IV started at 4:40 am that has an infusion time of 9 hr 42 min.  _____

2. An IV medication started at 7:30 am that has an infusion time of 45 min.  _____

3. An IV with an infusion time of 7 hr 7 min that was restarted at 10:42 am. _____

4. An IV with a restart time of 9:07 pm has an infusion time of 6 hr 27 min. _____

5. An IV with an infusion time of 3 hr 30 min was started at 11:49 pm. _____

6. An IV started at 2:43 pm to infuse in 40 min. _____

7. An IV medication started at 10:15 am to complete in 90 min. _____

8. An infusion started at 7:05 pm to complete in 8 hr. _____

9. An IV started at 5:47 am to complete in 5 hr. _____

10. An IV started at 4:20 am to complete in 12 hr. _____

**Answers** **1.** 2:22 pm **2.** 8:15 am **3.** 5:49 pm **4.** 3:34 am **5.** 3:19 am **6.** 3:23 pm **7.** 11:45 am **8.** 3:05 am **9.** 10:47 am **10.** 4:20 pm

## LABELING SOLUTION BAGS WITH INFUSION AND COMPLETION TIMES

IV bags/bottles are calibrated so that the amount of fluid remaining can be checked at any time. In the majority of clinical facilities it is routine to label bags when they are hung with start, progress, and finish times to provide a visual reference of the status of the infusion. Commercially prepared labels are available for this purpose; however, you can prepare one using any tape available.

Refer to Figure 17-1, where you can see closeup the calibrations on a 1000 mL bag. Notice that each 50 mL is calibrated but that only the 100 mL calibrations are numbered: 1, 2, 3 (for 100, 200, 300), etc. Also, notice that the calibrations on the IV bag are not all the same width. They are somewhat wider at the bottom because gravity and the pressure of the solution force more fluid to the bottom of the bag.

The tape on the IV solution bag in Figure 17-1 is for an 8 hr infusion, from 9 am to 5 pm. The 9A represents the start time of 9 am, and the 5P at the bottom represents the completion time of 5 pm. An 8 hr infusion time for 1000 mL means that 125 mL are to be infused per hour (1000 mL ÷ 8 hr = 125 mL/hr). Each 125 mL is labeled on the calibrated scale along with the hour the IV should be at this level. This tape allows for constant visual

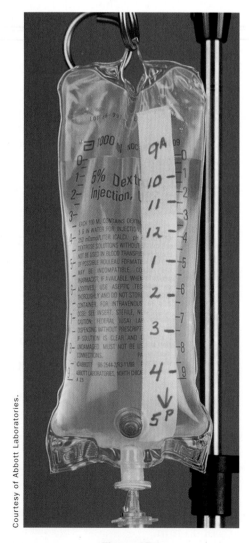

Courtesy of Abbott Laboratories.

**Figure 17-1**

monitoring of the IV. Regardless of your clinical responsibility, develop the habit of reading infusion time labeling, particularly if you have been giving personal care that involves movement or repositioning of the patient.

Let's look at an example of how you could label an IV that is just being started.

**EXAMPLE 1**   An IV of **1000 mL** has been ordered to run at **150 mL/hr**. It was started at **1:40 pm** Tape the bag with start, progress, and completion times.

**Add the tape to the bag/bottle so that it is near but does not cover the calibrations**. Enter the start time as 1:40 pm at the 1000 mL level. Next, mark each 150 mL from top to bottom with the successive hours the IV will run.

| | | |
|---|---|---|
| 1000 mL − 150 mL = 850 mL | Label 850 mL for 2:40 pm |
| 850 mL − 150 mL = 700 mL | Label 700 mL for 3:40 pm |
| 700 mL − 150 mL = 550 mL | Label 550 mL for 4:40 pm |
| 550 mL − 150 mL = 400 mL | Label 400 mL for 5:40 pm |
| 400 mL − 150 mL = 250 mL | Label 250 mL for 6:40 pm |
| 250 mL − 150 mL = 100 mL | Label 100 mL for 7:40 pm |

**Calculate the infusion time for the remaining 100 mL.**

$$100 \text{ mL} \div 150 \text{ mL/hr} = 0.66 = \textbf{0.67 hr}$$

$$60 \text{ min/hr} \times 0.67 \text{ hr} = 40.2 = \textbf{40 min}$$

$$7{:}40 \text{ pm} + \textbf{40 min} = \textbf{8:20 pm}$$

**The completion time is 8:20 pm.**

**EXAMPLE 2**   An infiltrated IV with **625 mL** remaining is restarted at **5:30 pm** to run at **150 mL/hr**. Relabel the bag with the new start, progress, and completion times.

**Label the 625 mL level with the 5:30 pm restart time.**

| | |
|---|---|
| 625 mL − 150 mL = 475 mL | Label 475 mL for 6:30 pm |
| 475 mL − 150 mL = 325 mL | Label 325 mL for 7:30 pm |
| 325 mL − 150 mL = 175 mL | Label 175 mL for 8:30 pm |
| 175 mL − 150 mL =  25 mL | Label  25 mL for 9:30 pm |

**Calculate the infusion time for the remaining 25 mL.**

$$25 \text{ mL} \div 150 \text{ mL/hr} = 0.166 = \textbf{0.17 hr}$$

$$60 \text{ min/hr} \times 0.17 \text{ hr} = 10.2 = \textbf{10 min}$$

$$9{:}30 \text{ pm} + \textbf{10 min} = \textbf{9:40 pm}$$

**The completion time is 9:40 pm.**

**EXAMPLE 3**   An infiltrated IV with **340 mL** remaining is restarted at **4:15 am** to run at **70 mL/hr**. Relabel the bag with the new start, progress, and completion times.

**Label the 340 mL level with the 4:15 am restart time.**

| | |
|---|---|
| 340 mL − 70 mL = 270 mL | Label 270 mL for 5:15 am |
| 270 mL − 70 mL = 200 mL | Label 200 mL for 6:15 am |
| 200 mL − 70 mL = 130 mL | Label 130 mL for 7:15 am |
| 130 mL − 70 mL = 60 mL | Label  60 mL for 8:15 am |

**Calculate the infusion time for the remaining 60 mL.**

60 mL ÷ 70 mL/hr = 0.857 = **0.86 hr**

60 min/hr × 0.86 hr = 51.6 = **52 min**

8:15 am + **52 min** = **9:07 am**

**The completion time is 9:07 am.**

Problems 17.4

Calculate the infusion and completion times. Label the IV bags provided with start, progress, and completion times. Have your instructor check your labeling.

1. The IV in Figure 17-2 of 1000 mL was started at 0710 to run at 75 mL/hr.

Infusion time _____   Completion time _____

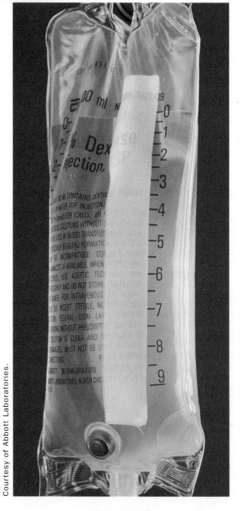

Courtesy of Abbott Laboratories.

**Figure 17-2**

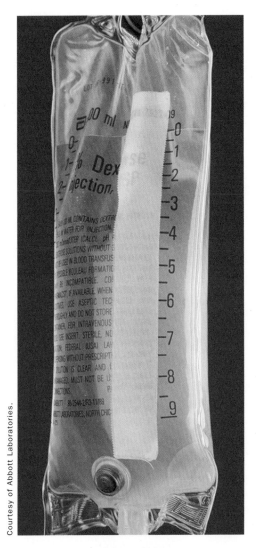

**Figure 17-3**                                        **Figure 17-4**

2. The 1000 mL IV in Figure 17-3 has an ordered rate of 125 mL/hr. It was started at 6:30 pm.

           Infusion time _____   Completion time _____

3. The IV in Figure 17-4 of 1000 mL has an ordered rate of 80 mL/hr. It was started at 5:40 am.

           Infusion time _____   Completion time _____

**Answers**   **1.** 13 hr 20 min; 2030   **2.** 8 hr; 2:30 am   **3.** 12 hr 30 min; 6.10 pm

## Summary

**This concludes the chapter on calculation of infusion and completion times and labeling of IV bags/bottles with start, progress, and completion times. The important points to remember from this chapter are:**

- The infusion time is the time required for an IV to infuse completely.

- The infusion time is calculated by dividing the total volume to infuse by the mL/hr rate ordered.

- The completion time is calculated by adding the infusion time to the start time.

- When the min calculated are 60 or more, an additional hr is added to the completion time and 60 min are subtracted from the total min.

- Calculating completion times provides an opportunity to plan ahead and have the next solution ordered ready to hang or to discontinue an IV when it has completed.

- Most clinical facilities label IV solution bags/bottles with start, progress, and finish times to provide a visual record of the infusion status.

## Summary Self-Test

**Calculate the infusion and completion times.**

1. The order is for 50 mL to infuse at 50 mL/hr. The infusion was started at 10:10 am.

   Infusion time _____   Completion time _____

2. An infusion of 950 mL is ordered at 80 mL/hr. It was started at 8:02 am.

   Infusion time _____   Completion time _____

3. A total of 280 mL remain in an IV bag. The flow rate is 70 mL/hr. It is now 11:03 am.

   Infusion time _____   Completion time _____

4. The order is to infuse 500 mL at 90 mL/hr. The IV was started at 2:40 pm.

   Infusion time _____   Completion time _____

5. An infiltrated IV with 850 mL remaining is restarted at 10 am at a rate of 150 mL/hr.

   Infusion time _____   Completion time _____

6. At 4:04 am, an IV of 500 mL is started at a rate of 50 mL/hr.

   Infusion time _____   Completion time _____

7. An IV medication with a volume of 150 mL is started at 1:45 pm to infuse at 60 mL/hr.

   Infusion time _____   Completion time _____

8. An IV of 520 mL is restarted at 0420 at a rate of 125 mL/hr.

   Infusion time _____   Completion time _____

9. It is 12:00 pm, and an IV of 900 mL is to infuse at a rate of 100 mL/hr.

   Infusion time _____   Completion time _____

10. An IV of 1000 mL is started at 0550 to infuse at 130 mL/hr.

    Infusion time _____   Completion time _____

11. An infusion of 250 mL is started at 11:20 am to infuse at a rate of 20 mL/hr.

    Infusion time _____   Completion time _____

12. The flow rate ordered for 1 L is 80 mL/hr. It was started at 8:07 pm.

    Infusion time _____   Completion time _____

13. A 250 mL volume is started at 3:40 pm to be infused at 90 mL/hr.

Infusion time _____   Completion time _____

14. A medication volume of 100 mL is started at 4:00 pm to infuse at 42 mL/hr.

Infusion time _____   Completion time _____

15. At 11:00 pm, 200 mL remain in an IV. The rate is 120 mL/hr.

Infusion time _____   Completion time _____

16. An infusion of 350 mL is to run at 150 mL/hr. It is now 9:47 am.

Infusion time _____   Completion time _____

17. An IV medication of 25 mL is started at 8:17 am to run at 25 mL/hr.

Infusion time _____   Completion time _____

18. An IV of 425 mL is restarted at 0814 to infuse at 90 mL/hr.

Infusion time _____   Completion time _____

19. At 10:30 pm, there are 180 mL left in an IV that is infusing at 25 mL/hr.

Infusion time _____   Completion time _____

20. At 1400, 500 mL is started to run at a rate of 60 mL/hr.

Infusion time _____   Completion time _____

21. An infusion of 250 mL is started at 3:04 am to run at 100 mL/hr.

Infusion time _____   Completion time _____

22. With 525 mL remaining, a rate change to 108 mL/hr is ordered. It is 2:10 am.

Infusion time _____   Completion time _____

23. A liter is started at 8:42 am at a rate of 120 mL/hr.

Infusion time _____   Completion time _____

24. An infusion of 1000 mL is to run at 200 mL/hr. It is started at 6:40 pm.

Infusion time _____   Completion time _____

25. An IV medication of 100 mL is started at 7:50 am to run at 150 mL/hr.

Infusion time _____   Completion time _____

26. A volume of 500 mL is started at 4:04 pm at a rate of 75 mL/hr.

Infusion time _____   Completion time _____

27. An IV of 950 mL is restarted at 2:10 am at 100 mL/hr.

Infusion time _____   Completion time _____

28. An IV medication of 30 mL is started at 0915 at a rate of 60 mL/hr.

Infusion time _____   Completion time _____

29. A medication volume of 90 mL was started at 6:15 am to be infused at 90 mL/hr.

Infusion time _____   Completion time _____

30. A rate of 80 mL/hr is set at 4:20 pm to infuse a medication with a volume of 100 mL.

Infusion time _____   Completion time _____

31. A volume of 750 mL is started at 0303 at a rate of 96 mL/hr.

Infusion time _____   Completion time _____

Label the following solution bags for the times and rates indicated. Have your instructor check your labeling.

32.
Started: 10:47 am
Rate: 80 mL/hr

33.
Started: 1315
Rate: 100 mL/hr

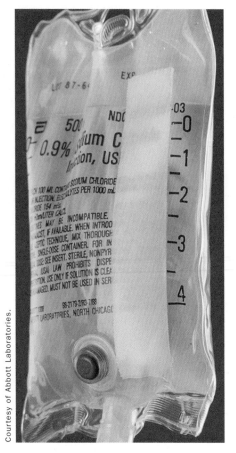

34.
Started: 2:10 pm
Rate: 90 mL/hr

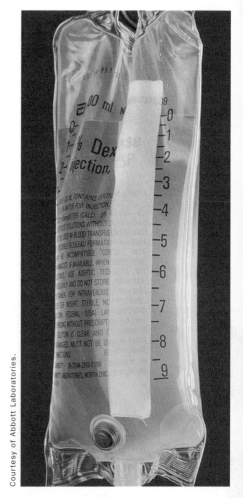

Courtesy of Abbott Laboratories.

Courtesy of Abbott Laboratories.

Courtesy of Abbott Laboratories.

35.
Started: 0440
Rate: 75 mL/hr

36.
Started: 0730
Rate: 50 mL/hr

37.
Started: 6:20 pm
Rate: 25 mL/hr

38.
Started: 3:03 am
Rate: 50 mL/hr

39.
Started: 0744
Rate: 125 mL/hr

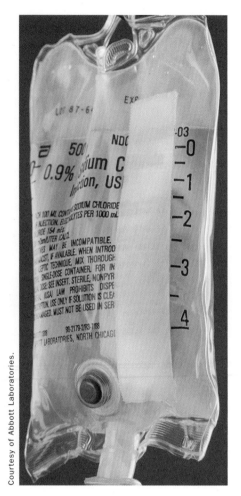

40.
Started: 2140
Rate: 100 mL/hr

**Answers**

1. 1 hr; 11:10 am
2. 11 hr 53 min; 7:55 pm
3. 4 hr; 3:03 pm
4. 5 hr 34 min; 8:14 pm
5. 5 hr 40 min; 3:40 pm
6. 10 hr; 2:04 pm
7. 2 hr 30 min; 4:15 pm
8. 4 hr 10 min; 0830
9. 9 hr; 9 pm
10. 7 hr 41 min; 1331
11. 12 hr 30 min; 11:50 pm
12. 12 hr 30 min; 8:37 am
13. 2 hr 47 min; 6:27 pm
14. 2 hr 23 min; 6:23 pm
15. 1 hr 40 min; 12:40 am
16. 2 hr 20 min; 12:07 pm
17. 1 hr; 9:17 am
18. 4 hr 43 min; 1257
19. 7 hr 12 min; 5:42 am
20. 8 hr 20 min; 2220
21. 2 hr 30 min; 5:34 am
22. 4 hr 52 min; 7:02 am
23. 8 hr 20 min; 5:02 pm
24. 5 hr; 11:40 pm
25. 40 min; 8:30 am
26. 6 hr 40 min; 10:44 pm
27. 9 hr 30 min; 11:40 am
28. 30 min; 0945
29. 1 hr; 7:15 am
30. 1 hr 15 min; 5:35 pm
31. 7 hr 49 min; 1052
32-40. Verify your answers with your instructor.

**Note:** Answers may vary slightly due to rounding.

# 18

# IV MEDICATION AND TITRATION CALCULATIONS

## Objectives

**The learner will calculate:**

1. flow rates to infuse ordered dosages.

2. dosages and flow rates based on kg body weight.

3. dosage and flow rate ranges for titrated medications.

Many IV drugs are used in critical and life-threatening situations to alter or maintain vital physiologic functions; for example, heart rate, cardiac output, blood pressure (BP), and respiration. In general, these drugs have a very rapid action and short duration. They are frequently administered diluted in 250–500 mL of IV solution, most commonly D5W.

Intravenous medications may be ordered by dosage (mcg/mg/units per min/hr) or based on body weight (mcg/mg/units per kg per min/hr). They may also be ordered to infuse within a specific dosage range—for example, 1–3 mcg/min—to elicit a measurable physiologic response; an example would be to maintain a systolic BP above 100 mm Hg. This adjustment of rate is called **titration**, and dosage increments are made within the ordered range until the desired response has been established. IV drugs require close and continuous monitoring, and an electronic infusion device (EID), either a volumetric pump or a syringe pump, is used for their administration. If an EID is not used, a microdrip set calibrated at 60 gtt/mL or a dosage controlled Soluset®/Buretrol®/Volutrol® burette is used.

All calculations in this chapter are for an EID or microdrip, and the mL/hr and gtt/min rates are therefore interchangeable. Calculations include converting ordered dosages to the flow rates necessary to administer them, and using flow rates to calculate the dosage infusing at any given moment. Body weight is often a critical factor in IV dosages, and its use in calculations will also be covered. A number of EIDs display, and can be set to deliver, dosage and flow rate equivalents, but you must know how to do these calculations in case you encounter a situation in which you will have to do one. IV drugs that alter a basic physiologic function generally have narrow margins of safety, and accuracy is imperative in their calculation. Double-checking of math is both mandatory and routine. As a general rule, dosages are calculated to the nearest tenth and flow rates are rounded to the nearest mL or gtt. When an EID is used, flow rates can be programmed to deliver tenths of a mL.

All calculations assume the use of an EID or microdrip infusion set; therefore, the mL/hr and gtt/min rates are identical and interchangeable.

## CALCULATING mL/hr RATE FOR DOSAGE ORDERED

One common IV critical care calculation is to determine the mL/hr flow rate for a specific drug dosage ordered. Let's start by looking at some examples of these.

**EXAMPLE 1**

A cardiac medication with a strength of **125 mg/100 mL** is to infuse at a rate of **20 mg/hr**. Calculate the **mL/hr** flow rate.

$$\frac{mL}{hr} = \frac{100\ mL}{125\ mg} \times \frac{20\ mg}{1\ hr}$$

$$= \frac{100\ mL}{125\ mg} \times \frac{20\ mg}{1\ hr}$$

$$= 16\ mL\ /\ hr$$

**To infuse 20 mg/hr, set the flow rate at 16 mL/hr.**

**EXAMPLE 2**

A dosage of **2 mcg/min** has been ordered using an **8 mg in 250 mL** solution. Calculate the **mL/hr** flow rate.

This equation will need a 60 min = 1 hr and a 1 mg = 1000 mcg conversion.

$$\frac{mL}{hr} = \frac{250\ mL}{8\ mg} \times \frac{1\ mg}{1000\ mcg} \times \frac{2\ mcg}{1\ min} \times \frac{60\ min}{1\ hr}$$

$$= \frac{250\ mL}{8\ mg} \times \frac{1\ mg}{1000\ mcg} \times \frac{2\ mcg}{1\ min} \times \frac{60\ min}{1\ hr}$$

$$= 3.75 = 4\ mL\ /\ hr$$

*(handwritten in margin:)* $\frac{250\ ml}{8\ mg}$  $\frac{1\ mg}{1000\ mcg}$  $\frac{2\ mg}{hr}$  $\frac{60}{1\ hr}$

**To infuse 2 mcg/min, set the flow rate at 4 mL/hr.**

**EXAMPLE 3**

A medication with a strength of **50 mg in 250 mL** is used to infuse a dosage of **200 mcg/min**. Calculate the flow rate in **mL/hr**.

This equation will need a 60 min = 1 hr and 1 mg = 1000 mcg conversion.

$$\frac{mL}{hr} = \frac{250\ mL}{50\ mg} \times \frac{1\ mg}{1000\ mcg} \times \frac{200\ mcg}{1\ min} \times \frac{60\ min}{1\ hr}$$

$$= \frac{250\ mL}{50\ mg} \times \frac{1\ mg}{1000\ mcg} \times \frac{200\ mcg}{1\ min} \times \frac{60\ min}{1\ hr}$$

$$= 60\ mL/hr$$

**To infuse 200 mcg/min, set the flow rate at 60 mL/hr.**

## Problems 18.1

Calculate the mL/hr flow rates. Express answers to the nearest whole mL/hr.

$\dfrac{100 \text{ mL}}{100 \text{ mg}} , \dfrac{20 \text{ mg}}{1 \text{ hr}} = 20 \text{ mL/hr}$

1. A 20 mg/hr dosage is ordered using a 100 mg/100 mL solution.  _____

2. A medication is ordered at the rate of 3 mcg/min. The solution strength is 8 mg in 250 mL.  _____

$\dfrac{500 \text{ mL}}{1500 \text{ mg}} , \dfrac{3 \text{ mg}}{\text{min}} , \dfrac{60 \text{ min}}{1 \text{ hr}}$

3. A solution of 2 g medication in 500 mL is used to administer a dosage of 2 mg/min.  _____

4. A 2 mcg/min infusion is ordered. The solution strength is 1 mg/250 mL.  _____

$\dfrac{250 \text{ mL}}{10000 \text{ mcg}} , \dfrac{20 \text{ mcg}}{\text{min}} , \dfrac{60}{1} =$

5. An initial dose of a drug is ordered at 25 mg/hr. The solution strength is 125 mg/100 mL.  _____

6. A 100 mg/250 mL solution strength is ordered at a rate of 15 mg/hr.  _____

$\dfrac{100 \text{ mL}}{250 \text{ mg}} , \dfrac{30 \text{ mcg}}{1 \text{ hr}}$

7. A solution strength of 10 mg/250 mL is to infuse at 5 mcg/min.  _____

8. A 500 mL/1.5 g solution is to infuse at 3 mg/min.  _____

9. A 10 mg/250 mL solution is to infuse at 20 mcg/min.  _____

10. A 250 mg/100 mL solution is to infuse at 30 mg/hr.  _____

**Answers   1.** 20 mL/hr   **2.** 6 mL/hr   **3.** 30 mL/hr   **4.** 30 mL/hr   **5.** 20 mL/hr   **6.** 38 mL/hr
**7.** 8 mL/hr   **8.** 60 mL/hr   **9.** 30 mL/hr   **10.** 12 mL/hr

## CALCULATING mL/hr RATE FOR DOSAGE PER kg ORDERED

Many IV medication infusions are calculated based on body weight; for example, 95.9 mcg/kg/hr. **Body weight to the nearest tenth kg** is used for the calculations. There are two ways the flow rate can be calculated. The first method requires two steps.

## TWO-STEP FLOW RATE CALCULATION FOR DOSAGE PER kg ORDERED

The dosage for the body weight is calculated to the nearest tenth, then used to determine the flow rate.

> **EXAMPLE 1**

Medication is ordered at the rate of **3 mcg/kg/min** for an adult weighing **95.9 kg**. The solution strength is **400 mg** in **250 mL**. Calculate the flow rate.

- **Calculate the 3 mcg/min dosage for 95.9 kg.**

  3 mcg/kg/min $\times$ 95.9 kg = **287.7 mcg/min**

- **Calculate the mL/hr flow rate for 287.7 mcg/min.**

$$\frac{mL}{hr} = \frac{250\ mL}{400\ mg} \times \frac{1\ mg}{1000\ mcg} \times \frac{287.7\ mcg}{1\ min} \times \frac{60\ min}{1\ hr}$$

$$= \frac{250\ mL}{400\ \cancel{mg}} \times \frac{1\ \cancel{mg}}{1000\ \cancel{mcg}} \times \frac{287.7\ \cancel{mcg}}{1\ \cancel{min}} \times \frac{60\ \cancel{min}}{1\ hr}$$

$$= 10.79 = \mathbf{11\ mL/hr}$$

**To infuse 3 mcg/kg/min, set the flow rate at 11 mL/hr.**

---

**EXAMPLE 2**

A solution strength of **2.5 g in 250 mL** has been ordered at a rate of **100 mcg/kg/min** for an adult weighing **104.6 kg**. Calculate the flow rate.

- **Calculate the dosage for 104.6 kg.**

$$100\ mcg/kg/min \times 104.6\ kg = 10{,}460\ mcg/min = \mathbf{10.5\ mg/min}$$

- **Calculate the flow rate for 10.5 mg/min.**

$$\frac{mL}{hr} = \frac{250\ mL}{2.5\ g} \times \frac{1\ g}{1000\ mg} \times \frac{10.5\ mg}{1\ min} \times \frac{60\ min}{1\ hr}$$

$$= \frac{250\ mL}{2.5\ \cancel{g}} \times \frac{1\ \cancel{g}}{1000\ \cancel{mg}} \times \frac{10.5\ \cancel{mg}}{1\ \cancel{min}} \times \frac{60\ \cancel{min}}{1\ hr}$$

$$= 63 = \mathbf{63\ mL/hr}$$

**To infuse 100 mcg/kg/min, set the flow rate at 63 mL/hr.**

---

**EXAMPLE 3**

A medication has been ordered at **4 mcg/kg/min** from a solution of **50 mg in 250 mL**. The body weight is **107.3 kg**.

- **Calculate the dosage for 107.3 kg.**

$$4\ mcg/kg/min \times 107.3\ kg = \mathbf{429.2\ mcg/min}$$

- **Calculate the flow rate for 429.2 mcg/min.**

$$\frac{mL}{hr} = \frac{250\ mL}{50\ mg} \times \frac{1\ mg}{1000\ mcg} \times \frac{429.2\ mcg}{1\ min} \times \frac{60\ min}{1\ hr}$$

$$= \frac{250\ mL}{50\ \cancel{mg}} \times \frac{1\ \cancel{mg}}{1000\ \cancel{mcg}} \times \frac{429.2\ \cancel{mcg}}{1\ \cancel{min}} \times \frac{60\ \cancel{min}}{1\ hr}$$

$$= 128.7 = \mathbf{129\ mL/hr}$$

**To infuse 4 mcg/kg/min, set the flow rate at 129 mL/hr.**

18

## Problems 18.2

Calculate the mcg/min and mL/hr flow rates.

262.2 mcg/min

$\frac{250 mL}{50000} \cdot \frac{262.2}{1 min} \cdot \frac{60}{1 hr}$

$\frac{250 mL}{400000} \cdot \frac{369.6}{1} \cdot \frac{60}{1}$

|  | mcg/min | mL/hr |
|---|---|---|
| 1. A 3 mcg/kg/min dosage has been ordered for an adult weighing 87.4 kg. The solution being used has a strength of 50 mg in 250 mL. | 262.2 | 79 |
| 2. IV medication has been ordered to infuse at 4 mcg/kg/min using a 400 mg/250 mL solution. The body weight is 92.4 kg. | 369.6 | 14 mL |
| 3. A 2.5 mcg/kg/min dosage has been ordered. The solution strength is 0.5 g/250 mL. The body weight is 80.7 kg. | _____ | _____ |
| 4. A rate of 150 mcg/kg/min has been ordered for a body weight of 92.1 kg. The solution strength is 2.5 g in 250 mL. | _____ | _____ |
| 5. A 5 mcg/kg/min infusion has been ordered for a body weight of 80.3 kg. The solution to be used has 1 g in 500 mL. | _____ | _____ |
| 6. A 2 mcg/kg/min dosage has been ordered for an adult weighing 79.9 kg. The solution strength available is 50 mg/250 mL. | _____ | _____ |
| 7. A dosage of 3 mcg/kg/min has been ordered using a 350 mg/250 mL solution strength. The body weight is 86.9 kg. | _____ | _____ |
| 8. An adult weighing 84.3 kg has a dosage of 3 mcg/kg/min ordered. The solution to be used is 0.75 g/300 mL. | _____ | _____ |
| 9. A 4.5 mcg/kg/min dosage is ordered for an 84.9 kg adult. The solution strength is 1.2 g/500 mL. | _____ | _____ |
| 10. A 6 mcg/kg/min dosage is ordered for an adult weighing 85.8 kg. The solution strength is 800 mg/500 mL. | _____ | _____ |

**Answers  1.** 262.2 mcg/min; 79 mL/hr  **2.** 369.6 mcg/min; 14 mL/hr  **3.** 201.8 mcg/min; 6 mL/hr
**4.** 13,815 mcg/min; 83 mL/hr  **5.** 401.5 mcg/min; 12 mL/hr  **6.** 159.8 mcg/min; 48 mL/hr
**7.** 260.7 mcg/min; 11 mL/hr  **8.** 252.9 mcg/min; 6 mL/hr  **9.** 382.1 mcg/min; 10 mL/hr
**10.** 514.8 mcg/min; 19 mL/hr

## ONE-STEP mL/hr FLOW RATE CALCULATION FOR DOSAGE FOR kg ORDERED

The one-step method of flow rate calculation requires very careful entry of ratios and equally careful cancellation of measurement units to verify accuracy in ratio entry. Let's look at the entire equation step by step. Express flow rates to the nearest mL.

**EXAMPLE 1**

Medication is ordered at the rate of **3 mcg/kg/min** for an adult weighing **95.9 kg**. The solution strength is **400 mg** in **250 mL**. Calculate the flow rate.

**The first two ratios entered are the same as in the two-step method.**

$$\frac{mL}{hr} = \frac{250\ mL}{400\ mg} \times \frac{1\ mg}{1000\ mcg}$$

**The denominator to be matched next is mcg. This is provided by the 3 mcg/kg/min dosage. Enter this with 3 mcg as the numerator; two measures, kg and min, become the new denominators.**

$$\frac{mL}{hr} = \frac{250\ mL}{400\ mg} \times \frac{1\ mg}{1000\ mcg} \times \frac{3\ mcg}{kg\ /\ min}$$

**Both kg and min must be matched in the next numerators. Either can be entered first, but min is the best choice because a conversion ratio is needed to change min to the hr being calculated. Enter the 60 min = 1 hr conversion, with 60 min as the numerator, to match the previous min denominator.**

$$\frac{mL}{hr} = \frac{250\ mL}{400\ mg} \times \frac{1\ mg}{1000\ mcg} \times \frac{3\ mcg}{kg\ /\ min} \times \frac{60\ min}{1\ hr}$$

**Only one measure remains to be entered: the 95.9 kg body weight. Enter this as the final numerator to match the remaining kg denominator. This completes the equation.**

$$\frac{mL}{hr} = \frac{250\ mL}{400\ mg} \times \frac{1\ mg}{1000\ mcg} \times \frac{3\ mcg}{kg\ /\ min} \times \frac{60\ min}{1\ hr} \times \frac{95.9\ kg}{}$$

**Cancel the alternate denominator/numerator measures. Only mL and hr remain in the equation. Do the math.**

$$\frac{mL}{hr} = \frac{250\ mL}{400\ mg} \times \frac{1\ mg}{1000\ mcg} \times \frac{3\ mcg}{kg\ /\ min} \times \frac{60\ min}{1\ hr} \times \frac{95.9\ kg}{}$$

$$= 10.79 = 11\ mL/hr$$

**The 11 mL/hr answer is identical to the 11 mL/hr answer obtained in the two-step calculation previously demonstrated.**

**EXAMPLE 2**

A dosage of **2.5 g in 250 mL** has been ordered at a rate of **100 mcg/kg/min** for an adult weighing **104.6 kg**. Calculate the flow rate.

**Enter the mL/hr being calculated. The first mL numerator is provided by the 250 mL containing 2.5 g medication. Enter it now.**

$$\frac{mL}{hr} = \frac{250 \ mL}{2.5 \ g}$$

**The dosage ordered is in mcg, so g to mg and mg to mcg conversion ratios are needed. Enter these now.**

$$\frac{mL}{hr} = \frac{250 \ mL}{2.5 \ g} \times \frac{1 \ g}{1000 \ mg} \times \frac{1 \ mg}{1000 \ mcg}$$

**Enter the 100 mcg/kg/min dosage next, with mcg as the numerator to match the previous mcg denominator.**

$$\frac{mL}{hr} = \frac{250 \ mL}{2.5 \ g} \times \frac{1 \ g}{1000 \ mg} \times \frac{1 \ mg}{1000 \ mcg} \times \frac{100 \ mcg}{kg/min}$$

**Enter the min/hr conversion ratio.**

$$\frac{mL}{hr} = \frac{250 \ mL}{2.5 \ g} \times \frac{1 \ g}{1000 \ mg} \times \frac{1 \ mg}{1000 \ mcg} \times \frac{100 \ mcg}{kg \ / \ min} \times \frac{60 \ min}{1 \ hr}$$

**Enter the 104.6 kg body weight to complete the equation.**

$$\frac{mL}{hr} = \frac{250 \ mL}{2.5 \ g} \times \frac{1 \ g}{1000 \ mg} \times \frac{1 \ mg}{1000 \ mcg} \times \frac{100 \ mcg}{kg \ / \ min} \times \frac{60 \ min}{1 \ hr} \times \frac{104.6 \ kg}{}$$

**Cancel the alternate denominator/numerator entries to double-check the accuracy of ratio entry. Do the math.**

$$\frac{mL}{hr} = \frac{250 \ mL}{2.5 \ \cancel{g}} \times \frac{1 \ \cancel{g}}{1000 \ \cancel{mg}} \times \frac{1 \ \cancel{mg}}{1000 \ \cancel{mcg}} \times \frac{100 \ \cancel{mcg}}{\cancel{kg} \ / \ \cancel{min}} \times \frac{60 \ \cancel{min}}{1 \ hr} \times \frac{104.6 \ \cancel{kg}}{}$$

$$= 62.76 = \mathbf{63 \ mL/hr}$$

The 63 mL/hr answer is identical to the 63 mL/hr answer obtained in the two-step calculation.

**EXAMPLE 3**

A medication has been ordered at 4 mcg/kg/min from a solution of **50 mg** in **250 mL**. The body weight is **107.3 kg**.

$$\frac{mL}{hr} = \frac{250\ mL}{50\ mg}$$

$$\frac{mL}{hr} = \frac{250\ mL}{50\ mg} \times \frac{1\ mg}{1000\ mcg}$$

$$\frac{mL}{hr} = \frac{250\ mL}{50\ mg} \times \frac{1\ mg}{1000\ mcg} \times \frac{4\ mcg}{kg/min}$$

$$\frac{mL}{hr} = \frac{250\ mL}{50\ mg} \times \frac{1\ mg}{1000\ mcg} \times \frac{4\ mcg}{kg/min} \times \frac{60\ min}{1\ hr}$$

$$\frac{mL}{hr} = \frac{250\ mL}{50\ mg} \times \frac{1\ mg}{1000\ mcg} \times \frac{4\ mcg}{kg/min} \times \frac{60\ min}{1\ hr} \times \frac{107.3\ kg}{}$$

$$= 128.76 = \textbf{129 mL/hr}$$

**The 129 mL/hr answer is identical to the 129 mL/hr rate calculated in the two-step method.**

## Problems 18.3

**Calculate the mL/hr flow rates. Express answers to the nearest whole mL/hr.**

1. A 3.5 mcg/kg/min dosage has been ordered for an adult weighing 90.3 kg. The solution being used has a strength of 40 mg in 150 mL.  _____

2. IV medication has been ordered to infuse at 3 mcg/kg/min using a 250 mg/250 mL solution. The body weight is 87.3 kg.  _____

3. A 4 mcg/kg/min dosage has been ordered. The solution strength is 600 mg/250 mL. The weight is 90.3 kg.  _____

4. A rate of 200 mcg/kg/min has been ordered for a 83.3 kg weight. The solution strength is 3.5 g in 250 mL.  _____

5. A 4.5 mcg/kg/min infusion has been ordered for a 79.9 kg body weight. The solution to be used has 1.5 g in 200 mL.  _____

6. A 4 mcg/kg/min dosage has been ordered for an adult weighing 83.8 kg. The solution strength available is 50 mg/150 mL.  _____

7. A dosage of 5 mcg/kg/min has been ordered using a 300 mg/250 mL solution strength. The body weight is 86.6 kg.  _____

8. An adult weighing 91.4 kg has a dosage of 4 mcg/kg/min ordered. The solution to be used is 700 mg/500 mL.  _____

9. A 175 mcg/kg/min dosage is ordered for an 84.9 kg adult. The solution strength is 4 g/250 mL.  _____

10. A 5 mcg/kg/min dosage is ordered for an adult weighing 78.9 kg. The solution strength is 2 g/250 mL.  _____

## CALCULATING INFUSION TITRATIONS

Titration refers to the **adjustment of dosage within a specific range to obtain a measurable physiologic response**; for example, a drug at 2–4 mcg/min to maintain systolic BP above 100 mm Hg. The dosage is increased or decreased within the ordered range until the desired response is obtained. The **lowest dosage is set first and adjusted upward and downward as necessary.** The **upper dosage is never exceeded** unless a new order is obtained.

Volumetric or syringe pumps are used for administration. Flow rates are calculated in mL/hr for the lowest and highest dosage ordered and adjusted within this range to elicit the desired physiologic response. Let's look at some examples.

**EXAMPLE 1**

A **2–4 mcg/min** dosage has been ordered. The solution being titrated has **8 mg** in **250 mL**. Calculate the flow rate of medication for the **2–4 mcg range**.

**Calculate the lower 2 mcg/min flow rate first.**

$$\frac{mL}{hr} = \frac{250\ mL}{8\ mg} \times \frac{1\ mg}{1000\ mcg} \times \frac{2\ mcg}{1\ min} \times \frac{60\ min}{1\ hr}$$

$$= \frac{250\ mL}{8\ mg} \times \frac{1\ mg}{1000\ mcg} \times \frac{2\ mcg}{1\ min} \times \frac{60\ min}{1\ hr}$$

$$= 3.75 = \mathbf{4\ mL\ /\ hr}$$

**The upper 4 mcg/min flow rate is exactly double the 2 mcg/min rate.**

$$4\ mL/hr \times 2 = \mathbf{8\ mL/hr}$$

**A dosage of 2–4 mcg/min is delivered by a flow rate of 4–8 mL/hr.**

**EXAMPLE 2**

A medication is to be titrated between **415–830 mcg/min**. The solution concentration is **100 mg** in **40 mL**. Calculate the **mL/hr** flow rate range.

**Calculate the flow rate for the lower 415 mcg/min dosage.**

$$\frac{mL}{hr} = \frac{40\ mL}{100\ mg} \times \frac{1\ mg}{1000\ mcg} \times \frac{415\ mcg}{1\ min} \times \frac{60\ min}{1\ hr}$$

$$= \frac{40\ mL}{100\ mg} \times \frac{1\ mg}{1000\ mcg} \times \frac{415\ mcg}{1\ min} \times \frac{60\ min}{1\ hr}$$

$$= 9.96 = \mathbf{10mL\ /\ hr}$$

**The 830 mcg dosage is exactly double 415 mcg.**

$$10 \text{ mL/hr} \times 2 = \textbf{20 mL/hr}$$

A dosage of 415–830 mcg/min requires a flow rate of 10–20 mL/hr.

### EXAMPLE 3

An adult weighing **103.1 kg** has dosage orders for **0.3–3 mcg/kg/min**. The solution concentration is **50 mg in 250 mL**.

Calculate the dosage range for 103.1 kg.

**Lower dosage:**  $0.3 \text{ mcg/kg/min} \times 103.1 \text{ kg} = 30.93 = \textbf{30.9 mcg/min}$

**Upper dosage:**  $3 \text{ mcg/kg/min} \times 103.1 \text{ kg} = \textbf{309.3 mcg/min}$

The dosage range for this 103.1 kg adult is 30.9–309.3 mcg/min.

Calculate the flow rate for the lower 30.9 mcg/min dosage.

$$\frac{\text{mL}}{\text{hr}} = \frac{250 \text{ mL}}{50 \text{ mg}} \times \frac{1 \text{ mg}}{1000 \text{ mcg}} \times \frac{30.9 \text{ mcg}}{1 \text{ min}} \times \frac{60 \text{ min}}{1 \text{ hr}}$$

$$= \frac{250 \text{ mL}}{50 \text{ mg}} \times \frac{1 \text{ mg}}{1000 \text{ mcg}} \times \frac{30.9 \text{ mcg}}{1 \text{ min}} \times \frac{60 \text{ min}}{1 \text{ hr}}$$

$$= 9.2 = \textbf{9 mL/hr}$$

Calculate the flow rate for the upper 309.3 mcg/min dosage.

$$\frac{\text{mL}}{\text{hr}} = \frac{250 \text{ mL}}{50 \text{ mg}} \times \frac{1 \text{ mg}}{1000 \text{ mcg}} \times \frac{309.3 \text{ mcg}}{1 \text{ min}} \times \frac{60 \text{ min}}{1 \text{ hr}}$$

$$= \frac{250 \text{ mL}}{50 \text{ mg}} \times \frac{1 \text{ mg}}{1000 \text{ mcg}} \times \frac{309.3 \text{ mcg}}{1 \text{ min}} \times \frac{60 \text{ min}}{1 \text{ hr}}$$

$$= 92.7 = \textbf{93 mL/hr}$$

To deliver 0.3–3 mcg/kg/min, the flow rate must be titrated from 9–93 mL/hr.

### Problems 18.4

Calculate the mL/hr flow rate ranges. Express answers to the nearest whole mL/hr.

1. A 2 g in 500 mL solution is ordered to titrate at 1–2 mg/min.  _____

2. A drug is ordered to titrate between 1–3 mcg/min. The solution strength is 1 mg per 250 mL.  _____

3. The dosage range is 5–8 mcg/kg/min. The body weight is 103.7 kg, and the solution strength is 100 mg in 40 mL.  _____

4. A drug is to titrate between 50–100 mcg/kg/min. The body weight is 78.7 kg, and the solution strength is 2500 mg in 250 mL.  _____

5. An adult weighing 73.2 kg has a solution of 500 mg medication in 250 mL ordered to titrate between 3–10 mcg/kg/min.  _____

6. A 2–3 mg/min dosage has been ordered. The solution strength available is 1.5 g/400 mL. _____

7. A dosage of 6–7 mcg/min has been ordered using a 5 mg/500 mL solution strength. _____

8. An adult weighing 101.6 kg has a dosage of 4–7 mcg/kg/min ordered. The solution to be used is 75 mg/50 mL. _____

9. A 30–70 mcg/kg/min dosage is ordered for an 80.4 kg adult. The solution strength is 3 g/250 mL. _____

10. A 4–8 mcg/kg/min dosage is ordered for an adult weighing 72.1 kg. The solution strength is 400 mg/250 mL. _____

**Answers** **1.** 15–30 mL/hr  **2.** 15–45 mL/hr  **3.** 12–20 mL/hr  **4.** 24–47 mL/hr  **5.** 7–22 mL/hr **6.** 32–48 mL/hr  **7.** 36–42 mL/hr  **8.** 16–28 mL/hr  **9.** 12–28 mL/hr  **10.** 11–22 mL/hr

## Summary

**This concludes the chapter on titration of IV medications. The important points to remember about these medications are:**

- They have a rapid action and short duration.

- They have a narrow margin of safety, and continuous monitoring is required in their use.

- They are frequency-titrated within a specific dosage/flow rate to elicit a measurable physiologic response.

- When titrated, they are initiated at the lowest dosage ordered and increased or decreased slowly to obtain the desired response.

- They are infused using an EID or 60 gtt/mL microdrip set.

- The mL/hr flow rate for EIDs and the gtt/min microdrip rate are identical and interchangeable.

## Summary Self-Test

**Calculate dosages to the nearest tenth, and flow rates to the nearest whole number.**

1. A 6 mcg/kg/min dosage is ordered for an adult weighing 75.4 kg. The solution available is 500 mg in 250 mL.

     mcg/min dosage _____  mL/hr flow rate _____

2. The order is to infuse a solution of 50 mg in 250 mL at 0.8 mcg/kg/min. Calculate the dosage and flow rate for a 65.9 kg adult.

     mcg/min dosage _____  mL/hr flow rate _____

3. A solution of 250 mg in 500 mL is to infuse between 0.5 and 0.7 mg/kg/hr. The adult weighs 82.4 kg.

     mg/hr dosage range _____  mL/hr flow rate range _____

4. A solution of 400 mg in 250 mL is infusing at 20 mL/hr.

     mcg/min dosage _____

5. A 1-6 mg/min dosage is ordered. The solution strength is 2 g/500 mL.

    mL/hr flow rate range _____

6. An infusion of 2 g in 500 mL is ordered at 60 mL/hr.

    mg/min dosage _____        mg/hr dosage _____

7. The solution available is 25 mg in 50 mL. The order is to infuse at 8 mg/hr.

    mL/hr flow rate _____

8. A solution of 100 mg in 40 mL is ordered to infuse at 5 mcg/kg/min for an adult weighing 77.1 kg.

    mL/hr flow rate _____

9. A drug is ordered at 4 mcg/min. The solution available is 1 mg in 250 mL.

    mL/hr flow rate _____

10. An adult weighing 80 kg has an infusion ordered at 8 mcg/kg/min. The solution strength is 800 mg in 500 mL.

    mcg/min dosage _____        mL/hr flow rate _____

11. A dosage of 400 mg is added to 250 mL and infused at 45 mL/hr. Calculate the mcg/min and mg/hr infusing.

    mcg/min dosage _____        mg/hr dosage _____

12. An adult has orders for a dosage of 1 mg/min. The solution strength is 250 mg in 250 mL.

    mL/hr flow rate _____

13. An adult weighing 77.9 kg is to receive 80 mcg/kg/min. The solution strength is 2.5 g in 250 mL.

    mcg/min dosage _____        mL/hr flow rate _____

14. A dosage of 4 mcg/min has been ordered using an 8 mg in 250 mL solution.

    mL/hr flow rate _____

15. An adult who weighs 81.7 kg has orders for 8-10 mcg/kg/min. The solution strength is 400 mg in 250 mL.

    mcg/min dosage range _____

16. A 6 mcg/kg/min dosage has been ordered for a 90.7 kg adult. The solution strength is 50 mg in 250 mL.

    mcg/min dosage _____        mL/hr flow rate _____

17. A dosage of 5 mcg/kg/min is ordered. The solution available is 400 mg in 250 mL. The adult weighs 70.7 kg.

    mcg/min dosage _____        mL/hr flow rate _____

18. A 3 mg/min dosage is ordered. The solution strength is 2 g in 500 mL.

    mL/hr flow rate _____

19. A solution of 50 mg/250 mL is infusing at 15 mL/hr.

    mcg/min infusing _____

20. A 2 g in 500 mL solution is to infuse at a rate of 2 mg/min.

    mL/hr flow rate _____

21. An adult whose weight is 102.4 kg is to receive a dosage of 2 mg/kg/hr. The solution strength is 1 g in 500 mL.

    mg/hr dosage _____    mL/hr flow rate _____

22. A solution strength of 1 g in 100 mL is to infuse at a rate of 15 mcg/kg/min. The body weight is 94.4 kg.

    mcg/min dosage _____    mL/hr flow rate _____

23. An adult is receiving 4 mL/hr of a solution that contains 8 mg in 250 mL.

    mcg/min infusing _____

24. A drug is ordered to titrate between 5 and 10 mcg/kg/min. The body weight is 97.1 kg, and the solution strength is 100 mg/40 mL.

    mcg/min range _____    mL/hr flow rate range _____

25. A 500 mg in 250 mL solution is ordered for a 101.2 kg adult to titrate between 3 and 10 mcg/kg/min.

    mcg/min dosage range _____    mL/hr flow rate range _____

26. An infusion of 500 mg in 250 mL is infusing at a rate of 14 mL/hr.

    mcg/min infusing _____

27. A 5-10 mcg/kg/min dosage is to be titrated for an adult patient weighing 79.6 kg. The solution strength is 100 mg in 40 mL.

    mcg/min dosage range _____    mL/hr flow rate range _____

28. A 400 mg in 250 mL solution is to be titrated at 2-20 mcg/kg/min. The body weight is 62.3 kg.

    mcg/min dosage range _____    mL/hr flow rate range _____

29. A drug has been ordered for an adult weighing 84.9 kg to titrate at 2.5-10 mcg/kg/min. The solution strength is 500 mg in 250 mL.

    mcg/min dosage range _____    mL/hr flow rate range _____

30. A drug is ordered at a rate of 1-4 mg/min. The solution strength is 2 g in 500 mL.

    mL/hr flow rate range _____

31. A 10 mcg/min dosage is ordered using an 8 mg/250 mL solution.

    mL/hr flow rate _____

32. A 2 g in 500 mL dosage is to infuse at 3 mg/min.

    mL/hr flow rate _____

33. A 250 mL solution with 1 mg of medication is to be infused at 5 mcg/min.

    mL/hr flow rate _____

34. A 4 mcg/min dosage is ordered. The solution is 250 mL with 8 mg of medication.

    mL/hr flow rate _____

35. A 2 g in 500 mL solution is ordered to infuse at a rate of 6 mg/min.

    mL/hr flow rate _____

36. A 2 g in 500 mL solution is ordered to infuse at 4 mg/min.

    mL/hr flow rate _____

37. A 12 mcg/min dosage using an 8 mg in 250 mL of solution is ordered.

    mL/hr flow rate _____

38. A 40 mg/hr dosage is ordered, and a 100 mg in 100 mL solution is ordered.

     mL/hr flow rate _____

39. The order is to infuse 4 mcg/min from a 250 mL solution containing 1 mg of medication.

     mL/hr flow rate _____

40. Infuse 10 mg/hr from a 125 mg/l00 mL solution.

     mL/hr flow rate _____

**Answers**

1. 452.4 mcg/min; 14 mL/hr
2. 52.7 mcg/min; 16 mL/hr
3. 41.2–57.7 mg/hr; 82–115 mL/hr
4. 533.3 mcg/min
5. 15–90 mL/hr
6. 4 mg/min; 240 mg/hr
7. 16 mL/hr
8. 9 mL/hr
9. 60 mL/hr
10. 640 mcg/min; 24 mL/hr
11. 1200 mcg/min; 72 mg/hr
12. 60 mL/hr
13. 6232 mcg/min; 37 mL/hr
14. 8 mL/hr
15. 653.6–817 mcg/min
16. 544.2 mcg/min; 163 mL/hr
17. 353.5 mcg/min; 13 mL/hr
18. 45 mL/hr
19. 50 mcg/min
20. 30 mL/hr
21. 204.8 mg/hr; 102 mL/hr
22. 1416 mcg/min; 8 mL/hr
23. 2.1 mcg/min
24. 485.5–971 mcg/min; 12–23 mL/hr
25. 303.6–1012 mcg/min; 9–30 mL/hr
26. 466.7 mcg/min
27. 398–796 mcg/min; 10–19 mL/hr
28. 124.6–1246 mcg/min; 5–47 mL/hr
29. 212.3–849 mcg/min; 6–25 mL/hr
30. 15–60 mL/hr
31. 19 mL/hr
32. 45 mL/hr
33. 75 mL/hr
34. 8 mL/hr
35. 90 mL/hr
36. 60 mL/hr
37. 23 mL/hr
38. 40 mL/hr
39. 60 mL/hr
40. 8 mL/hr

# HEPARIN INFUSION CALCULATIONS

## Objectives

The learner will calculate:

1. heparin dosages.

2. mL/hr flow rates for an EID.

3. hourly dosage infusing from mL/hr rate.

Heparin is a powerful anticoagulant drug that inhibits new blood clot formation, or the extension of already-existing clots. Heparin is commonly mixed in IV solutions for administration, especially postoperatively to prevent clot fomation from venous stasis. Heparin IV use is so frequent that it is prepared in ready-to-hang IV bags, such as the **1000 units (2 units/mL) strength illustrated** in Figure 19-1. Notice on this bag that **heparin and its dosage strength is clearly printed in red**, as a safety factor to distinguish it from other intravenous solutions.

Heparin can also be administered subcutaneously in small dosages. Subcutaneous injections require **deep injection at a 45° angle** to discourage bleeding from medication leaking through the injection tract. Also, **subcutaneous sites are not massaged after injection**, again to prevent bleeding at the site.

Heparin dosages may be based on body weight in kg, or on a patient's clotting time. Because of heparin's potent anticoagulant action, clotting times are checked frequently during administration.

There is no essential difference in the calculations you have already prac-ticed for critical care dosages and those for heparin dosages, except that heparin dosages for subcutaneous injection are measured using a TB syringe. However, heparin's action is so critical that it does deserve to be addressed separately. In this chapter, you will be introduced to labels of a variety of heparin dosages, prac-tice measuring heparin dosages for addition to IV solutions, calculate units per hour infusing from mL/hr flow rates, and be reminded of the precautions used to main-tain patency of intravenous injection ports.

### HEPARIN IV AND VIAL LABELS

Let's start by taking a look at the heparin IV solution bag in Figure 19-1. This is an example of premixed IV solution. Notice the blue "Heparin Sodium 1,000 units in 0.9% Sodium Chloride Injection" labeling on this 500 mL bag and the red dosage labeling "Heparin 1,000 units (2 units/mL)" printed sideways on the top right. The red dosages draw particular attention to

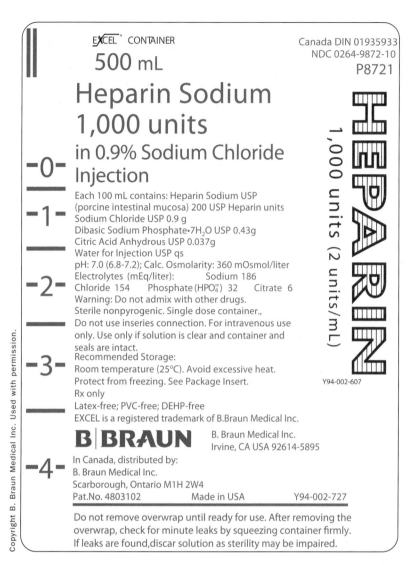

**Figure 19-1**

the fact that these bags contain heparin, and make the bags instantly recognizable. They serve as an important safety factor in solution identification.

If a commercially prepared IV heparin dosage strength that you require is not available, you may be required to prepare the solution yourself from **a number of available vial dosage strengths**. Let's stop and look at the vial labels in Figures 19-2 through 19-5, so that you can refresh your memory with some typical calculations.

## Problems 19.1

**Read the heparin labels provided to determine how many mL of heparin will be necessary to prepare the solutions indicated.**

1. Refer to the label in Figure 19-2 to determine how many mL will be required to add 20,000 units to an IV solution.         _____

2. Refer to the label in Figure 19-3 to determine how many mL will be required to add 20,000 units to an IV solution.         _____

**Figure 19-2**

**Figure 19-3**

**Figure 19-4**

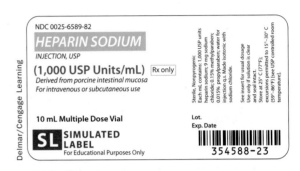

**Figure 19-5**

3. Refer to the label in Figure 19-4 to determine how many mL of heparin will be required to add 12,000 units to an IV solution. _____

4. Refer to the label in Figure 19-5 to determine how many mL will be required to add 10,000 units to an IV solution. _____

---

**Answers**  **1.** 4 mL  **2.** 2 mL  **3.** 6 mL  **4.** 10 mL

---

## CALCULATING mL/hr IV FLOW RATE FROM units/hr ORDERED

Because heparin is most frequently ordered in units/hr to be administered—for example, 1000 units/hr—and infused using an EID (electronic infusion device), a common calculation will be for the mL/hr flow rate needed for this dosage. Let's look at these calculations first, keeping in mind that **the mL/hr flow rate for an EID is identical to the gtt/min rate for a microdrip.**

**EXAMPLE 1**  The order is to infuse heparin **1000 units/hr** from a solution of **20,000 units in 500 mL** D5W. Calculate the **mL/hr** flow rate.

Enter the mL/hr being calculated first. Locate the ratio containing mL, the 20,000 units/500 mL strength, and enter this as the starting ratio with mL as the numerator, to match the mL numerator of the units being calculated; 20,000 units becomes the denominator.

$$\frac{mL}{hr} = \frac{500 \ mL}{20,000 \ units}$$

The starting ratio denominator, units, must be matched in the next numerator. Enter the 1000 units/hr rate ordered, with units as the numerator. This completes the equation.

$$\frac{mL}{hr} = \frac{500 \ mL}{20,000 \ units} \times \frac{1000 \ units}{1 \ hr}$$

Cancel alternate denominator/numerator units in the equation to double-check that the ratios have been entered correctly. Only mL and hr should remain. Do the math.

$$\frac{mL}{hr} = \frac{500 \ mL}{20,000 \ \cancel{units}} \times \frac{1000 \ \cancel{units}}{1 \ hr} = 25 \ \textbf{mL/hr}$$

**A rate of 25 mL/hr is required to infuse 1000 units/hr from a solution strength of 20,000 units in 500 mL.**

**EXAMPLE 2**  The order is for heparin **800 units/hr**. The solution available is **40,000 units in 1000 mL** D5W. Calculate the **mL/hr** flow rate.

Enter the mL/hr being calculated. Enter the 1000 mL/40,000 units ratio, with mL as the numerator.

$$\frac{mL}{hr} = \frac{1000 \ mL}{40,000 \ units}$$

Enter the next ratio, 800 units/hr, with 800 units as the numerator to match the starting ratio denominator.

$$\frac{mL}{hr} = \frac{1000 \ mL}{40,000 \ units} \times \frac{800 \ units}{1 \ hr}$$

Cancel to double-check for correct ratio entry, and do the math.

$$\frac{mL}{hr} = \frac{1000 \ mL}{40,000 \ \cancel{units}} \times \frac{800 \ \cancel{units}}{1 \ hr} = 20 \ \textbf{mL/hr}$$

**A rate of 20 mL/hr is required to infuse 800 units/hr from a solution strength of 40,000 units in 1000 mL.**

**EXAMPLE 3**  The order is to infuse heparin **1100 units/hr** from a solution strength of **60,000 units in 1 L** D5W. Calculate the **mL/hr** flow rate.

$$\frac{mL}{hr} = \frac{1000 \ mL}{60,000 \ units} \times \frac{1100 \ units}{1 \ hr}$$

$$\frac{mL}{hr} = \frac{1000 \ mL}{60,000 \ \cancel{units}} \times \frac{1100 \ \cancel{units}}{1 \ hr} = 18.33 = 18 \ \textbf{mL/hr}$$

**A rate of 18 mL/hr will be required to infuse 1100 units per hour from a 60,000 units in 1 L solution.**

19

## Problems 19.2

**Calculate the mL/hr flow rates.**

1. The order is to infuse 1000 units heparin per hour from an available solution strength of 25,000 units in 500 mL D5W.   _____

2. Heparin has been ordered at 2500 units per hour. The solution strength is 50,000 units in 1000 mL D5W.   _____

3. The order is to infuse 1100 units per hour from a 15,000 units in 1 L D5W solution.   _____

4. An adult has orders for 50,000 units of heparin in 1000 mL D5W to infuse at a rate of 2000 units per hour.   _____

5. Administer 1500 units per hour of heparin from an available strength of 40,000 units in 1 L.   _____

**Answers   1.** 20 mL/hr   **2.** 50 mL/hr   **3.** 73 mL/hr   **4.** 40 mL/hr   **5.** 38 mL/hr

## CALCULATING units/hr INFUSING FROM mL/hr FLOW RATE

On occasion it may be necessary to calculate the units/hr of heparin infusing from the mL/hr flow rate. This is done using the units/mL solution strength and mL/hr rate of infusion.

**EXAMPLE 1**   An IV of **1000 mL** containing **40,000 units** of heparin is running at **30 mL/hr**. Calculate the **units/hr** infusing.

$$\frac{units}{hr} = \frac{40,000\,units}{1000\ mL} \times \frac{30\ mL}{1\ hr}$$

$$\frac{units}{hr} = \frac{40,000\,units}{1000\ mL} \times \frac{30\ mL}{1\ hr} = \textbf{1200 units/hr}$$

**A 1000 mL solution containing 40,000 units heparin running at 30 mL/hr is infusing 1200 units/hr.**

**EXAMPLE 2**   A solution of **1 L** of D5W with **20,000 units** heparin is running at **80 mL/hr**. Calculate the **units/hr** infusing.

$$\frac{units}{hr} = \frac{20,000\ units}{1000\ mL} \times \frac{80\ mL}{1\ hr}$$

$$\frac{units}{hr} = \frac{20,000\ units}{1000\ mL} \times \frac{80\ mL}{1\ hr} = \textbf{1600 units/hr}$$

**A 1 L (1000 mL) solution containing 20,000 units heparin running at 80 mL/hr is infusing 1600 units/hr.**

**EXAMPLE 3**   An IV of D5W **500 mL** containing **10,000 units** heparin is
running at **40 mL/hr**. Calculate the **units/hr** infusing.

$$\frac{units}{hr} = \frac{10,000\ units}{500\ mL} \times \frac{40\ mL}{1\ hr}$$

$$\frac{units}{hr} = \frac{10,000\ units}{500\ mL} \times \frac{40\ mL}{1\ hr} = \textbf{800 units/hr}$$

**A 500 mL solution containing 10,000 units heparin running at
40 mL/hr is infusing 800 units/hr.**

## Problems 19.3

**Calculate the units/hr of heparin infusing in the IV administrations.**

1. An IV of 750 mL containing 30,000 units heparin running
   at 25 mL/hr.                                                   _____

2. A solution of 20,000 units in 500 mL running at 30 mL/hr.      _____

3. A 1 L volume of D5W containing heparin 30,000 units running
   at 40 mL/hr.                                                   _____

4. An IV of 1 L DNS containing 20,000 units heparin running
   at 30 mL/hr.                                                   _____

5. A 25,000 units heparin in 500 mL solution running at 30 mL/hr. _____

6. An IV of 1000 mL containing 40,000 units heparin running
   at 25 mL/hr.                                                   _____

7. A 1000 mL solution with 45,000 units heparin running
   at 25 mL/hr.                                                   _____

8. A solution of 1000 mL containing 25,000 units heparin running
   at 30 mL/hr.                                                   _____

9. A 1 L solution with 35,000 units heparin running at 45 mL/hr.  _____

10. A 20,000 units in 500 mL solution running at 20 mL/hr.        _____

**Answers  1.** 1000 units/hr  **2.** 1200 units/hr  **3.** 1200 units/hr  **4.** 600 units/hr  **5.** 1500 units/hr
**6.** 1000 units/hr  **7.** 1125 units/hr  **8.** 750 units/hr  **9.** 1575 units/hr  **10.** 800 units/hr

## HEPARIN FLUSH DOSAGE

As you learned in an earlier chapter, heparin flush solutions used to maintain patent
(open) indwelling IV infusion ports come in **two dosage strengths: 10 units/mL
and 100 units/mL.**

You have just learned that **heparin vial dosage strengths available for IV
dilution range from 1,000 to 50,000 units/mL.** So it is time now to be reminded
of the **enormous difference in dosage strengths between the 10 to 100 units/mL
flush solutions, and the 1,000 to 50,000 units/mL intravenous admixture dosage
strengths.**

**Misreading heparin labels can be life-threatening.** Too large a dosage used for a flush will cause systemic hemorrhage; too small a dosage added to an IV can lead to death from venous stasis and clot emboli.

 The average IV port heparin flush dosage is 10 units, and never exceeds 100 units.

## Summary

**This concludes the chapter on heparin administration. The important points to remember are:**

- Heparin is a potent anticoagulant that is frequently added to IV solutions.

- It is measured in USP units.

- Heparin therapy requires a frequent check of coagulation times.

- Subcutaneous heparin injections are given deep subcutaneously at a 45° angle in an attempt to reduce medication leakage through the injection track.

- Heparin injection sites are never massaged.

- IV heparin may be ordered by mL/hr flow rate or by units/hr to infuse.

- An EID or microdrip is used for heparin infusion.

- Commercially prepared IV heparin solutions are available in several strengths.

- Additional IV solution strengths may require the preparation of heparin from available 1000 to 50,000 units/mL vial strengths.

- Frequent blood tests for clotting time are required to monitor heparin dosage.

- Heparin IV port flushes never exceed 100 units.

## Summary Self-Test

**Calculate the mL/hr heparin flow rates.**

1. An adult is to receive heparin 1000 units/hr. The IV solution available has 25,000 units in 1 L D5W, and a pump will be used.    _____

2. A solution of 35,000 units heparin in 1 L D5W is to infuse via volumetric pump at 1200 units/hr.    _____

3. The order is for 1000 units heparin per hour. The solution strength is 20,000 units in 500 mL D5NS.    _____

4. The order is for 1250 units/hr heparin from a solution strength of 15,000 units in 500 mL D5W. A pump is used to monitor the infusion.    _____

5. A solution of 10,000 units heparin in 500 mL D5W is ordered to infuse at 1000 units/hr.    _____

6. An IV of 1000 mL D5W with 40,000 units heparin is to infuse at 1200 units/hr via a pump.  _____

7. The order is to infuse 500 mL D5W with 25,000 units heparin at 1500 units/hr.  _____

8. 500 mL D5W with 30,000 units of heparin is to infuse via a pump at 1500 units/hr.  _____

9. The order is to infuse 1 L D5W with 45,000 units of heparin at 1875 units/hr.  _____

10. A rate of 500 units/hr is ordered using a 250 mL with 10,000 units IV solution.  _____

11. A solution of 40,000 units in 1000 mL is to be used to infuse 1500 units/hr.  _____

12. A rate of 1500 units/hr is ordered using a 30,000 units in 500 mL solution.  _____

13. Heparin 750 units/hr is ordered using an IV solution of 500 mL containing 5000 units heparin.  _____

14. An IV solution of 10,000 units in 1000 mL heparin is to infuse 500 units/hr.  _____

15. Heparin 1500 units per hour is to be infused using a solution strength of 15,000 units in 500 mL.  _____

**Answers**

| | | |
|---|---|---|
| **1.** 40 mL/hr | **6.** 30 mL/hr | **12.** 25 mL/hr |
| **2.** 34 mL/hr | **7.** 30 mL/hr | **13.** 75 mL/hr |
| **3.** 25 mL/hr | **8.** 25 mL/hr | **14.** 50 mL/hr |
| **4.** 41.6 or 42 mL/hr | **9.** 41.6 or 42 mL/hr | **15.** 50 mL/hr |
| **5.** 50 mL/hr | **10.** 12.5 or 13 mL/hr | |
| | **11.** 37.5 or 38 mL/hr | |

# Pediatric Medication Calculations

**CHAPTER 20**

Pediatric Oral and Parenteral
Medications / 286

**CHAPTER 21**

Pediatric Intravenous
Medications / 292

# PEDIATRIC ORAL AND PARENTERAL MEDICATIONS

Two differences between adult and pediatric dosages will be immediately apparent: **Most oral drugs are prepared as liquids** because infants and small children cannot be expected to swallow tablets easily, if at all, and **dosages are dramatically smaller**. The oral route is used whenever possible, but when a child cannot swallow or the drug is ineffective given orally, drugs will be administered by a parenteral route.

Both the subcutaneous and intramuscular routes may be used depending on the type of drug to be administered. However, the smaller size of infants and children limits the use of both routes, as does the nature of the drug being used. For example, many antibiotics are administered intravenously rather than intramuscularly.

## ORAL MEDICATIONS

Most oral pediatric drugs are prepared as liquids to facilitate ease in swallowing. If the child is old enough to cooperate, these dosages may be measured in a medication cup. Solutions are also frequently measured using oral syringes, such as the ones shown in Figure 20-1. Notice that oral syringes have the same metric calibrations as hypodermic syringes, but they may also include household measures; for example, tsp. **Oral syringes have different-sized tips** to prevent use with hypodermic needles. On some oral syringes, the **tip is positioned off-center (termed *eccentric*)**, to further distinguish them from hypodermic syringes, or they may be **amber-colored**, as in Figure 20-1.

If oral syringes are not available, hypodermic syringes (**without the needle**) can also be used for dosage measurement. In addition to accuracy, syringes provide an excellent method of administering oral liquid drugs to infants and small children. Some oral liquid preparations incorporate a calibrated medication dropper as an integral part of the medication bottle. These may be **calibrated in mL** like the dropper shown in Figure 20-2 or in **actual dosage**; for example, 25 mg or 50 mg. Animal-shaped measures such as those shown in Figure 20-3 are also helpful in enticing reluctant toddlers to take necessary medications. In each instance, the goal is to ensure that the infant or child actually swallows the total dosage.

**Figure 20-1** | Oral syringes. Courtesy of Covidien.

Delmar/Cengage Learning

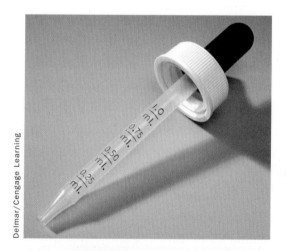

**Figure 20-2** | Calibrated dropper.

Delmar/Cengage Learning

**Figure 20-3** | Animal-shaped measures.

Care must be taken with liquid oral drugs to identify those prepared as **suspensions**. A **suspension consists of an insoluble drug in a liquid base**; for example, the cefaclor oral suspension in Figure 20-4. The drug in a suspension settles to the bottom of the bottle between uses, and **thorough mixing immediately prior to pouring** is mandatory. Suspensions must also be administered to the child promptly after measurement to prevent the drug from settling out again and an incomplete dosage being administered.

**Figure 20-4**

**Suspensions must be thoroughly mixed before measurement and promptly administered to prevent the settling out of their insoluble drugs.**

When a tablet or capsule is administered, the child's mouth must be checked to be certain the medication has actually been swallowed. If swallowing is a problem, some tablets can be crushed and given in a small amount of applesauce, ice cream, or juice if the child has no dietary restrictions to contraindicate this. Keep in mind, however, that **enteric-coated and timed-release tablets or capsules cannot be crushed** because this would destroy the coating that allows them to function on a delayed-action basis.

## INTRAMUSCULAR AND SUBCUTANEOUS MEDICATIONS

The drugs most often given subcutaneously are insulin, and immunizations that specifically require the subcutaneous route. Any site with sufficient subcutaneous tissue may be used, with the upper arm being the site of choice for immunizations. The intramuscular route is used most frequently for preoperative and postoperative medications for sedation and pain, and for immunizations such as DPT (diphtheria, pertussis, tetanus), which must be administered deep IM. The intramuscular site of choice for infants and small children is the vastus lateralis or rectus femoris of the thigh because the gluteal muscles do not develop until a child has learned to walk. Usually, not more than 1 mL is injected per site, and sites are rotated regularly.

Dosage calculation is the same as for adults, except **dosages are sometimes calculated to the nearest hundredth and measured using a tuberculin syringe** (refer to Chapter 8 if you need to review the calibrations and use of a TB syringe). There is less margin for error in pediatric dosages, and calculations and measurements are carefully double-checked.

# Summary

This concludes the introduction to pediatric oral, IM, and subcutaneous medication administrations. The important points to remember from this chapter are:

- Care must be taken when administering oral drugs to ensure that the child has actually swallowed the dosage.

- If liquid medications are prepared as suspensions, mix thoroughly prior to measurement, and administer promptly to prevent the settling out of their insoluble drugs.

- Care must be taken not to confuse oral syringes, which are unsterile, with hypodermic syringes, which are sterile.

- The IM site of choice for infants and small children is the vastus lateralis or rectus femoris of the thigh.

- Usually not more than 1 mL is injected per IM or subcutaneous site, and sites are rotated regularly.

- Pediatric parenteral dosages are frequently calculated to the nearest hundredth and measured using a TB syringe.

# Summary Self-Test

For Part I, use the pediatric medication labels provided to measure the following oral dosages. Indicate in the second column if the medication is a suspension.

PART I                                                                    mL          Suspension

1. Prepare a 20 mg dosage of fluoxetine.                    _____    _____

2. Prepare a 125 mg dosage of penicillin V potassium.    _____    _____

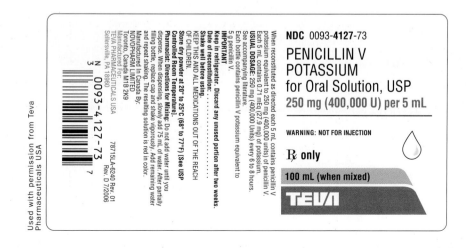

| | mL | Suspension |
|---|---|---|
| 3. Prepare 100 mg of amoxicillin. | _____ | _____ |
| 4. Prepare 100 mg of Vantin®. | _____ | _____ |
| 5. Prepare 5 mg of Lomotil®. | _____ | _____ |
| 6. Prepare cefpodoxime proxetil 60 mg. | _____ | _____ |
| 7. Prepared Depakene® 150 mg. | _____ | _____ |
| 8. Prepare 120 mg of acetaminophen. | _____ | _____ |
| 9. Prepare 187 mg of cefaclor. | _____ | _____ |

Used with permission of Ranbaxy Pharmaceuticals Inc.

**RANBAXY**
NDC 63304-955-04

**CEFACLOR**
For Oral Suspension USP

**187 mg/5 mL**

100 mL (when mixed)
SHAKE WELL BEFORE USE

Rx only

Manufactured for
Ranbaxy Pharmaceuticals Inc.
Jacksonville, FL 32216 USA
by Ranbaxy Laboratories Ltd.
New Delhi - 110 019, India

0903

**Usual Dosage:** Children; 20 mg/kg a day (40 mg/kg in otitis media) in three divided doses.
Adults: 250 mg three times a day. See literature for complete dosage information.
Contains Cefaclor monohydrate equivalent to 3.74 g cefaclor in a dry, pleasantly flavored mixture.
**Prior to Mixing:** Store at 20° - 25° C (68° - 77° F). (See USP Controlled Room Temperature). Protect from moisture.
**Directions for Mixing:** Add **70 mL** of water in two portions to the medium in the bottle. Shake well after each addition.
Each 5 mL (Approx. one teaspoonful) will then contain Cefaclor USP monohydrate equivalent to 187 mg anhydrous cefaclor.
Over size bottle provides extra space for shaking.
**Store in a refrigerator.** May be kept for 14 days without significant loss of potency. Keep tightly closed. Discard unused portion in 14 days.

Store dry powder at room temperature. Keep tightly closed. Shake well before using. Refrigeration preferable but not required. Discard suspension after 14 days.
**Directions for mixing:** Add **23 mL** of water Shake vigorously. Each mL will then contain amoxicillin trihydrate equivalent to 50 mg amoxicillin.

NDC 0025-6589-82

**AMOXICILLIN**

**50 mg/mL**    Rx only
*PEDIATRIC DROPS*
*FOR ORAL SUSPENSION*

**30 mL (when reconstituted)**

**SL** SIMULATED LABEL
For Educational Purposes Only

**Dosage:** 20 to 40 mg/kg/day in divided doses every 8 hours depending on age, weight, and infection severity. See accompanying prescribing information.
**Net contents:** Equivalent to 1.5 grams amoxicillin as the trihydrate.

Lot.
Exp. Date

354588-23

Used with permission from Bristol-Myers Squibb Company.

NDC 0087-0730-01

**DROPS**
**TEMPRA**®
**ACETAMINOPHEN**

**ANALGESIC**
**10% SOLUTION**
1/2 FL. OZ. (15 ML.)

**Mead Johnson**

P 7698-03

TO RELIEVE DISCOMFORT DUE TO COLDS, SIMPLE HEADACHES, MINOR ACHES AND PAINS.
Each 0.6 mL of TEMPRA® drops contains 60 mg. (1 grain) of acetaminophen and 10% alcohol.
Your physician is the best source of counsel and guidance in illness when pain or fever is present.
KEEP THIS AND ALL MEDICATIONS OUT OF THE REACH OF CHILDREN.
Made in U.S.A.          ©M.J.& Co.

MEAD JOHNSON NUTRITIONAL DIVISION
Mead Johnson & Company - Evansville, Indiana 47721 U.S.A.

Used with permission from Abbott Laboratories.

Do not accept if band on cap is broken or missing.

Each 5 mL contains equivalent of 250 mg valproic acid as the sodium salt.

See enclosure for prescribing information.

©Abbott

Abbott Laboratories
North Chicago,
IL60064, U.S.A.

Exp.

Lot

NDC 0074-5682-16
**16 fl oz Syrup**

**DEPAKENE**®

**VALPROIC ACID SYRUP, USP**

**250 mg per 5 mL**

Caution: Federal (U.S.A.) law prohibits dispensing without prescription.

**6505-01-094-9241**

Dispense in the original container or a glass, USP tight container.

Store below 86°F (30°C).

007456816

02-7538-2/R12

Used with permission from Pharmacia Corporation.

Rx only
See package insert for dosage and complete product information.
Warning: Not for injection
Store unconstituted product at controlled room temperature 20° to 25°C (68° to 77°F) [see USP]. Store constituted suspension in a refrigerator 2° to 8°C (36° to 46°F). Shake well before using. Keep container tightly closed. The mixture may be used for 14 days. Discard unused portion after 14 days.
**Directions for mixing:** Shake bottle to loosen granules. Add approximately 1/2 the total amount of distilled water required for constitution (total water = 57 mL). Shake vigorously to wet the granules. Add remaining water and shake vigorously.
Each 5 mL of suspension contains cefpodoxime proxetil equivalent to 100 mg cefpodoxime.
U.S. Patent No. 4,668,783
Licensed from Sankyo Company, Ltd., Japan
Made by
Pharmacia N.V./S.A., Puurs - Belgium
For
Pharmacia & Upjohn Company
A subsidiary of Pharmacia Corporation
Kalamazoo, MI 49001, USA
815 120 206
5Q7474

NDC 0009-3615-01

**Vantin**® *For Oral Suspension*
cefpodoxime proxetil
for oral suspension, USP

**100 mg per 5 mL**

Equivalent to 100 mg per 5 mL cefpodoxime when constituted

100 mL (when mixed)

**PHARMACIA**

Used with permission from Pfizer Inc.

2 Fl Oz          Rx only
NDC 0025-0066-02

**Lomotil**® **Cv**
**Liquid**

Each 5 ml contains:
diphenoxylate hydrochloride USP 2.5 mg
atropine sulfate USP 0.025 mg.
Ethyl alcohol 15%.

**Special Note:** Lomotil is not recommended for children under 2 years of age.

**PHARMACIA**

**Store below 77°F (25°C).**

**Pharmacist:** Caution patient not to exceed recommended dose and to keep out of the reach of children. Dispense only with calibrated dropper. Dispense only in this bottle.

**Usual Adult Dosage:** 10 ml (5 mg) four times daily.
**Children 2 to 12 years:** An initial total daily dosage of 0.3 to 0.4 mg/kg, administered in four divided doses or as recommended in attached literature.
**Children 13 to 16 years:** 10 ml (5 mg) three times daily. For maintenance, less according to response.

Dist. by: G.D. Searle LLC, Chicago, IL 60680, USA

**Use the labels provided to calculate the dosages for Parts II and III. Calculate all dosages to hundredths.**

PART II

10. Prepare a 20 mg dosage of meperidine.   _____

11. A dosage of morphine 10 mg has been ordered.   _____

12. Draw up a 100 mg dosage of clindamycin.   _____

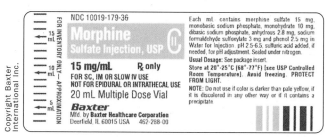

PART III

13. Prepare a 40 mg dosage of meperidine.   _____

14. A dosage of Dilantin® 50 mg has been ordered.   _____

15. Prepare a 6 mg dosage of morphine.   _____

| Answers | | | |
|---|---|---|---|
| **1.** 5 mL; no | **4.** 5 mL; suspension | **8.** 1.2 mL; no | **12.** 0.67 mL |
| **2.** 2.5 mL; no | **5.** 10 mL; no | **9.** 5 mL; suspension | **13.** 0.8 mL |
| **3.** 2 mL; suspension | **6.** 3 mL; suspension | **10.** 0.8 mL | **14.** 1 mL |
| | **7.** 3 mL; no | **11.** 0.67 mL | **15.** 0.6 mL |

# PEDIATRIC INTRAVENOUS MEDICATIONS

## Objectives

The learner will:

1. list the steps in preparing and administering IV medications from a solution bag.

2. list the steps in preparing and administering IV medications using a calibrated burette.

3. explain why a flush is included in IV medication administration.

4. calculate flow rates for the administration of pediatric IV medications.

5. use normal daily and hourly dosage ranges to calculate and assess dosages ordered.

## Prerequisites

Chapters 13–16

Pediatric IV medication administration involves a challenge and a responsibility that is multifaceted. Infants and children, particularly under the age of 4, are incompletely developed physiologically, and drug tolerance, absorption, and excretion are ongoing concerns. In addition, infants and acutely ill children can tolerate only a narrow range of hydration, making administration of IV drugs, which are diluted for administration, a critical and exact skill. Drug dilution protocols may specify a range for dilution, and on many occasions, the smallest possible volume may have to be used in order not to overhydrate a child. Dosage and dilution decisions may have to be made on a day-to-day or even a dose-to-dose basis, and will involve the team effort of nurse, physician, and pharmacist. In addition, the suitability of any flow rate calculated for administration must be made on an individual basis. For example, a calculated flow rate of 100 gtt/min for a 2-year-old child is too high a rate to administer.

The fragility of infants' and children's veins, and the irritating nature of many medications, mandate careful site inspection for signs of inflammation and infiltration. This should be done immediately before, during, and after each infusion. Signs of inflammation include redness, heat, swelling, and tenderness. Signs of infiltration include swelling, coolness, pain or discomfort, and lack of blood return in the IV tubing. Either complication necessitates discontinuance of the IV and a restart at a new site.

**IV medication guidelines are always used to determine drug dosages, dilutions, and administration rates.**

Let's start by looking at the different methods of IV medication administration.

## METHODS OF IV MEDICATION ADMINISTRATION

Intravenous medications may be administered over a period of several hours or on an **intermittent** basis involving several dosages in a 24-hour period. When ordered to infuse over several hours, medications are usually added to an IV solution bag. Adding the drug to the IV bag may be a hospital pharmacy or nurse responsibility. The steps for adding the drug to the solution are as follows:

**STEP 1**   Locate the type and volume of IV solution ordered.

**STEP 2**   Measure the dosage of drug to be added.

**STEP 3**   Use strict aseptic technique to add the drug to the solution bag through the medication port.

**STEP 4**   Mix the drug thoroughly in the solution.

**STEP 5**   Label the IV solution bag with the name and dosage of the drug added.

**STEP 6**   Add your initials and the time and date you added the drug.

**STEP 7**   Hang the IV and then set the flow rate for the infusion. Chart the administration when it has completed.

For intermittent administrations, the medication may also be prepared in small-volume solution bags, or using a calibrated burette such as the one illustrated in Figure 21-1. Because the total capacity of burettes is between 100 and 150 mL, calibrated in 1 mL increments, the exact measurement of small volumes is possible.

Regardless of the method of intermittent administration, the medication infusion is **routinely followed by a flush** to make sure the medication has cleared the tubing and that the total dosage has been administered. The volume of the flush will vary depending on the length of IV tubing from the medication source—that is, the burette or syringe—to the infusion site. If a primary line exists, the medication may be administered by IVPB (IV piggyback) via a secondary line. If no IV is infusing, a saline or heparin lock (heplock) is frequently in place and used for intermittent administration.

When IV medications are diluted for administration, it is necessary to determine hospital policy on **inclusion of the medication volume as part of the volume specified for dilution.** For example, if 20 mg has a volume of 2 mL, and it is to be diluted in 30 mL, does this mean you must add 28 mL of diluent to the burette or 30 mL?

**Hospital policies may vary,** but in all examples and problems in this chapter, **the drug volume will be treated as part of the total diluent volume.** The sequencing of medication and flush administration covered next for burette use is also representative of the procedure that might be followed for IVPB administrations.

Delmar/Cengage Learning

**Figure 21-1 |**
Calibrated burette.

21

## MEDICATION ADMINISTRATION VIA BURETTE

When a burette is used for medication administration, the entire preparation is usually done by nurses. Volumetric and syringe pumps are used extensively to administer intermittent IV medications to infants and children. When these are used, the alarm will sound each time the burette or syringe empties to signal when each successive step is necessary. For example, it will alarm when the medication has infused and the flush must be started and again when the flush is completed.

Let's look at some sample orders and go step by step through one procedure that may be used.

**EXAMPLE 1**

A dosage of **250 mg** in **15 mL** of D5 1/2NS is to be infused in **30 min**. It is to be followed with a **5 mL** D5 1/2NS flush. A volumetric pump will be used, and the tubing is a **microdrip** burette.

**STEP 1**  Read the drug label to determine what volume the 250 mg dosage is contained in. Let's assume this is 1 mL.

**STEP 2**  The dilution is to be 15 mL. Run a total of 14 mL of D5 1/2NS into the burette, then add the 1 mL containing the medication dosage of 250 mg. This gives the ordered volume of 15 mL. Roll the burette between your hands to mix the drug thoroughly with the solution.

**STEP 3**  Calculate the flow rate for this microdrip using dimensional analysis.

Total volume = **15 mL**      Infusion time = **30 min**

$$\frac{mL}{hr} = \frac{15\ mL}{30\ min} \times \frac{60\ min}{1\ hr} = 30\ mL/hr$$

**STEP 4**  Set the pump to infuse 30 mL/hr.

**STEP 5**  Label the burette to identify the drug and dosage added. Attach a label that states "medication infusing." This makes it possible for others to know the status of the administration if you are not present when the infusion is complete and the pump alarms.

**STEP 6**  When the medication has infused, add the 5 mL D5 1/2NS flush. Remove the "medication infusing" label and attach a "flush infusing" label. Continue to infuse at the 30 mL/hr rate until the burette empties for the second time.

**STEP 7**  When the flush has been completed, restart the primary IV or disconnect from the saline/heparin lock. Remove the "flush infusing" label. Chart the dosage and time.

**EXAMPLE 2**

An antibiotic dosage of **125 mg in 1 mL** is to be **diluted in 20 mL** of D5 1/4NS and infused over **30 min**. A **flush of 15 mL** D5 1/4NS is to follow. A volumetric pump will be used.

**STEP 1**   125 mg has a volume of 1 mL. Add 19 mL of D5 1/4NS to the burette, add the 1 mL of medication, and mix thoroughly.

**STEP 2**   Calculate the mL/hr flow rate using dimensional analysis.

Total volume = **20 mL**      Infusion time = **30 min**

$$\frac{mL}{hr} = \frac{20 \text{ mL}}{30 \text{ min}} \times \frac{60 \text{ min}}{1 \text{ hr}} = \textbf{40 mL/hr}$$

**STEP 3**   Set the pump to infuse 40 mL/hr.

**STEP 4**   Label the burette with the drug and dosage, and attach a "medication infusing" label.

**STEP 5**   When the medication has infused, start the 15 mL flush. Remove the "medication infusing" label and add the "flush infusing" label.

**STEP 6**   When the flush has completed, restart the primary IV or disconnect from the saline lock. Remove the "flush infusing" label. Chart the dosage and time.

If a 60 gtt/mL calibrated burette is used without a pump, the gtt/min rate will be the same as the mL/hr rate.

**EXAMPLE 3**

An antibiotic dosage of **50 mg** has been ordered diluted in **20 mL** of D5W to infuse over **20 min**. A **15 mL flush** of D5W is to follow. A **microdrip** will be used, but an infusion control device will not be used.

**STEP 1**   Read the medication label to determine what volume contains 50 mg. You determine that 50 mg is contained in 2 mL.

**STEP 2**   Run 18 mL of D5W into the burette and add the 2 mL containing 50 mg of drug. Roll between your hands to mix thoroughly.

**STEP 3**   Calculate the flow rate in gtt/min necessary to deliver the medication.

Total volume = **20 mL**      Infusion time = **20 min**

$$\frac{gtt}{min} = \frac{60 \text{ gtt}}{1 \text{ mL}} \times \frac{20 \text{ mL}}{20 \text{ min}} = \textbf{60 gtt/min}$$

**STEP 4**    The mL/hr and gtt/min rates are identical for a microdrip. Set the rate at 60 gtt/min.

**STEP 5**    Label the burette with drug name and dosage, and attach a "medication infusing" label.

**STEP 6**    When the medication has cleared the burette, add the 15 mL D5W flush. Continue to run at 60 gtt/min. Remove the "medication infusing" label and replace with a "flush infusing" label.

**STEP 7**    When the burette empties for the second time, restart the primary IV or disconnect from the saline lock. Remove the "flush infusing" label. Chart the dosage and time administered.

**EXAMPLE 4**

An IV medication dosage of **100 mcg** has been ordered diluted in **35 mL** of NS and infused in **50 min**. A **10 mL** flush is to follow. A **microdrip** burette will be used.

**STEP 1**    Read the medication label to determine what volume contains 100 mcg: 100 mcg = 1.5 mL

**STEP 2**    Run 33.5 mL of NS into the burette, and add the 1.5 mL of medication. Roll the burette between your hands to mix thoroughly.

**STEP 3**    Calculate the gtt/min flow rate.

$$\frac{\text{gtt}}{\text{min}} = \frac{60\ \text{gtt}}{1\ \text{mL}} \times \frac{35\ \text{mL}}{50\ \text{min}} = \textbf{42 gtt/min}$$

**STEP 4**    Set the flow rate at 42 gtt/min.

**STEP 5**    Label the burette with the drug name and dosage and "medication infusing" label.

**STEP 6**    When the medication has cleared the burette, add the 10 mL flush. Continue to run at 42 gtt/min. Replace the "medication infusing" label with the "flush infusing" label.

**STEP 7**    When the burette empties of the flush solution, restart the primary IV or disconnect from the saline lock. Remove the "flush infusing" label, and chart the dosage and time administered.

## Problems 21.1

Determine the volume of solution that must be added to a burette to mix the following IV drugs. Then, calculate the flow rate in gtt/min for each administration using a microdrip, and indicate the mL/hr setting for a pump.

1. An IV medication of 75 mg in 3 mL is ordered diluted to 55 mL to infuse over 45 min.

   Dilution volume _____ gtt/min _____ mL/hr_____

2. A dosage of 100 mg in 2 mL is diluted to 30 mL of D5W to infuse in 20 min.

   Dilution volume _____ gtt/min _____ mL/hr_____

3. The volume of a 10 mg dosage of medication is 1 mL. Dilute to 40 mL and administer over 50 min.

   Dilution volume _____ gtt/min _____ mL/hr_____

4. A dosage of 15 mg with a volume of 3 mL is to be diluted to 70 mL and administered in 50 min.

   Dilution volume _____ gtt/min _____ mL/hr_____

5. A medication of 1 g in 4 mL is to be diluted to 60 mL and infused over 90 min.

   Dilution volume _____ gtt/min _____ mL/hr_____

**Answers   1.**  52 mL; 73 gtt/min; 73 mL/hr   **2.**  28 mL; 90 gtt/min; 90 mL/hr
**3.** 39 mL; 48 gtt/min; 48 mL/hr   **4.** 67 mL; 84 gtt/min; 84 mL/hr   **5.** 56 mL; 40 gtt/min; 40 mL/hr

## COMPARING IV DOSAGES ORDERED WITH AVERAGE DOSAGES

Knowing how to compare dosages ordered with average dosages for a particular medication is a nursing responsibility.

Dosages of IV medications are calculated on the basis of body weight or BSA (body surface area).

Average dosages may be listed in terms of mg, mcg, or units per day or per hour. BSA in $m^2$ is most often used to calculate chemotherapeutic drugs, which are administered only by certified nursing staff. The following examples will demonstrate how to use average dosage to check dosages ordered.

**EXAMPLE 1**

A child weighing **22.6 kg** has an order for **500 mg** of medication in **100 mL** of D5W **every 12 hours**. The normal dosage range is **40–50 mg/kg/day**. Determine if the dosage ordered is within the normal range.

**STEP 1**  Calculate the normal daily dosage range for this child.

40 mg/day $\times$ 22.6 kg = **904 mg**
50 mg/day $\times$ 22.6 kg = **1130 mg**

**STEP 2**  Calculate the dosage infusing in 24 hr.

500 mg in 12 hr = **1000 mg in 24 hr**

**STEP 3**  Assess the accuracy of the dosage ordered.

The 500 mg in 12 hr is within the 904–1130 mg/day dosage range.

**EXAMPLE 2**

A child with a body weight of **18.4 kg** is to receive a medication with a dosage range of **100–150 mg/kg/day**. The order is for **600 mg** in **75 mL** of D5W **every 6 hours**. Determine if the dosage is within normal range.

**STEP 1**  Calculate the normal daily dosage range.

100 mg/day $\times$ 18.4 kg = **1840 mg/day**
150 mg/day $\times$ 18.4 kg = **2760 mg/day**

**STEP 2**  Calculate the daily dosage ordered.

The dosage ordered is 600 mg every 6 hours (4 doses/24 hours)

600 mg $\times$ 4 = **2400 mg/day**

**STEP 3**  Assess the accuracy of the dosage ordered.

The dosage ordered, 2400 mg/day, is within the normal range of 1840–2760 mg/day.

**EXAMPLE 3**

A child weighing **17.7 kg** is receiving an IV of **250 mL** of D5W containing **2000 units** of medication, which is to infuse at **50 mL/hr**. The dosage range is **10–25 units/kg/hr**. Assess the accuracy of this dosage.

**STEP 1**  Calculate the dosage range per hour.

10 units/kg/hr $\times$ 17.7 kg = **177 units/hr**

25 units/kg/hr $\times$ 17.7 kg = **442.5 units/hr**

**STEP 2**   Calculate the dosage infusing per hour.

$$\frac{\text{units}}{\text{hr}} = \frac{2000 \text{ units}}{250 \text{ mL}} \times \frac{50 \text{ mL}}{1 \text{ hr}} = \textbf{400 units/hr}$$

**STEP 3**   Assess the accuracy of the dosage ordered.

The IV is infusing at a rate of 50 mL per hour, which is 400 units/hr. The normal dosage range is 177–442.5 units/hr. The dosage is within normal range.

**EXAMPLE 4**

A child weighing **32.7 kg** has an IV of **250 mL** of D5 1/4S containing **400 mcg** of medication to infuse in **5 hours**. The normal range for this drug is **1–3 mcg/kg/hr**. Determine if this dosage is within the normal dosage range.

**STEP 1**   Calculate the hourly dosage range.

1 mcg/kg/hr × 32.7 kg = **32.7 mcg/hr**
3 mcg/kg/hr × 32.7 kg = **98.1 mcg/hr**

**STEP 2**   Calculate the dosage infusing per hour.

400 mcg ÷ 5 hr = **80 mcg/hr**

**STEP 3**   Assess the accuracy of the dosage ordered.

The dosage of 80 mcg/hr infusing is within the normal range of 32.7–98.1 mcg/hr.

## Problems 21.2

Calculate the normal dosage range to the nearest tenth and the dosage being administered for the following medications. Assess the dosages ordered.

1. A child weighing 24.4 kg has an IV of 250 mL of D5W containing 2500 units of a drug. The dosage range for this drug is 15–25 units/kg/hr. The pump is set to deliver 50 mL/hr.

    Dosage range per hr _____   Dosage infusing per hr _____

    Assessment _____

2. A solution of D5W containing 25 mg of a drug is to infuse in 30 min. The dosage range is 4–8 mg/kg/day every 6 hours. The child weighs 18.7 kg.

    Dosage range per day _____   Daily dosage ordered _____

    Assessment _____

3. An IV solution containing 125 mg of medication is infusing. The dosage range is 5–10 mg/kg/dose, and the child weighs 14.2 kg.

        Dosage range per dose _____      Assessment _____

4. A child weighing 14.3 kg is to receive an IV drug with a dosage range of 50–100 mcg/kg/day in two divided doses. An infusion of 50 mL of D5W containing 400 mcg to run 30 min has been ordered.

        Daily dosage range _____      Daily dosage ordered _____

                                                        Assessment _____

5. A dosage of 4 mg (4000 mcg) of drug in 500 mL of D5 1/2S is to infuse in 4 hours. The dosage range of the drug is 24–120 mcg/kg/hr, and the child weighs 16.1 kg.

        Dosage range per hr _____      Dosage infusing per hr _____

                                                        Assessment _____

6. A child weighing 20.9 kg is to receive a medication with a normal dosage range of 80–160 mg/kg/day in divided doses every 6 hours. The IV ordered contains 500 mg.

        Dosage range per day _____      Daily dosage ordered _____

                                                        Assessment _____

7. A child weighing 22.3 kg is to receive 750 mL of D5 1/4S containing 6 g of a drug, which is to run for 24 hours. The dosage range of the drug is 200–300 mg/kg/day.

        Dosage range per day _____      Assessment _____

8. An IV of 50 mL of D5W containing 55 mcg of a drug is infusing in a 30-min period. The child weighs 14.9 kg and the dosage range is 6–8 mcg/kg/day, every 12 hours.

        Dosage range per day _____      Daily dosage ordered _____

                                                        Assessment _____

9. A child weighing 27.1 kg is to receive a medication with a normal range of 0.5–1 mg/kg/dose. An IV containing 20 mg of medication has been ordered.

        Dosage per dose _____      Assessment _____

10. An IV medication of 60 mcg in 200 mL is ordered to infuse in 2 hr. The normal dosage range is 1.5–3 mcg/kg/hr. The child weighs 16.7 kg.

        Dosage range per hr _____      Dosage infusing per hr _____

                                                        Assessment _____

**Answers** **1.** 366–610 units/hr; 500 units/hr; normal range **2.** 74.8–149.6 mg/day; 100 mg/day; normal range **3.** 71–142 mg/dose; normal range **4.** 715–1430 mcg/day; 800 mcg; normal range **5.** 386.4–1932 mcg/hr; 1000 mcg; normal range **6.** 1672–3344 mg/day; 2000 mg; normal range **7.** 4460–6690 mg/day; normal range **8.** 89.4–119.2 mcg/day; 110 mcg; normal range **9.** 13.6–27.1 mg/dose; normal range **10.** 25.1–50.1 mcg/hr; 30 mcg; normal range

## Summary

**This concludes the chapter on administration of IV drugs to infants and children. The important points to remember from this chapter are:**

- IV medications may be ordered to infuse in several hours or minutes.

- IV medications are diluted for administration, and it is important to determine hospital policy on inclusion of the medication volume as part of the total dilution volume.

- A flush is used following medication administration to make sure the medication has cleared the tubing and the total dosage has been administered.

- The volume of flush solution on intermittent infusions will vary depending on the amount needed to clear the infusion line.

- Average dosage ranges are used to assess dosages ordered.

- Pediatric IV medication administration requires constant assessment of the child's ability to tolerate dosage, dilution, and rate of administration.

- Children's veins are very fragile, and intravenous sites must be checked for inflammation and infiltration immediately before, during, and after each medication administration.

## Summary Self-Test

**Determine the volume of solution that must be added to a calibrated burette to mix the following IV drugs. The medication volume is included in the total dilution volume. Calculate the flow rate in gtt/min for each infusion. A microdrip with a calibration of 60 gtt/mL is used.**

|  | Volume of diluent | gtt/min rate |
|---|---|---|
| 1. An IV antibiotic of 750 mg in 3 mL has been ordered diluted to a total of 25 mL of D5W to infuse in 40 minutes. | _____ | _____ |
| 2. A dosage of 500,000 units of a penicillin preparation with a volume of 4 mL has been ordered diluted to 50 mL D5 1/2NS to infuse in 60 min. | _____ | _____ |
| 3. A dosage of 1.5 g/2 mL of an antibiotic is to be diluted to a total of 40 mL of D5W and administered in 40 min. | _____ | _____ |
| 4. An antibiotic dosage of 200 mg in 4 mL is to be diluted to 50 mL and administered in 70 min. | _____ | _____ |
| 5. A dosage of 20 mg in 2 mL has been ordered diluted to 30 mL to be infused in 35 min. | _____ | _____ |
| 6. A dosage of 25 mg in 5 mL has been ordered diluted to 40 mL and administered in 50 min. | _____ | _____ |
| 7. A 10 mg in 2 mL dosage has been ordered diluted to 20 mL to infuse in 30 min. | _____ | _____ |

8. A medication dosage of 800 mg in 4 mL is to be diluted to 60 mL and infused in 80 min.   _____   _____

9. A dosage of 0.5 g in 2 mL is to be diluted to 40 mL and run in 30 min.   _____   _____

10. A medication of 1000 mg in 1 mL is to be diluted to 15 mL and administered in 20 min.   _____   _____

**The following IV drugs are to be administered using a volumetric or syringe pump. Determine the amount of diluent to be added and the flow rate in mL/hr to set the pumps.**

|  | **Volume of diluent** | **mL/hr rate** |
|---|---|---|
| 11. A dosage of 40 mg in 4 mL is to be diluted to 50 mL and administered in 90 min. | _____ | _____ |
| 12. A 2 g in 5 mL dosage has been ordered diluted to a total of 90 mL and administered in 45 min. | _____ | _____ |
| 13. An 80 mg dosage with a volume of 2 mL is to be diluted to 80 mL and administered in 60 min. | _____ | _____ |
| 14. A 60 mg dosage with a volume of 4 mL is ordered diluted to 30 mL and run in 20 min. | _____ | _____ |
| 15. A 5 mg per 2 mL dosage is to be diluted to 80 mL and administered in 50 min. | _____ | _____ |
| 16. The dosage ordered is 0.75 g in 3 mL to be diluted to 30 mL and infused in 40 min. | _____ | _____ |
| 17. A medication of 100 mg in 2 mL is ordered diluted to 30 mL and run in 25 min. | _____ | _____ |
| 18. The dosage ordered is 100 mg in 1 mL to be diluted to 50 mL and infused in 45 min. | _____ | _____ |
| 19. A 30 mg dosage in 1 mL has been ordered diluted to 10 mL to infuse in 10 min. | _____ | _____ |
| 20. A dosage of 250 mg in 5 mL has been ordered diluted to 40 mL and infused in 60 min. | _____ | _____ |

**Calculate the normal dosage range to the nearest tenth and the dosage being administered for the following medications. Assess the dosages ordered.**

21. A child weighing 15.4 kg is to receive a dosage with a range of 5–7.5 mg/kg/dose. The solution bag is labeled 100 mg.

   Dosage range _____   Assessment _____

22. The order is for 200 units in 75 mL. The child weighs 13.1 kg, and the dosage range is 15–20 units/kg per dose.

   Dosage range _____   Assessment _____

21

23. A dosage of 1.5 mg in 20 mL has been ordered. The normal
    dosage range is 0.1–0.3 mg/kg/day in two divided doses.
    The child's weight is 12.4 kg.          Dosage range per day _____

               Daily dosage ordered _____   Assessment _____

24. A dosage of 400 mg in 75 mL of medication is to be infused
    every 8 hours. The normal range is 15–45 mg/kg/day, and the
    child weighs 27.9 kg.                    Dosage range per day _____

               Daily dosage ordered _____   Assessment _____

25. A child weighing 15.7 kg is to receive a medication with a normal
    hourly range of 3–7 mcg/kg. A 250 mL solution bag containing
    350 mcg is infusing at a rate of 50 mL/hr.

               Dosage range per hr _____   Dosage infusing per hr _____

               Assessment _____

26. A child weighing 19.6 kg is to receive a medication with a normal
    dosage range of 60–80 mg/kg/day. A 90 mL infusion containing
    375 mg has been ordered every 6 hours.   Dosage range per day _____

               Daily dosage ordered _____   Assessment _____

27. Two infusions of 250 mL each containing 300 mg of medication are to
    infuse continuously over a 24-hr period. The child receiving the infusion
    weighs 11.7 kg, and the normal dosage range of the drug is
    50–100 mg/kg/day.

               Dosage range per day _____   Daily dosage ordered _____

               Assessment _____

28. The order is for 100 mL of D5W containing 150 mg of medication
    to infuse every 8 hours. The normal dosage range is 3–12 mg/kg/day,
    and the child weighs 40.1 kg.            Dosage range per day _____

               Daily dosage ordered _____   Assessment _____

29. A child has an infusion of 250 mL containing 500 units of
    medication to run at 50 mL/hr. The normal dosage range
    is 10–25 units/kg/hr. The child weighs 10.3 kg.   Dosage range per hr _____

               Dosage infusing per hr _____   Assessment _____

30. The normal dosage range of a drug is 0.5–1.5 units/kg/hr.
    A child weighing 10.7 kg has a 150 mL volume of solution
    containing 45 units infusing at a rate of 20 mL/hr.

               Normal dosage range per hr _____

               Dosage infusing per hr _____   Assessment _____

31. A child weighing 12.5 kg is receiving an IV of 2500 units of
    medication in 250 mL of D5W at 40 mL/hr. The normal
    dosage range is 10–25 units/kg/hr.       Normal dosage range per hr _____

               Dosage infusing per hr _____   Assessment _____

32. A child with a weight of 10 kg is to receive a medication with a
    normal dosage range of 60–80 mg/kg/day. The order is for
    200 mg every 6 hours.                    Normal dosage range per hr _____

                         Daily dosage ordered _____   Assessment _____

33. The order is for 0.5 g in 100 mL of D5W every 6 hours. The normal
    dosage range is 100–200 mg/kg/day. The child weighs 15 kg.

                                                     Normal dosage range per hr _____

                         Daily dosage ordered _____   Assessment _____

34. A continuous IV of 500 mL with 20 mEq KCl is infusing at 30 mL/hr.
    The dosage for potassium chloride is not to exceed 40 mEq/day.

                                                   Dosage infusing per hr _____

                     Dosage infusing per day _____   Assessment _____

35. A 24 kg child is receiving 116 mg of medication via IV 3 times each day (every 8 hours).
    Dosage range for this drug is 10–20 mg/kg/day.

                                         Normal dosage range per day _____

               Dosage received after 3 doses _____   Assessment _____

36. A child weighing 15 kg has an order for 40 mcg of medication in 75 mL D5W to infuse every
    12 hours. The normal dosage range is 8–10 mcg/kg/day.

               Normal dosage per day _____   Dosage ordered _____

                                                   Assessment _____

37. The usual dosage for children is 50 mg/kg/24 hr in equally divided doses. The order is to
    infuse 50 mL with 290 mg every 6 hours. The child weighs 51 lb.

               Normal dosage per day _____   Daily dosage ordered _____

                                                   Assessment _____

38. Order: 500 mL D5RL with 30 mEq KCl to infuse at 40 mL/hr. A maximum of 10 mEq/hr of
    KCl should not be exceeded, and the total 24 hr dosage should not exceed 40 mEq/day.

               Dosage infusing per hr _____   Dosage infusing per day _____

                                                   Assessment _____

39. A child weighing 30 kg has an IV of 100 mL of D5W containing 600 mcg of medication to
    infuse in 2 hours. The normal range for this drug is 2–4 mcg/kg/hr.

                                         Normal dosage range per hr _____

                 Dosage infusing per hr _____   Assessment _____

40. 150 mL with 18 mg of medication is ordered to infuse in 10 hours. The normal range for this
    drug is 0.2 mg–0.6 mg/kg/hr. The child weighs 9 kg.

                                         Normal dosage range per hr _____

                 Dosage infusing per hr _____   Assessment _____

# ISMP's List of *Error-Prone Abbreviations, Symbols,* and *Dose Designations* (continued)

| Dose Designations and Other Information | Intended Meaning | Misinterpretation | Correction |
|---|---|---|---|
| Drug name and dose run together (especially problematic for drug names that end in "l" such as Inderal40 mg; Tegretol300 mg) | Inderal 40 mg<br><br>Tegretol 300 mg | Mistaken as Inderal 140 mg<br><br>Mistaken as Tegretol 1300 mg | Place adequate space between the drug name, dose, and unit of measure |
| Numerical dose and unit of measure run together (e.g., 10mg, 100mL) | 10 mg<br><br>100 mL | The "m" is sometimes mistaken as a zero or two zeros, risking a 10- to 100-fold overdose | Place adequate space between the dose and unit of measure |
| Abbreviations such as mg. or mL. with a period following the abbreviation | mg<br><br>mL | The period is unnecessary and could be mistaken as the number 1 if written poorly | Use mg, mL, etc. without a terminal period |
| Large doses without properly placed commas (e.g., 100000 units; 1000000 units) | 100,000 units<br><br>1,000,000 units | 100000 has been mistaken as 10,000 or 1,000,000; 1000000 has been mistaken as 100,000 | Use commas for dosing units at or above 1,000, or use words such as 100 "thousand" or 1 "million" to improve readability |

| Drug Name Abbreviations | Intended Meaning | Misinterpretation | Correction |
|---|---|---|---|
| ARA A | vidarabine | Mistaken as cytarabine (ARA C) | Use complete drug name |
| AZT | zidovudine (Retrovir) | Mistaken as azathioprine or aztreonam | Use complete drug name |
| CPZ | Compazine (prochlorperazine) | Mistaken as chlorpromazine | Use complete drug name |
| DPT | Demerol-Phenergan-Thorazine | Mistaken as diphtheria-pertussis-tetanus (vaccine) | Use complete drug name |
| DTO | Diluted tincture of opium, or deodorized tincture of opium (Paregoric) | Mistaken as tincture of opium | Use complete drug name |
| HCl | hydrochloric acid or hydrochloride | Mistaken as potassium chloride (The "H" is misinterpreted as "K") | Use complete drug name unless expressed as a salt of a drug |
| HCT | hydrocortisone | Mistaken as hydrochlorothiazide | Use complete drug name |
| HCTZ | hydrochlorothiazide | Mistaken as hydrocortisone (seen as HCT250 mg) | Use complete drug name |
| MgSO4** | magnesium sulfate | Mistaken as morphine sulfate | Use complete drug name |
| MS, MSO4** | morphine sulfate | Mistaken as magnesium sulfate | Use complete drug name |
| MTX | methotrexate | Mistaken as mitoxantrone | Use complete drug name |
| PCA | procainamide | Mistaken as patient controlled analgesia | Use complete drug name |
| PTU | propylthiouracil | Mistaken as mercaptopurine | Use complete drug name |
| T3 | Tylenol with codeine No. 3 | Mistaken as liothyronine | Use complete drug name |
| TAC | triamcinolone | Mistaken as tetracaine, Adrenalin, cocaine | Use complete drug name |
| TNK | TNKase | Mistaken as "TPA" | Use complete drug name |
| ZnSO4 | zinc sulfate | Mistaken as morphine sulfate | Use complete drug name |

| Stemmed Drug Names | Intended Meaning | Misinterpretation | Correction |
|---|---|---|---|
| "Nitro" drip | nitroglycerin infusion | Mistaken as sodium nitroprusside infusion | Use complete drug name |
| "Norflox" | norfloxacin | Mistaken as Norflex | Use complete drug name |
| "IV Vanc" | intravenous vancomycin | Mistaken as Invanz | Use complete drug name |

| Symbols | Intended Meaning | Misinterpretation | Correction |
|---|---|---|---|
| ʒ | Dram | Symbol for dram mistaken as "3" | Use the metric system |
| ♏ | Minim | Symbol for minim mistaken as "mL" | |
| x3d | For three days | Mistaken as "3 doses" | Use "for three days" |
| > and < | Greater than and less than | Mistaken as opposite of intended; mistakenly use incorrect symbol; "< 10" mistaken as "40" | Use "greater than" or "less than" |
| / (slash mark) | Separates two doses or indicates "per" | Mistaken as the number 1 (e.g., "25 units/10 units" misread as "25 units and 110" units) | Use "per" rather than a slash mark to separate doses |
| @ | At | Mistaken as "2" | Use "at" |
| & | And | Mistaken as "2" | Use "and" |
| + | Plus or and | Mistaken as "4" | Use "and" |
| ° | Hour | Mistaken as a zero (e.g., q2° seen as q 20) | Use "hr," "h," or "hour" |

**These abbreviations are included on TJC's "minimum list" of dangerous abbreviations, acronyms and symbols that must be included on an organization's "Do Not Use" list, effective January 1, 2004. Visit www.jointcommission.org for more information about this TJC requirement.

© ISMP 2009

# INDEX

## A

Abbreviations
    error(s) in, 81
    error-prone, ISMP's list of,
      307–310
    metric, 38
Addition, of decimals, 7–8
ADD-Vantage System, 217
Alaris SE Dual pump, 221–222
Apothecary measures, 49, 306

## B

B. Braun Outlook 200, 222
Basic equation, 161–166
B-D SafetyGlide syringes, 89
Body surface area (BSA), dosage
      calculation based on,
      203–212
    assessing orders, 206–210
    from kg and cm, 203–205
    from lb and in., 205–206
Body weight dosage calculation,
      188–202
    conversions, lb to kg,
      188–190
    from drug label information,
      190–192
    from drug literature, 192–196
BSA. See Body surface area (BSA)
Burette(s)
    pediatric medications vs.,
      294–297
    volume-controlled, 219

## C

Calculator(s), using, 17
Capsule(s), labels, 53–57
Centi-, 37
    abbreviation for, 38
Centimeters (cm), BSA calculated
      from, 203–205
Children. See Pediatric Dosages
      and Pediatric
      Medication(s)

Clinical ratios, 160
Conversion(s)
    body weight dosage
      calculation, lb to kg,
      188–190
    metric, equations requiring,
      166–169
    units, 160–186. See also
      Dimensional analysis

## D

Decimal(s)
    addition of, 7–8
    multiplication of, 11–13
    relative value of, 2–6
    subtraction of, 7–8
Decimal fraction(s), division of, 13
Decimal fraction equations, 25–28
Decimal points, elimination of,
      13–14
Denominator, 13, 161
Dimensional analysis, 160–186
    basic equation, 161–166
    described, 160
    equations requiring metric
      conversions, 166–169
Division, of decimal fractions, 13
Division factor method, in flow
      rate calculation, 237–239
Dosage(s)
    insulin
      combining, 151–152
      measuring, 138–157
    metric, errors in, 43, 81–82
    oral, size of, 52
    right, 78
Dosage calculations, 159–186
    body weight—based, 188–202.
      See also Body weight
      dosage calculation
    BSA—based, 203–212. See also
      Body surface area (BSA),
      dosage calculation based on
    capsules, 57–61
    oral, 52–74

parenteral medications,
      105–108
    tablets, 57–61
Dram, 306
Drip chamber, 214
Drop, 306
Drug(s)
    powdered, reconstitution of,
      122–137
    right, 78
    See also Powdered
      drugs, reconstitution of
Drug literature, calculating
      dosages from, 192–196
Drug measures, 35–50
Drug names, errors in, 81
Drug orders, assessing, BSA in,
      206–210

## E

Equation(s)
    basic, 161–166
    decimal fraction, 25–28
    fraction, solving, 22–33
    multiple-number, 28–31
    requiring metric conversions,
      166–169
    whole-number, 22–25
Error(s), medication
      administration—
      related, 81–83. See
      also Medication
      administration, errors
      associated with
Error-prone pediatric abbreviations,
      ISMP's list of, 307–310

## F

Flow rate, regulation of,
      240–241
Flow rate calculation, 229–246
    calculating gtt/min flow
      rates from mL/hr ordered,
      231–234

correcting off-schedule rates, 241–244
division factor method, 237–239
formula method, 234–237
regulating flow rate, 240–241
tubing calibration, 229–230
Fluid(s), IV. *See* Intravenous (IV) fluids
Formula method, in flow rate calculation, 234–237
Fraction(s)
decimal, division of, 13
reduction of, 14–16
Fraction equations
decimal, 25–28
solving, 22–33

## G

Grain, 306
Gram, abbreviation for, 38

## H

Heparin
flush dosage, 281–282
infusion calculations, 276–283
mL/hr IV flow rate from units/hr ordered, 278–280
units/hr infusing from mL/hr flow rate, 280–281
IV labels, 276–278
Heparin infusion dosage alert, 220
Heplocks, 219
Household measures, 49
Hundredth, nearest, expressing to, 18–19
Hypodermic syringes, measurement, 85–99
5 mL, 93–95
large, 96–97
safety, 89–90
TB, 90–93
10 mL, 93–95
3 mL, 85–89
20 mL, 96–97

## I

Identa-Band, 80
Inches (in), BSA calculated from, 205–206

Indwelling infusion ports/ intermittent locks, 219
Infusion(s), heparin, calculations of, 276–283. *See also* Heparin, infusion calculations
Infusion port adapter, 219
Infusion titrations, calculating, 270–275
Injection port, 215
Institute for Safe Medication Practices (ISMP), 75, 82
list of error-prone abbreviations, 307–310
Insulin, 138–157
action times, 145–146
dosages of
combining, 151–152
measuring of, 138–157
immediate-acting, 146
injection sites and techniques, 152
label identification, 139–145
long-acting, 146
rapid-acting, 145
short-acting, 145
syringes, 146–150
types of, 138–139
International/military time calculations, 249–250
International Units (U), 46–47
solutions measured in, 105–106
Intramuscular medications, 288
Intravenous (IV) calculations, 213–283
Intravenous (IV) completion times, calculating, 247–261. *See also* Intravenous (IV) therapy, calculating infusion/completion times
Intravenous (IV) flow rate calculation, 229–246. *See also* Flow rate calculation; Intravenous (IV) therapy
Intravenous (IV) fluids
introduction to, 225
percentages in, 226
preparation of, 225
Intravenous (IV) infusion times, calculating infusion/ completion times,

247–261. *See also* Intravenous (IV) therapy, calculating infusion/ completion times
Intravenous (IV) pediatric medications, 292–305. *See also* Pediatric medications, intravenous
Intravenous (IV) therapy, 214–228
calculating infusion/completion times, 247–261
international/military time calculations, 249–250
from mL/hr ordered, 247–249
standard time calculations, 250–252
flow rate calculation, 229–246. *See also* Flow rate calculation
fluids, 225–226
heparin, 276–283. *See also* Heparin
heparin infusion dosage alert, 220
indwelling infusion ports/ intermittent locks, 219
labeling solution bags with infusion and completion times, 252–255
medication/titration calculations, 262–275
infusion titrations, 270–275
mL/hr for dosage ordered, 263–264
mL/hr for dosage/kg ordered, 264–270
parenteral nutrition, 226
PCA devices, 223–224
primary line, 214–216,
secondary line, 216–217
syringe pumps, 223
volume-controlled burettes, 219
volumetric pumps, 221–222
ISMP. *See* Institute for Safe Medication Practices (ISMP)
IV fluids. *See* Intravenous (IV) fluids
IVPB, 216–217
IV piggybacks, 216–217,
IV therapy. *See* Intravenous (IV) therapy

**IMPORTANT! READ CAREFULLY**: This End User License Agreement ("Agreement") sets forth the conditions by which Cengage Learning will make electronic access to the Cengage Learning-owned licensed content and associated media, software, documentation, printed materials, and electronic documentation contained in this package and/or made available to you via this product (the "Licensed Content"), available to you (the "End User"). BY CLICKING THE "I ACCEPT" BUTTON AND/OR OPENING THIS PACKAGE, YOU ACKNOWLEDGE THAT YOU HAVE READ ALL OF THE TERMS AND CONDITIONS, AND THAT YOU AGREE TO BE BOUND BY ITS TERMS, CONDITIONS, AND ALL APPLICABLE LAWS AND REGULATIONS GOVERNING THE USE OF THE LICENSED CONTENT.

## 1.0 SCOPE OF LICENSE

1.1 *Licensed Content.* The Licensed Content may contain portions of modifiable content ("Modifiable Content") and content which may not be modified or otherwise altered by the End User ("Non-Modifiable Content"). For purposes of this Agreement, Modifiable Content and Non-Modifiable Content may be collectively referred to herein as the "Licensed Content." All Licensed Content shall be considered Non-Modifiable Content, unless such Licensed Content is presented to the End User in a modifiable format and it is clearly indicated that modification of the Licensed Content is permitted.

1.2 Subject to the End User's compliance with the terms and conditions of this Agreement, Cengage Learning hereby grants the End User, a nontransferable, nonexclusive, limited right to access and view a single copy of the Licensed Content on a single personal computer system for noncommercial, internal, personal use only. The End User shall not (i) reproduce, copy, modify (except in the case of Modifiable Content), distribute, display, transfer, sublicense, prepare derivative work(s) based on, sell, exchange, barter or transfer, rent, lease, loan, resell, or in any other manner exploit the Licensed Content; (ii) remove, obscure, or alter any notice of Cengage Learning's intellectual property rights present on or in the Licensed Content, including, but not limited to, copyright, trademark, and/or patent notices; or (iii) disassemble, decompile, translate, reverse engineer, or otherwise reduce the Licensed Content.

## 2.0 TERMINATION

2.1 Cengage Learning may at any time (without prejudice to its other rights or remedies) immediately terminate this Agreement and/or suspend access to some or all of the Licensed Content, in the event that the End User does not comply with any of the terms and conditions of this Agreement. In the event of such termination by Cengage Learning, the End User shall immediately return any and all copies of the Licensed Content to Cengage Learning.

## 3.0 PROPRIETARY RIGHTS

3.1 The End User acknowledges that Cengage Learning owns all rights, title and interest, including, but not limited to all copyright rights therein, in and to the Licensed Content, and that the End User shall not take any action inconsistent with such ownership. The Licensed Content is protected by U.S., Canadian and other applicable copyright laws and by international treaties, including the Berne Convention and the Universal Copyright Convention. Nothing contained in this Agreement shall be construed as granting the End User any ownership rights in or to the Licensed Content.

3.2 Cengage Learning reserves the right at any time to withdraw from the Licensed Content any item or part of an item for which it no longer retains the right to publish, or which it has reasonable grounds to believe infringes copyright or is defamatory, unlawful, or otherwise objectionable.

## 4.0 PROTECTION AND SECURITY

4.1 The End User shall use its best efforts and take all reasonable steps to safeguard its copy of the Licensed Content to ensure that no unauthorized reproduction, publication, disclosure, modification, or distribution of the Licensed Content, in whole or in part, is made. To the extent that the End User becomes aware of any such unauthorized use of the Licensed Content, the End User shall immediately notify Cengage Learning. Notification of such violations may be made by sending an e-mail to infringement@cengage.com.

## 5.0 MISUSE OF THE LICENSED PRODUCT

5.1 In the event that the End User uses the Licensed Content in violation of this Agreement, Cengage Learning shall have the option of electing liquidated damages, which shall include all profits generated by the End User's use of the Licensed Content plus interest computed at the maximum rate permitted by law and all legal fees and other expenses incurred by Cengage Learning in enforcing its rights, plus penalties.

## 6.0 FEDERAL GOVERNMENT CLIENTS

6.1 Except as expressly authorized by Cengage Learning, Federal Government clients obtain only the rights specified in this Agreement and no other rights. The Government acknowledges that (i) all software and related documentation incorporated in the Licensed Content is existing commercial computer software within the meaning of FAR 27.405(b)(2); and (2) all other data delivered in whatever form, is limited rights data within the meaning of FAR 27.401. The restrictions in this section are acceptable as consistent with the Government's need for software and other data under this Agreement.

## 7.0 DISCLAIMER OF WARRANTIES AND LIABILITIES

7.1 Although Cengage Learning believes the Licensed Content to be reliable, Cengage Learning does not guarantee or warrant (i) any information or materials contained in or produced by the Licensed Content, (ii) the accuracy, completeness or reliability of the Licensed Content, or (iii) that the Licensed Content is free from errors or other material defects. THE LICENSED PRODUCT IS PROVIDED "AS IS," WITHOUT ANY WARRANTY OF ANY KIND AND CENGAGE LEARNING DISCLAIMS ANY AND ALL WARRANTIES, EXPRESSED OR IMPLIED, INCLUDING, WITHOUT LIMITATION, WARRANTIES OF MERCHANTABILITY OR FITNESS FOR A PARTICULAR PURPOSE. IN NO EVENT SHALL CENGAGE LEARNING BE LIABLE FOR: INDIRECT, SPECIAL, PUNITIVE OR CONSEQUENTIAL DAMAGES INCLUDING FOR LOST PROFITS, LOST DATA, OR OTHERWISE. IN NO EVENT SHALL CENGAGE LEARNING'S AGGREGATE LIABILITY HEREUNDER, WHETHER ARISING IN CONTRACT, TORT, STRICT LIABILITY OR OTHERWISE, EXCEED THE AMOUNT OF FEES PAID BY THE END USER HEREUNDER FOR THE LICENSE OF THE LICENSED CONTENT.

## 8.0 GENERAL

8.1 *Entire Agreement.* This Agreement shall constitute the entire Agreement between the Parties and supercedes all prior Agreements and understandings oral or written relating to the subject matter hereof.

8.2 *Enhancements/Modifications of Licensed Content.* From time to time, and in Cengage Learning's sole discretion, Cengage Learning may advise the End User of updates, upgrades, enhancements and/or improvements to the Licensed Content, and may permit the End User to access and use, subject to the terms and conditions of this Agreement, such modifications, upon payment of prices as may be established by Cengage Learning.

8.3 *No Export.* The End User shall use the Licensed Content solely in the United States and shall not transfer or export, directly or indirectly, the Licensed Content outside the United States.

8.4 *Severability.* If any provision of this Agreement is invalid, illegal, or unenforceable under any applicable statute or rule of law, the provision shall be deemed omitted to the extent that it is invalid, illegal, or unenforceable. In such a case, the remainder of the Agreement shall be construed in a manner as to give greatest effect to the original intention of the parties hereto.

8.5 *Waiver.* The waiver of any right or failure of either party to exercise in any respect any right provided in this Agreement in any instance shall not be deemed to be a waiver of such right in the future or a waiver of any other right under this Agreement.

8.6 *Choice of Law/Venue.* This Agreement shall be interpreted, construed, and governed by and in accordance with the laws of the State of New York, applicable to contracts executed and to be wholly preformed therein, without regard to its principles governing conflicts of law. Each party agrees that any proceeding arising out of or relating to this Agreement or the breach or threatened breach of this Agreement may be commenced and prosecuted in a court in the State and County of New York. Each party consents and submits to the nonexclusive personal jurisdiction of any court in the State and County of New York in respect of any such proceeding.

8.7 *Acknowledgment.* By opening this package and/or by accessing the Licensed Content on this Web site, THE END USER ACKNOWLEDGES THAT IT HAS READ THIS AGREEMENT, UNDERSTANDS IT, AND AGREES TO BE BOUND BY ITS TERMS AND CONDITIONS. IF YOU DO NOT ACCEPT THESE TERMS AND CONDITIONS, YOU MUST NOT ACCESS THE LICENSED CONTENT AND RETURN THE LICENSED PRODUCT TO CENGAGE LEARNING (WITHIN 30 CALENDAR DAYS OF THE END USER'S PURCHASE) WITH PROOF OF PAYMENT ACCEPTABLE TO CENGAGE LEARNING, FOR A CREDIT OR A REFUND. Should the End User have any questions/comments regarding this Agreement, please contact Cengage Learning at Delmar.help@cengage.com.

**System Requirements for: Dimensional Analysis CD**

**Minimum System Requirements:**

**PC:**
- Operating System: XP w/ SP2, Vista w/ SP1
- Processor: Minimum required by operating system
- Memory: Minimum required by operating system, 1.5GB Recommended
- Screen resolution: 1024 x 768 minimum
- CD-ROM drive
- Sound card and listening device required for audio features

**Mac:**
- Operating System: Mac OS X 10.4, 10.5
- Processor: Minimum required by operating system
- Memory: Minimum required by operating system, 1.5GB Recommended
- Screen resolution: 1024 x 768 minimum
- CD-ROM drive
- Sound card and listening device required for audio features

**PC Setup Instructions:**
1. Insert disc into CD-ROM drive. The program should start automatically. If it does not, go to step 2.
2. From My Computer, double-click the icon for the CD drive.
3. Double-click the *click_me.exe* file to start the program.

**Mac Setup Instructions:**
1. Insert disc into CD-ROM drive. The CD icon will pop up on your desktop
2. Double-click the icon for the CD.
3. Double-click the *click_me* file to start the program.

**Technical Support:**
Telephone: 1-800-648-7450
8:30 AM - 6:30 PM Eastern Time
E-mail: delmar.help@cengage.com

Microsoft®, Windows®, Windows XP® and Windows Vista® are trademarks of the Microsoft Corporation.

Mac® and Mac OS X® are trademarks of Apple Inc., registered in the U.S. and other countries.